Introduction to
Biochemical Toxicology

Introduction to Biochemical Toxicology

Edited by

Ernest Hodgson and **Frank E. Guthrie**

Interdepartmental Program in Toxicology
North Carolina State University, Raleigh, North Carolina

Elsevier
New York • Amsterdam • Oxford

Elsevier Science Publishing Co., Inc.
52 Vanderbilt Avenue, New York, N.Y. 10017

Distributors outside the United States and Canada:

Blackwell Scientific Publications
Osney Mead
Oxford, England OX2 0EL

Library of Congress Cataloging in Publication Data

Main entry under title.

Introduction to biochemical toxicology.

    Includes bibliographies and index.
    1. Toxicology. 2. Poisons—Metabolism. 3. Poisons—Physiological effect.
    I. Hodgson, Ernest, 1932- II. Guthrie, Frank Edwin, 1923- [DNLM:
    1. Poisoning—Metabolism. 2. Poisons—Metabolism. QV600 I68]
RA1216.I55   615.9   80-11374
ISBN 0-444-00347-9

Editorial Services Barbara Conover
Design Edmée Froment
Art Editor Virginia Kudlak
Production Manager Joanne Jay
Compositor Bi-Comp, Inc.
Printer Halliday Lithograph

Manufactured in the United States of America

Contents

Chapter 3. Toxicokinetics   40
Daniel B. Tuey

Chapter 4. Metabolism of Toxicants: Phase I Reactions   67
Ernest Hodgson and Walter C. Dauterman

Preface

As a result of a training program in environmental and biochemical toxicology, funded by National Institute of Environmental Health Sciences Training Grant ES-07046, a course in Biochemical Toxicology has been taught at North Carolina State University for the past several years. A disadvantage to both students and teachers has been the lack of an adequate textbook for this subject. Although several pharmacology texts contain much excellent material, they are not directed toward considerations of toxicants per se. The present book is aimed at the senior–beginning graduate student level and is largely confined to considerations of the biochemistry of toxicants, their uptake, distribution, metabolism, mode of action, and elimination.

The editors share the view that an introductory text must present fundamental information in as uncomplicated a manner as possible. For this reason, the book may seem too simple to the advanced student. To further readability, references have been deleted. However, a list of suggested readings at the end of each chapter will permit students to extend their knowledge in any of the areas covered. For a reference work with an extensive bibliography the reader is directed to *Biochemical Toxicology* by A. de Bruins (Elsevier, 1976).

The book should be easily understood by any student with adequate background in biology and chemistry, including biochemistry. It has been our experience that when a fundamental understanding of biochemistry is lacking, the student should be advised to postpone an undertaking in biochemical toxicology.

Because this is a new venture in a field not previously covered by a separate text, future editions might well be quite different from the present one. To ensure improvement as well as change the editors would welcome constructive criticism and suggestions not only on the material presented but also on the choice of material to present. The views of those using the book for instructional purposes would be of especial value.

In addition to authors reviewing each other's chapters the following colleagues were kind enough to act as reviewers during the course of preparation and their efforts are gratefully acknowledged: J. R. Bend, E. McConnell, R. M. Philpot, B. R. Smith, L. Valcovic, and A. Wilson of the National Institute of Environmental Health Sciences; F. E. Bell, S. G. Chaney, J. L. Irvin, P. G. Kaufman, H. C. Smith, and J. H. Wilson of the University of North Carolina at Chapel Hill; C. E. Anderson, E. V. Caruolo, R. C. Fites, H. R. Horton, S. C. Huber, D. Huisingh, R. G. Noggle, J. F. Roberts, P. V. Shah, and D. S. Smith of North Carolina State University; C. F. Arntzen and H. M. Hall of the U. S. Department of Agriculture; F. E. Hastings of the U. S. Forest Service; H. M. Mehendale of the University of Mississippi Medical Center; L. G. Tate of the University of South Alabama; and B. A. Pappas of Carleton University, Ottawa. The expert typing and editorial assistance of Faye Lloyd are gratefully acknowledged.

Ernest Hodgson
Frank E. Guthrie

Raleigh, North Carolina

Contributors

DAUTERMAN, WALTER C.
Department of Entomology and Toxicology Program, North Carolina State University, Raleigh, N. C. 27650

de SERRES, FREDERICK J.
Office of the Director, National Institute of Environmental Health Sciences, P. O. Box 12233, Research Triangle Park, N. C. 27709

DONALDSON, WILLIAM E.
Department of Poultry Science and Toxicology Program, North Carolina State University, Raleigh, N. C. 27650

GRALLA, EDWARD J.
Chemical Industry Institute of Toxicology, P. O. Box 12137, Research Triangle Park, N. C. 27709

GROSCH, DANIEL S.
Department of Genetics and Toxicology Program, North Carolina State University, Raleigh, N. C. 27650

GUTHRIE, FRANK E.
Department of Entomology and Toxicology Program, North Carolina State University, Raleigh, N. C. 27650

HODGSON, ERNEST
Department of Entomology and Toxicology Program, North Carolina State University, Raleigh, N. C. 27650

HOLBROOK, DAVID J., JR.
Department of Biochemistry and Nutrition, School of Medicine, University of North Carolina, Chapel Hill, N. C. 27514

KULKARNI, ARUN P.
Department of Entomology and Toxicology Program, North Carolina State University, Raleigh, N. C. 27650

MAILMAN, RICHARD B.
Department of Psychiatry and Biological Sciences Research Center, University of North Carolina School of Medicine, Chapel Hill, N. C. 27514

MAIN, A. RUSSELL
Department of Biochemistry and Toxicology Program, North Carolina State University, Raleigh, N. C. 27650

MATTHEWS, H. B.
Pharmacokinetics Branch, National Institute of Environmental Health Sciences, P. O. Box 12233, Research Triangle Park, N. C. 27709

MORELAND, DONALD E.
U. S. Department of Agriculture, Departments of Crop Science and Botany and Toxicology Program, North Carolina State University, Raleigh, N. C. 27650

TUEY, DANIEL B.
Biometry Branch, National Institute of Environmental Health Sciences, P. O. Box 12233, Research Triangle Park, N. C. 27709

Abbreviations

These abbreviations are used throughout the book. Abbreviations used in a single chapter are not included but are defined on initial use.

ACTH	adrenocorticotropic hormone
AChE	acetylcholinesterase
ATP	adenosine triphosphate
AMP	adenosine monophosphate
BuCh	butyrylcholine
BuChE	butyrylcholinesterase
cAMP	cyclic AMP
cGMP	cyclic GMP
ChE	cholinesterase
CoA	coenzyme A
CoQ	coenzyme Q
DAO	diamine oxidase
DNP	2,4-dinitrophenol
DPIP	2,6-dichlorophenolindophenol
ED_{50}	median effective dose
EF-2	elongation factor 2
EPA	Environmental Protection Agency
FAD	flavin adenine dinucleotide
FDA	Food and Drug Administration
FFA	free fatty acids
FMN	flavin mononucleotide
FP	flavoprotein
GABA	γ-aminobutyric acid
GMP	guanosine monophosphate
GSH	reduced glutathione
GTP	guanosine triphosphate
LD_{50}	lethal dose for 50% of population
MAO	monoamine oxidase
PAM	pyridine aldoxime methiodide
PCB	polychlorinated biphenyl
Pi	inorganic phosphate
PMS	phenazine methosulfate
TCDD	2,3,7,8-tetrachlorodibenzo-p-dioxin
UDP	uridine diphosphate
UDPGA	uridine diphosphate glucuronic acid
UMP	uridine monophosphate
UTP	uridine triphosphate
VLDLP	very low density lipoprotein

Introduction to
Biochemical Toxicology

Ernest Hodgson and
Frank E. Guthrie

1

Biochemical Toxicology
Definition and Scope

1.1. Introduction

Toxicology can be defined quite simply as the branch of science dealing with poisons. Having said that, it must be admitted that attempts to define all of the various parameters lead to difficulties. The first difficulty is seen in the definition of a poison. Broadly speaking, a poison is any substance causing harmful effects in an organism to which it is administered, either deliberately or by accident. Clearly, this effect is dose related since any substance, at a low enough dose, is without effect, while many, if not most, substances have deleterious effects at some higher dose. Much of toxicology deals with compounds exogenous to the normal metabolism of the organism, such compounds being referred to as foreign compounds or, more recently, as xenobiotics. However, many compounds endogenous to the organism, e.g., metabolic intermediates such as glutamate, and hormones such as thyroxine, are toxic when administered in unnaturally high doses. Similarly, trace elements such as selenium, which are essential in the diet in low concentrations, are frequently toxic at higher levels. Such effects are properly included in toxicology, while the endogenous generation of high levels of metabolic intermediates due to disease or metabolic defect is not, although the effects on the organism may be similar. Whether the harmful effects of physical phenomena such as irradiation, sound, temperature, and humidity are included in toxicology appears to be largely dependent on the preference of the writer. It is convenient, however, to include them under the broad definition of toxicology.

The method of assessing toxic effects is another parameter of considerable complexity. Acute toxicity, usually measured as mortality and expressed as the LD_{50}—the dose required to kill 50% of a population of the organism in question under specified conditions—is probably the simplest measure of toxicity. Even so, reproducibility of LD_{50} values is highly dependent upon the extent to which many variables are controlled. These include the age, sex, and physiological condition of the animals, their diet, the environmental temperature and humidity, and the method of administering the toxicant.

Chronic toxicity may be manifested in a variety of ways—carcinomas, cataracts, peptic ulcers, and reproductive effects, to name only a few. Furthermore, compounds may have different effects at different doses. Vinyl chloride, a potent hepatotoxin at high doses, is a carcinogen with a very long latent period at low doses. Most drugs have therapeutic effects at low doses but are toxic at higher levels. The relatively nontoxic acetylsalicyclic acid (aspirin) is a useful analgesic at low doses, is toxic at high doses, and may cause peptic ulcers with chronic use.

Considerable variation also exists in the toxic effects of the same compound administered to different animals, or even to the same animal by different routes. The insecticide malathion has a low toxicity to mammals, whereas it is toxic enough to insects to be a widely used commercial insecticide. The route of entry of toxicants into the animal body is frequently oral, in the food or drinking water in the case of many chronic environmental contaminants such as lead or insecticide residues, or directly as in the case of accidental or deliberate acute poisoning. Other routes for nonexperimental poisoning include dermal absorption and pulmonary absorption. The above routes of administration are all used experimentally, and, in addition, several types of injection are also common— intravenous, intraperitoneal, intramuscular, and subcutaneous. The toxicity of many compounds varies tenfold or greater depending upon the method of administration.

1.2. Relationship of Toxicology to Other Sciences

Toxicology is frequently said to be a branch of pharmacology, a science that deals primarily with the therapeutic effects of exogenous substances and with all the chemical and biochemical ramifications involved in those effects. Since the therapeutic dose range of pharmacological compounds is usually quite small, and most of these compounds are toxic at higher doses, it may be more appropriate to consider pharmacology a branch of toxicology. This apparently frivolous idea is reinforced when one considers that the number of known therapeutic agents is small compared to the number of known toxic compounds and that many clinical drugs have toxic side effects even at recommended doses.

Toxicology is clearly related to the two applied biologies—medicine and agriculture. In the former, clinical diagnosis and treatment of poisoning as well as the management of toxic side effects are areas of significance, while in the latter the development of agricultural biocides such as insecticides, herbicides, nematocides, and fungicides is of great importance. The detection and management of the off-target effects of such compounds is also an area of increasing importance that is essential to their continued use. Toxicology may also be considered an area of fundamental biology since the adaptation of organisms to toxic environments has important implications for ecology and evolution.

The tools of chemistry and biochemistry are the primary ones of toxicology, and progress in toxicology is closely related to the development of new methodology. Those of chemistry provide analytical methods for toxic compounds, particularly for forensic toxicology and residue analysis, and those of biochemistry provide the techniques to investigate the metabolism and mode of action of toxic compounds. On the other hand, studies of the chemistry of toxic compounds have contributed to fundamental organic chemistry, and studies of the enzymes involved in detoxication and toxic action have contributed to our basic knowledge of biochemistry.

1.3. Scope of Toxicology

Toxicology in the most general sense may be one of the oldest practical sciences. From his earliest beginnings, man must have been aware of numerous toxins such as snake venoms and those of poisonous plants. From the earliest written records it is clear that the ancients had considerable knowledge of poisons. The Greeks made use of hemlock as a method of execution, and they and, more particularly, the Romans made much use of poisons for political and other assassinations. Indeed, it was Dioscorides, a Greek at the court of Nero, who made the earliest known attempt to classify poisons. Although poisoning has enjoyed a considerable vogue at many times and places since, the scientific study of toxicology can probably be dated from Paracelsus, who, in the sixteenth century, put forward the necessity for experimentation and included much in his range of interests that would today be classified as toxicology.

The modern study of toxicology is usually dated from the Spaniard, Orfila (1787–1853), who, at the University of Paris, identified toxicology as a separate science. Among his many contributions, he devised chemical methods for the detection of poisons and stressed the value of chemical analysis to provide legal evidence. He was also the author, in 1815, of the first book devoted entirely to the toxic effects of chemicals.

Toxicology can be subdivided in a variety of ways. Loomis refers to the three "basic" subdivisions as environmental, economic, and forensic. Environmental toxicology is further divided into such areas as pollution, residues, and industrial hygiene; economic toxicology is said to be devoted to the development of drugs, food additives, and pesticides; and forensic toxicology is concerned with diagnosis, therapy, and medicolegal considerations. Clearly, these categories are not mutually exclusive; for example, the off-target effects of pesticides are considered to be environmental, while the development of pesticides is economic.

Environmental toxicology is the most rapidly growing branch of the science. Public concern over environmental pollutants and their possible chronic effects, particularly carcinogenicity, has given rise, in the United States, to new research and regulatory agencies and recently to the Toxic Substances Control Act. Similar developments are also taking place in many other countries. The range of environmental pollutants is enormous, including industrial and domestic effluents, combustion products of fossil fuels, agricultural chemicals, and many other compounds that may be found in food, air, and water. Such compounds as food additives and cosmetics are also being subjected to the same scrutiny.

Other subspecialties are frequently mentioned that do not fit into the above divisions. Behavioral toxicology, an area of increasing importance, could be involved in any of these and is usually treated as a separate subspecialty. Analytical toxicology provides the methods used in essentially every branch of the subject, while biochemical toxicology, the subject of this text, provides the fundamental basis for all branches of toxicology.

1.4. Biochemical Toxicology

1.4.1. General Description

Biochemical toxicology is that branch of the science that deals with events at the molecular level when toxic compounds interact with living organisms. It is fundamental to our understanding of toxic processes, both acute and chronic, and is essential for the rational development of new therapies, for the determination of toxic hazards, and for the development of new biocides for agriculture and medicine. The poisoning process may be thought of as a series of several more or less distinct phases, and biochemical toxicology is intimately involved with all but one of these. *Exposure,* or the way in which an organism becomes part of an environment containing the toxicant, is properly the domain of epidemiology and industrial hygiene. *Uptake,* however, involves the biochemistry of cell membranes in the portals of entry and the structure–function relationships of toxicant absorption. *Distribution* involves the mechanism of transport throughout the body and the distribution between tissues. *Metabolism,* which may take place at the portal of entry or in such organs as the liver, involves the study of the enzymes that detoxify and/or activate xenobiotics. Compounds with intrinsic toxicity or activated metabolites are involved in the *action* phase, in which they interact with cellular components at their site of action to initiate the toxic effect. The study of mode of action is a critical area of biochemical toxicology; many of the chronic effects of toxicants are poorly described and understood, and much work is needed. A further distribution phase brings metabolic products to the organs of *excretion,* primarily the kidneys, gall bladder, and lungs, again involving processes that are proper subjects for biochemical toxicology.

This introductory chapter is a general guide to the overall process and also to the appropriate section of the book for the discussion of a particular body locus or metabolic process. The organization follows the route that a typical toxicant might take through the mammalian body. Occasional digressions refer to organisms of other phyla—plants, insects, fish, or birds.

1.4.2. Portals of Entry

The principal portals of entry are the skin, the gastrointestinal tract, and the lungs. The structure of these organs is discussed in Chapter 2. In Chapter 2 the fact is stressed that in all cases the toxicant must pass through a number of biological membranes before it can be distributed throughout the body and that uptake depends on the nature of the membrane as well as the physical properties of the toxicant. The structure of cell membranes, basically bimolecular lipid leaflets with associated proteins, and their various modifications are presented in some detail since their nature is responsible for the fact that lipophilicity is the most important determinant of the rate of uptake of exogenous molecules. Active transport, pinocytosis, etc. are much less common than diffusion across the lipid membranes.

The insect, with its waxy epicuticle, and plants, with a waxy cuticle and a stomatal system, represent important special cases, which are also discussed in Chapter 2.

1.4.3. Distribution

Various facets of the distribution of toxicants throughout the body are discussed in Chapters 2 and 3. Section 2.2 is concerned primarily with the binding of toxicants to blood proteins, particularly lipoproteins. Lipoproteins are an important class of protein, particularly in the vascular fluids. They vary in molecular weight from 200,000 to 10,000,000, and the lipid content varies from 4% to 95%, being composed of triglycerides, phospholipids, and free and esterified cholesterol. Although they are classified into groups based on their flotation constants, each group is, in fact, a mixture of many similar lipoproteins.

The nature and importance of various types of ligand–protein interactions are assessed, including covalent binding, ionic binding, hydrogen bonding, van der Waals forces, and hydrophobic interactions. Many of the same binding forces are also important in toxicant–receptor interactions, as discussed in Chapter 10.

Chapter 3 deals with the mathematical approach to the distribution of toxicants, or toxicokinetics. It provides a simplified, but still mathematically rigorous, treatment of distribution data, including both analysis and the formulation of mathematical models.

1.4.4. Metabolism

The majority of xenobiotics that enter the body do so because they are lipophilic. The metabolism of xenobiotics, which is carried out by a wide range of relatively nonspecific enzymes, serves to increase their water solubility and make possible their elimination from the body. This process is generally held to consist of two phases. In phase I, which is considered in Chapter 4, a reactive polar group is introduced into the molecule, rendering it a suitable substrate for phase II reactions. Phase I reactions include the well-known cytochrome P-450–dependent mixed-function oxidations as well as reductions, hydrolyses, etc. Phase II reactions (Chapter 5) include all of the conjugation reactions in which a polar group on the toxicant is combined with an endogenous compound such as glucuronic acid, glutathione, etc. to form a highly water-soluble conjugate that can be eliminated from the body.

It should be pointed out at this early stage that these metabolic reactions are not all detoxications since many foreign compounds are metabolized to highly reactive products that are responsible for their toxic effects. These include the activation of thiophosphates to potent phosphate cholinesterase inhibitors (Chapter 11) and the activation of carcinogens (Chapter 16) and hepatotoxicants (Chapter 18).

Although the liver is the most studied organ with regard to xenobiotic metabolism, several other organs are known to be active in this respect, although neither the specific activity nor the range of substrates metabolized is as large as in the liver. These organs include the lungs and the gastrointestinal tract, as one might expect of organs that are important sites for the entry of xenobiotics into the body, and to a lesser extent, the other important portal of entry, the skin. Other organs, such as the kidney, may also be important sites for xenobiotic metabolism. The distribution of xenobiotic-metabolizing enzymes between different organs is touched upon in several chapters, including chapters 4, 5, 6, 7, and 18.

Because toxicants are both activated and inactivated metabolically, physiological factors affecting metabolic rates can have dramatic effects on the expression of toxicity. These effects, including age, sex, pregnancy, and diet are considered in Chapter 7.

Comparative toxicology is of considerable importance from the point of view of selectivity, resistance to toxic action, and environmental studies of toxicants, as well as of some academic importance from the evolutionary viewpoint. Although only a few generalizations can be made on the basis of phylogenetic relationships, there have been many comparisons between species of toxicological interest. These are summarized in Chapter 6, and resistance to toxic action is outlined in Chapter 19.

Foreign compounds can be substrates, inhibitors, or inducers of the enzymes that metabolize them and, not infrequently, serve in more than one of these roles. Since the enzymes in question are nonspecific, numerous interactions

Figure 1. Diagrammatic cross-section of a mammalian liver cell.
SOURCE: *Lentz, Cell Fine Structure. Philadelphia: W. B. Saunders, 1971.*

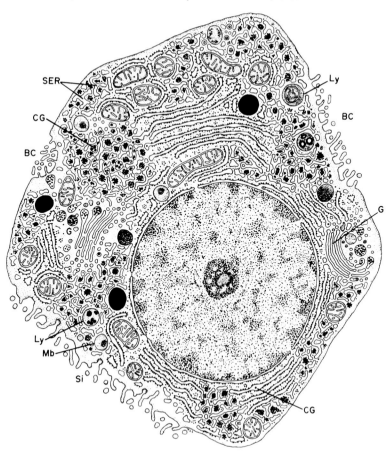

between foreign compounds are possible. These may be synergistic or antagonistic and may have a profound effect on the expression of toxicity. Depending upon the compounds and the enzymes involved in a particular interaction, the effect can be an increase or a decrease in either acute or chronic toxicity. The basic principles of such interactions are summarized in Chapter 8, while various specific effects are noted in other chapters, such as Chapter 16 on chemical carcinogenesis and Chapter 18 on hepatotoxicity.

The cell type that has been studied most intensively in biochemical toxicology is the hepatocyte, the cell that forms the bulk of the liver. A diagrammatic cross section of a liver cell is shown in Figure 1.1. These cells are highly active metabolically, both in normal intermediary metabolism and in reactions involving xenobiotics. The principal cell organelles shown in the diagram almost all play some role of importance in biochemical toxicology.

The *nucleus,* the chromosomes of which contain the DNA responsible for the code for most of the proteins synthesized in the cell, is the site for the primary reaction of carcinogenesis, since carcinogens react with DNA, as described in Chapter 16. Depending upon the toxicant, the organ, and the cell type involved, similar reactions are involved in mutagenesis and other reproductive effects (Chapter 15) as well as in teratogenesis. The nuclear envelope has recently been shown to have an active aryl hydrocarbon hydroxylase system.

Mitochondria are the site of electron transport and oxidative phosphorylation, pathways that provide sites for the action of many acute toxicants (Chapter 13).

The *endoplasmic reticulum* exists in two forms: rough, which has associated with protein synthesis (Chapter 14), and, while both rough and smooth are active in the oxidation of xenobiotics, the latter usually has the highest specific activity. After disruption of the cells, followed by differential centrifugation, the two types are isolated as rough and smooth microsomes.

The enzymes and metabolic pathways associated with the metabolism of toxicants are discussed in detail in Chapters 4–8.

1.4.5. Sites of Action

Compounds of intrinsic toxicity and active metabolites produced in the body ultimately arrive either at a site of action or an excretory organ. Although almost any organ can show the effects of toxicity, some are more easily affected than others by particular classes of toxicants, and some have been studied in greater detail than others. In all cases, however, toxicant–receptor interactions are of importance. The fundamentals of such interactions are discussed in Chapter 10.

Acute toxicants tend to affect either oxidative metabolism, as discussed in Chapter 13, the synapses of the nervous system, or the neuromuscular junction. Toxic effects on the central nervous system are discussed in Chapter 12, and the most studied class of toxicants affecting synapses, the cholinesterase inhibitors, are discussed in Chapter 11. Figure 12.2 shows a typical nerve synapse.

The commonest modes of chronic toxicity (Chapter 21) involve interaction with nucleic acids, causing carcinogenesis (Chapter 14 and 16) or reproductive effects (Chapter 15). A synopsis of short-term tests for mutagenicity is presented in Chapter 22. Although specific organ damage is known for several organs and toxicants, the central role of the liver in studies of toxic action is acknowledged in a separate chapter on hepatotoxicity (Chapter 18).

While toxicants can be classified in many ways, based either on natural distribution, commercial use patterns, or chemistry, only two such groups are accorded separate treatment, nutritional trace elements in Chapter 17 and natural toxins in Chapter 20.

Many metabolic pathways are affected by toxicants, but space limitations preclude their detailed description in this introductory chapter. They include glycolysis, the tricarboxylic acid cycle, the pentose cycle, the electron transport system and oxidative phosphorylation, nucleic acid synthesis, protein synthesis, and many others, as well as such specialized systems as photosynthesis in plants. Some of these pathways are discussed in other chapters, and the remainder can be found in any adequate general textbook of biochemistry. Because it is important in numerous aspects of biochemical toxicology and it is relevant to several chapters of this book, a simplified scheme for protein synthesis is shown in Figure 1.2.

In vivo testing for chronic toxicity in animals and short-term mutagenicity tests are both somewhat remote from a strictly biochemical treatment of the mechanisms involved in toxicology. However, the addition of Chapters 21 and 22 was the result of consideration of their current general interest and the necessity to take a biochemical approach to the mechanisms involved in these important procedures.

1.4.6. Excretion

Either the unmetabolized toxicants or their metabolic products are ultimately excreted, the latter usually as conjugated products resulting from phase II reac-

Figure 1.2 Simplified scheme for protein synthesis in animals.
SOURCE: *Watson, Molecular Biology of the Gene. New York: W. A. Benjamin, 1965.*

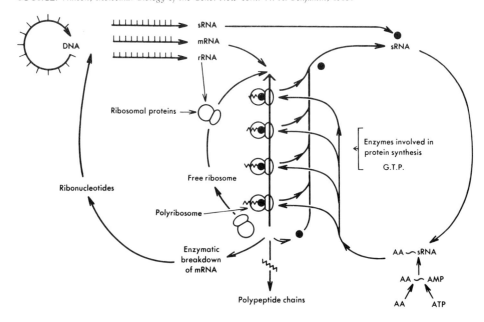

tions. The two primary routes of excretion (the urinary system and the biliary system), minor routes (such as the lungs, sweat glands, sebaceous glands, hair, feathers, and nails), and sex-related routes (such as milk, eggs, and fetus) are discussed in Chapter 9.

1.5. Conclusions

The preceding description of the nature and scope of biochemical toxicology should make it clear that the biochemistry of toxic action is a many-faceted subject, covering all aspects from the initial environmental contact with a toxicant to its ultimate excretion back into the environment. A considerable amount of material is summarized in the following chapters and, in general, the authors assume a competent knowledge of basic biochemistry. Much essential information is still missing—to be discovered, one might hope, by some of the students who use this book.

Suggested Reading

Ariens, E. J., Simonis, A. M., Offermeier, J. Introduction to General Toxicology. New York: Academic Press, 1976.

Casarett, L. J. Origin and scope of toxicology. In Casarett, L. J., Doull, J. (Eds.). Toxicology, The Basic Science of Poisons. New York: Macmillan, 1975.

Hayes, W. J. Toxicology of Pesticides. Baltimore: Williams & Wilkins, 1975.

Loomis, T. A. Essentials of Toxicology. Philadelphia: Lea & Febiger, 1974.

Frank E. Guthrie

2

Absorption and Distribution

2.1. Absorption

Absorption is the process whereby a toxicant moves through body membranes and enters the circulation. The biological effects initiated by a xenobiotic are not related simply to the inherent toxic properties of the toxicant; the initiation, intensity, and duration of response are a function of numerous factors intrinsic to the biological system as well as the administered dose. Each factor has a role related to the ultimate interaction of toxicant and active site. Only when the molecule has reached that specific site can the inherent toxicity be realized. The route a toxicant follows from the point of administration to the site of action involves a number of tissue transformations. For example, in the case of absorption of a toxicant through the gastrointestinal tract, the chemical proceeds from the intestinal lumen into the epithelial cells. Following intracellular transport, it passes through the basement membrane and lamina propria and enters the blood or lymph capillaries for transport to the site of action (or perhaps inaction). At that site, the toxicant is released from the capillaries, probably into an interstitial area, and finally through various membranes to its site of action, which may be a specific receptor, an enzyme, a nerve membrane, or many other possible sites.

2.1.1. Membranes

Transfer to and passage into a cell organelle are usually necessary to effect the molecular interaction of toxicant and macromolecule. Because there is often multitransfer through membranes, it is important to understand membrane characteristics and the factors that permit passage of foreign compounds through them.

Whether a toxicant initiates action through the dermal, oral, or vapor route, membranes are initially encountered. These may be associated with several layers of cells or a single cell, and both living and dead protoplasm may be involved. Each area of entry may have specific modifications, but a unifying concept of biology is the basic similarity of all membranes—tissue, cell, and organelle.

The basic model postulated by Davson and Danielli in 1935 is the most generally accepted one, and a body of data (microscopic and biochemical) has confirmed this hypothesis with relatively minor modifications, although membranes are now believed to have greater fluidity than originally proposed. The majority of biochemical experiments have been performed with mammalian red blood cell stroma, but more limited experiments with other cells suggest considerable similarity. All membranes appear to be bimolecular lipid leaflets closely associated with proteins. The leaflets are oriented on opposing sides such that each is a mirror image of the other. The average width of a membrane is approximately 75 Å. Figure 2.1A illustrates a current concept of a biological membrane.

Several types of lipids are found in biological membranes, phospholipids and cholesterol predominating, with lesser amounts of sphingolipids. Phosphatidylcholine, -serine, and -ethanolamine are the primary phosphatides with the two fatty acid hydrocarbon chains (typically 16–18 but varying from 12–22 carbons) comprising the nonpolar regions. One of these chains may be saturated while the other is unsaturated. Proteins are intimately associated with the membrane and may be located on the surface or within the membrane, or extend completely through the membrane. Hydrophobic forces are responsible for maintaining structural integrity of both proteins and lipids within the mem-

Figure 2.1 (A– F)   Some features of cells and tissues related to penetration of toxicants.

A.   Schematic diagram of biological membrane. Head groups of lipids (as phosphatidylcholine) represented by spheres, tail ends by zig-zag lines. Black, white, or stippled spheres indicate different kinds of lipids and illustrate asymmetry in certain cases. Large bodies are associated proteins.
SOURCE: *Modified from Singer and Nicolson. Science 175 (1972), 720. Copyright 1972 by The American Association for the Advancement of Science.*

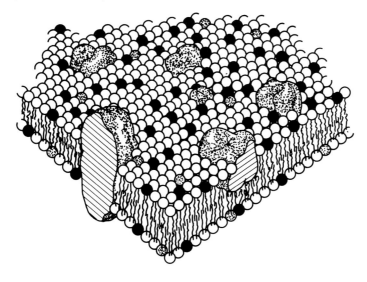

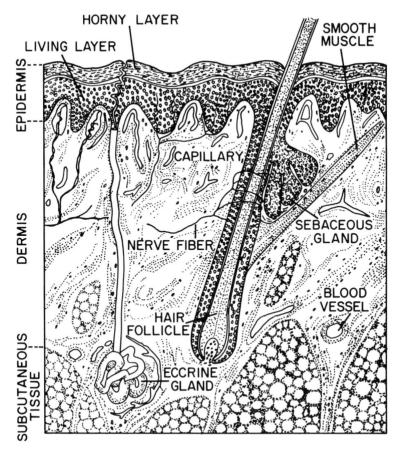

B. Zones of skin in idealized section. Dermis supported by fat-rich, subcutaneous zone intermingled with other tissues.
SOURCE: *Modified from Sci. Am., 212 (1965), 56.*

C. Structure of fish gill. Magnified section along dashed line of filament.
SOURCE: *Modified from Webster, Comparative Vertebrate Morphology. New York: Academic Press, Inc., 1974.*

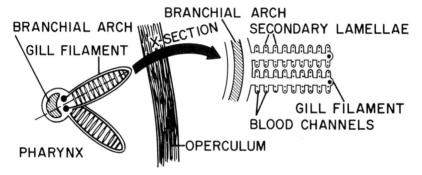

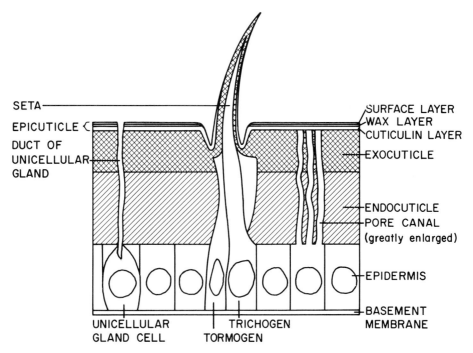

D. Diagrammatic section of insect cuticle illustrating primary layers of accessory components. Pore canals purposefully out of proportion.
SOURCE: *Modified from Richards, in Rockstein, Biochemistry of Insects, 1978.*

brane structure. The ratio of lipid to protein varies from 5 : 1 for myelin to 1 : 5 for the inner membrane of mitochondria. A more important feature may be the proportion of the membrane surface consisting of lipid bilayer. The inner membrane of the mitochondria has 40% lipid bilayer surface, whereas 100% of the myelin is lipid bilayer. The membrane is not static but has fluid characteristics.

E. Schematic diagram of cross section of a leaf.

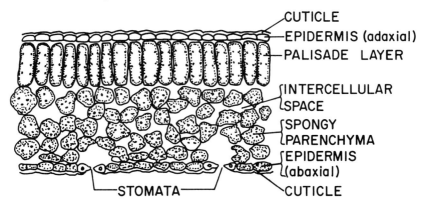

There are presumed to be a number of pores (approximately 4 Å) located in the membrane that permit water and small molecules (molecular weight 100 or less) to penetrate the charged, highly lipid barrier. More specialized membranes such as those found in the kidney, where the pore size may be 40 Å, permit passage of compounds with molecular weight greater than 50,000.

The amphipathic nature of the membrane creates a barrier for ionized, highly polar compounds, although it does not completely exclude them. The importance of favorable nonionic, lipid-soluble characteristics will be illustrated later. It should be noted that changes in lipids, makeup of surface membranes, alterations of shape and size of proteins, and physical features of bonding may cause changes in permeability characteristics of membranes. It has been suggested that 0.06% of the membrane surface has characteristics different from the rest of the membrane, which may account for the enhanced permeability of some toxicants.

2.1.1a. Ionization

Evidence that membranes are more permeable to the nonionized than the ionized form of a toxicant was first shown with alkaloids. When strychnine, nicotine, and other alkaloids were introduced into the strongly acid gastrointestinal area, absorption was extremely low, and toxic effects were not observed because the compounds did not penetrate in the highly ionized state. If the stomach contents were made alkaline, the toxicant (now nonionized) was readily absorbed and animals were killed. Ionization becomes particularly important when toxicants are introduced into the gastrointestinal tract, where a variety of pH conditions are manifest. Although many drugs are in a potentially ionizable form, most toxicants are in an un-ionized form and are unaffected by pH. The obvious exception to this generalization is nitrogen-containing toxicants, especially alkaloids.

The amount of a toxicant in the ionized or un-ionized form depends upon the pKa (negative logarithm of the acidic dissociation constant) of the toxicant and the pH of the bathing medium. Where the pH of a solution is equal to the pKa of the dissolved compound, one-half exists in the ionized and one-half in the un-ionized (free) form. The degree of ionization is given by the Henderson-Hasselbalch equation:

$$\log \frac{\text{un-ionized form}}{\text{ionized form}} = pKa - pH \text{(for acids)}$$

$$\log \frac{\text{ionized form}}{\text{un-ionized form}} = pKa - pH \text{(for bases)}$$

Since the lipid-soluble (un-ionized) form of a weak electrolyte is the diffusible constituent, weak organic acids diffuse most readily in an acidic environment and organic bases in a basic environment (Table 2.1). There is some degree of penetration even when toxicants are not in the most lipid-soluble form, and a small amount of absorption can produce serious effects if a compound is very toxic. Moreover, in isolated instances very highly ionized compounds, such as pralidoxime (2-PAM), paraquat, and diquat, are absorbed to an appreciable extent in the gastrointestinal tract. The mechanisms whereby such ionized, lipid-insoluble compounds are absorbed are not clear.

Table 2.1 Intestinal Absorption of Weak Bases and Acids at Various pH Values in the Rat

		Percent intestinal absorption at pH			
	pKa	3.6–4.3	4.7–5.0	7.2–7.1	8.0–7.8
Bases					
Aniline	4.6	40	48	58	61
Aminopyrene	5.0	21	35	48	52
Quinine	8.4	9	11	41	54
Acids					
5-Nitrosalicyclic	2.3	40	27	< 2	< 2
Salicyclic	3.0	64	35	30	10
Benzoic	4.2	62	36	35	5

Source: Hogben et al., J. Pharmacol. Exp. Ther. 125 (1959), 275.

2.1.1b. Partition Coefficients

There have been a number of studies that correlate the partition coefficient (solubility in organic phase/solubility in water) of toxicants with the rate of penetration. One such study shows a generally good correlation between partition coefficient and rate of penetration (Figure 2.2A). However, such relationships are often less obvious (Figure 2.2B), and poorly lipid-soluble compounds (low partition coefficients) have often been found to penetrate easily. It appears that use of these measurements has become more rigidly accepted as indices of permeability characteristics than would be warranted by a consideration of membrane properties. Obviously, a general relationship exists, and a certain amount of lipid solubility is necessary. However, once initial penetration has occurred, the molecule must necessarily traverse a more polar region to dissociate from the membrane. Compounds with extremely high partition coeffi-

Figure 2.2 Contrast of correlation between partition coefficients and penetration. **A** shows a good correlation (*Chara*), whereas data for **B** show a less positive correlation in *Beggiatoa*.
SOURCE: *Modified from Callander, Trans. Faraday Soc. 31 (1937), 986; and Richland and Hoffman, Planta 1 (1925), 1.*

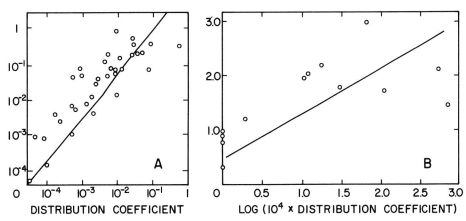

cients tend to remain in membranes rather than pass through them. This has been well authenticated for transport through skin, where water hydration of the stratum corneum creates an affinity for both water-soluble and lipid-soluble compounds. A partition coefficient around 1 is often taken as desirable for skin penetration. Chemical similarity, size of molecule, and conformational similarities all contribute to correlative features of partition coefficients. Therefore, correlations between partition coefficients and penetration seem poorest among groups of toxicants chemically unrelated and best for an analogous series of compounds.

The vehicles used to determine partition coefficients may also cause drastic differences in partitioning among compounds to seem apparent when, in fact, compounds penetrate similarly. Chloroform : water, ether : water, and olive oil : water may each give appreciably different partition coefficients for a series of compounds, but general agreement in penetration phenomena may be apparent. Although an organic solvent with a carbon chain of approximately 15–20 (such as olive oil) is most frequently chosen to mimic the natural membrane phospholipid side chain in the determination of partition coefficients, this may not be an appropriate system. The lipids on either side of the membrane may be different, different areas may have different lipids, and solubility characteristics cannot adequately duplicate the membrane lipids with any proven success.

2.1.2. Mechanisms of Transport

Although the mechanisms of absorption of drugs have received considerable attention, the transport of toxicants across membranes has been a neglected area of research. Four primary mechanisms seem to be operable to varying degrees.

2.1.2a. Passive Transport

Passive transport is generally conceded to be the primary mechanism for the passage of toxicants. The chemical moves across membranes by simple diffusion, and appropriate water : lipid partition coefficients are largely responsible for the rate of movement. Compounds in the ionized form have considerable difficulty moving in this fashion as lipid solubility is low, and there may be ionic interactions among xenobiotics, lipids, and proteins in the membrane.

2.1.2b. Filtration

Filtration via pores is an apt channel for relatively small molecules (molecular weight approximately 100), but larger molecules are excluded except in more porous tissues. Thus, compounds from "outside" the body have limited access via these pores.

2.1.2c. Special Transport

Special transport may be effected by systems that help transport endogenous compounds across membranes. Such processes may require energy and conduct the compound against a concentration gradient (active transport) or may not require energy and be unable to move compounds against a gradient (facilitated transport). The mechanisms are somewhat similar and will be considered together. Special transport is important for movement of toxicants into an animal only in relatively rare instances (5-fluorouracil is transported by the pyrimidine transport system, thallium is transported by an active mechanism normally absorbing iron, and lead may be absorbed by the system normally transporting calcium), but such mechanisms are important in the elimination of many toxicants after absorption has occured. A carrier molecule (postulated to be a protein) associates with the toxicant for both active and facilitated mechanisms, furthering movement across the membrane for ultimate release. This action would be particularly beneficial for compounds that lack sufficient lipid solubility to move rapidly through the membrane. Such penetration is more rapid than simple diffusion up to the point where concentrations are equal on both sides of the membrane.

2.1.2d. Endocytosis

Pinocytosis (liquids) and phagocytosis (solids) are specialized processes in which the cell membrane invaginates or flows around a toxicant to engulf it, thus enabling transfer across a membrane. Although of importance once the toxicant has gained entry into the animal, this mechanism does not appear to be of importance in the initial absorption of a toxicant into the animal except in isolated instances, such as absorption of carrageenens with molecular weight of approximately 40,000 in the gut.

2.1.3. Rate of Penetration

Movement of nonpolar toxicants can be predicted on the assumptions manifest from Fick's law of diffusion. Polar compounds and electrolytes of small molecular weight are believed to be subject to the same general treatment. A first-order equation, or slight deviation therefrom, appears to be applicable to the majority of toxicants. The rate of diffusion is related to the concentration gradient across the membrane ($C_1 - C_2$); the surface area available for transfer (A); the thickness of the membrane (d); and the diffusion constant (k). It may be stated as follows:

$$\text{Rate of diffusion} = k \; \frac{A(C_1 - C_2)}{d}.$$

As the toxicant is rapidly removed after absorption, C_2 can usually be ignored, i.e., $C_1 \gg C_2$. The rate of diffusion is related to the size of the molecule, the spatial configuration of the molecule, and the degree of ionization and lipid solubility. A plot of the logarithm of the amount unpenetrated versus time should be linear. The normal monophasic form of the curve is shown in Figure 2.3A. Deviations from first-order kinetics are known as shown in Figure 2.3B. Explanations for these slight deviations from pure diffusion include rapid penetration of nonpolar compounds through an initial fatty barrier, contributions of appendageal shunts, effects of carriers, injury to surface membranes, etc.

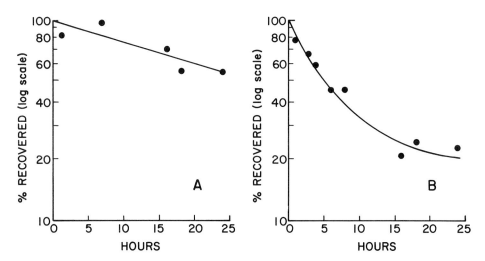

Figure 2.3 Monophasic (**A**—DDT) and multiphasic (**B**—dieldrin) penetration of toxicants through excised skin of rat.
SOURCE: *Modified from O'Brien, Insecticides: Action and Metabolism. New York: Academic Press, Inc., 1967.*

When relatively comparable methods have been used, determination of the half-time of penetration $T_{0.5}$ is a useful calculation. The rate constant of penetration, k, is derived as follows [also see Chapter 3, Equation (3.6)]:

$$k = \frac{0.693}{T_{0.5}}.$$

When oral and dermal administration in experiments in vitro with several environmental contaminants were compared (Table 2.2), the half-time penetration rates were found to vary considerably. It is obvious that rates of penetration through different routes in these mammals show little or no correlation.

Table 2.2 Half-time Penetration Rates of Some Insecticides Applied Dermally and Orally to Mammals

Compound	H₂O sol.	Partition coefficient, oliver oil/water	$T_{0.5}$ (min) Dermal (rat)	$T_{0.5}$ (min) Oral (mouse)
Carbaryl	40 ppm	38	870	49
Malathion	145 ppm	72	330	209
Dieldrin	110 ppb	281	210	2585
DDT	1.2 ppb	785	1560	1722
Nicotine	Miscible	21	—	125

Source: Data from Olson and O'Brien, J. Insect Physiol. 9 (1963), 777; and Shah and Guthrie, Comp. Gen. Pharmacol. 1 (1970), 391.

2.1.4. Route of Penetration in Mammals

The primary routes of entry of environmental contaminants are gastrointestinal, dermal, and respiratory. A number of methods of studying these routes have been developed; those concerned with respiration require highly specialized instrumentation. Appropriate chapters in Brodie et al.[1] or Hayes[2] describe a number of these special techniques.

2.1.4a. Skin Penetration

The skin is a complex, multilayered tissue comprising 18,000 cm^2 of surface in an average human male. It is a membrane that is relatively impermeable to aqueous solutions and most ions. However, it is permeable in varying degrees to a large number of xenobiotics—solid, liquid, and gaseous. Although one tends to think of most cases of poisoning as occurring through the oral or, less so, the respiratory route, the advent of organic chemicals has produced a large number of toxicants that can penetrate the dermal barrier. A striking recent example of the significance of absorption through the skin is the large number of agricultural workers who have experienced acute dermal poisoning from exposure to parathion (dermal $LD_{50} \cong 20$ mg/kg) directly during application or from more casual exposure such as worker contact with vegetation previously treated with such insecticides.

The gross features of the human skin are illustrated in Figure 2.1B. Three distinct layers and a number of associated appendages make up this non-homogenous organ. The epidermis is a multilayered tissue varying in thickness from 0.15 mm (eyelids) to 0.8 mm (palms). This tissue appears to afford the greatest deterrent to absorption. The epithelial tissues develop and grow differently from other tissues. Proliferative layers of the basal cells (stratum germinativum) differentiate and gradually replace cells above them as surface cells deteriorate and are sloughed from the epidermis. The germinal cell layer consists of nucleated columnar cells forming a layer approximately 6 μm in width. As it moves toward the surface, the basal cell loses its columnar shape, becoming rounded and ultimately flattened. Three loosely defined layers, the stratum spinosum, stratum granulosum, and stratum lucidum, are areas of considerable morphological and biochemical change, and, although variable, their width is several times that of the final layer. The primary morphological changes that occur as the cells progressively die are that they become greatly flattened, and the nucleus becomes progressively less obvious. In regard to penetration, the primary biochemical change is the production of fibrous, insoluble keratin that fills the cells, and a sulfur-rich amorphous protein that comprises the cell matrix and thickened cell membrane. It is the final layer, the stratum corneum, that provides the primary barrier to the penetration of foreign compounds. This barrier consists of 8–16 layers of flattened, stratified, highly keratinized cells.

---

[1] Brodie, B. B., Gillette, J. R., Ackerman, H. S. (Eds.). Handbook of Experimental Pharmacology, Vol. 28, Part 1, Concepts in Biochemical Pharmacology. Berlin: Springer, 1971.

[2] Hayes, W. J. Toxicology of Pesticides. Baltimore: Williams & Wilkins, 1975.

These cells are approximately 25–40 μm wide, lie tangential to the skin surface, and are oriented as relatively impermeable shingles to form a layer approximately 10 μm thick. The sequence of events from basal cell to stratum corneum requires about 4 weeks. Although highly water retarding, the dead, keratinized cells are highly water absorbent (hydrophilic), a property that keeps the skin supple and soft. A natural oil covering the skin, the sebum, appears to maintain the water-holding capacity of the epidermis but has no appreciable role in retarding the penetration of xenobiotics.

A number of investigations have shown that disruption of the stratum corneum removes all but a superficial deterrent to penetration. One line of evidence concerns "stripping" experiments, in which an adhesive is placed on the skin repeatedly, removing progressive sections of the corneum. At some critical point, the skin loses its ability to retard penetration. The stratum corneum has been calculated to afford 1000 times the resistance to penetration as the area under it.

The two other main areas of the skin (dermis and subcutaneous tissue) offer little resistance to penetration, and once a substance has penetrated the outer epithelium, these tissues are rapidly traversed. The dermis is a highly vascular area, providing ready access for distribution once the epithelial barrier has been passed. The blood supply in the dermis is under complex, interacting neural and humoral influences whose temperature-regulating function can have an effect on distribution by altering blood supply to this area. The subcutaneous tissue is highly lipoidal and serves as a shock absorber, insulator, and reserve depot of energy. Hydration markedly affects the pH of the skin, which varies between 4.2 and 7.3.

The appendages of the skin are found in the dermis and extend through the epidermis. The primary appendages are the sweat glands (eccrine and apocrine), hair, and sebaceous glands. Since these structures extend to the outer surface, they may play a role in penetration.

Anatomically, percutaneous absorption might occur through several routes, but the majority of nonionized, lipid-soluble toxicants appear to move directly through the cells of the stratum corneum, the rate-limiting barrier of the skin. Some arguments for transepidermal absorption are that epidermal damage or partial removal increases permeability, the epidermal penetration rate equals whole-skin penetration, epidermal penetration is markedly slower than dermal, and the epidermal surface area is 100–1000 times the surface area of the skin appendages. Very small and/or polar molecules appear to have more favorable penetration through appendages or other diffusion shunts, but only a small fraction of toxicants are represented by these molecules. Initial penetration particularly may be aided by appendages. Passage through the skin is passive, there being no evidence for active transport. Simple diffusion seems to account for penetration of the skin whether by gas, ion, or nonelectrolyte.

Polar substances, in addition to movement through shunts, may diffuse through the outer surface of the protein filaments of the hydrated stratum corneum, while nonpolar molecules dissolve in and diffuse through the nonaqueous lipid matrix between the protein filaments.

Variations in areas of the body. Penetration of the body regions will vary according to the polarity and size of the molecule, but it is generally accepted that for most nonionized toxicants the rate of penetration is in the following order: scrotal > forehead > axilla = scalp > back = abdomen > palm and plantar. The palm and plantar regions are highly diffuse, but their much greater thickness (100–400 times that of other regions) introduces an overall lag time in diffusion.

Effects of surfactants and solvents. Soaps and detergents are perhaps the most damaging substances routinely applied to skin. Whereas organic solvents must be applied in high concentrations to damage skin, 1% aqueous solutions of detergents increase the penetration of solute through human epidermis. Alteration of the stratum corneum appears to be the cause of increased penetration. Organic solvents can be divided into damaging and nondamaging categories. The damaging category includes methanol, acetone, ether, hexane, and mixed solvents such as chloroform : methanol or ether : ethanol. These solvents and mixtures are best able to extract lipids and proteolipids from tissues and would be expected to alter permeability for this reason. Although the mechanical strength of the stratum corneum is unaltered, delipidization produces a more porous, nonselective surface. Solvents such as higher alcohols, esters, olive oil, etc. do not appear to damage skin appreciably. To the contrary, the penetration rate of solutes dissolved in them is often reduced. Surprisingly, it has been found that lipid-soluble toxicants may be markedly resistant to washing within a short time after application. For example, 15 min after application, a substantial portion of parathion cannot be removed from exposed skin by soap and water.

Species differences. Although generalizations are tenuous at best, human skin appears to be more impermeable, or at least as impermeable, as the skin of the cat, dog, rat, mouse, or guinea pig. The skin of pigs and guinea pigs in particular serves as a useful approximation to human skin, but only after a comparison has been made for each specific substance.

Miscellaneous effects. Temperature, surface area of applied dose, simultaneous application of another toxicant, relative humidity, concentration of toxicant, occlusion, age, and hyperemia are among a number of chemical, physical, and physiological factors that may alter penetration.

2.1.4a. Gastrointestinal Penetration

Toxicants enter the physiological system through a variety of pathways, and the oral route is especially important for accidental or purposeful (suicide) ingestion of poisonous materials. Food additives, food toxins, airborne particles excluded from passage to alveoli, etc. are also introduced into the digestive system. The buccal cavity and, to a lesser extent, the rectum are occasionally used for the introduction of drugs, but toxicants would not be expected to be absorbed in those areas except under very unusual circumstances. Thus, the penetration of orally administered toxicants is primarily confined to the stomach and intestine.

The digestive tract is lined by a single layer of columnar cells, usually protected by mucous, which is thought to offer no appreciable deterrent to penetration. The circulatory system is closely associated with the intestinal tract (30–50 μm from membrane to vasculature), and once toxicants have crossed the epithelium of the intestinal tract, entry into capillaries is rapidly effected. Venous blood flow from the stomach and intestine introduces absorbed materials to the hepatic portal vein, resulting in transport to the liver, thereby favoring detoxication. On the other hand, compounds introduced through the skin or lungs follow more indirect routes to organs of detoxication. A major factor favoring absorption in the intestine is the presence of microvilli that increase the surface area to an estimated 2000 ft^2 in the small intestine, an increase of 600-fold over that of a tube that does not contain villi.

Because the intestinal area offers maximal opportunity for absorption, it is generally accepted that penetration is greater in this area of the gastrointestinal tract. However, it seems evident that this effect would depend largely on the length of time a toxicant is held in the stomach. If a toxicant that is readily absorbed remains in the stomach sufficiently long, considerable absorption will have already occurred before there is any opportunity for intestinal absorption. Thus, intestinal absorption may actually be responsible for a smaller proportion of the total penetration of some compounds.

The gastrointestinal tract has areas of highly variable pH, which can change the permeability characteristics of ionic compounds to a marked degree. For example, passive diffusion is greatly limited except for un-ionized, lipid-soluble compounds. Although variable according to secretory activity, the pH of the stomach is around 1–3 and the intestine approximates 6.0. The measured pH of the intestinal contents may not be the same as the pH of the epithelium at the site of absorption, which explains the entrance of compounds whose pKa would suggest a less absorbable condition. Table 2.1 illustrates the relationship between the ionization of bases and acids at different intestinal pH and shows clearly that absorption is increased as the degree of ionization is reduced.

In contrast to the skin, there is evidence for active transport of a few toxicants across the intestinal epithelium. These mechanisms are primarily utilized for the movement of amino acids, sugars, and ions. For toxicants that are structurally similar, active transport may permit entry of an otherwise poorly absorbed molecule. For example, 5-bromouracil is absorbed by the pyrimidine transport system and cobalt by the system normally transporting iron.

Another feature somewhat peculiar to intestinal absorption is the movement of some potentially toxic macromolecules by processes other than simple diffusion or active transport. Bacterial exotoxins, particles of azo dyes averaging 300 Å, polystyrene latex particles of 2200 Å, and carrageenens with molecular weight of approximately 40,000 are absorbed through the intestinal tract, probably by a mechanism similar to pinocytosis.

A number of other factors that contribute to gastrointestinal absorption should be mentioned. It is obvious that a toxicant must be dissolved before absorption can take place. Factors such as particle size, organic solvent, emulsifier, and rate of dissolution have obvious effects. In addition, the presence of microorganisms and hydrolytic-promoting pH conditions offer opportunities for the metabolism of many toxicants. Other factors affecting gastrointestinal absorption include binding to gut contents, intestinal motility, rate of emptying, temperature of food, dietary and health effects, and gastrointestinal secretion.

The secretion of conjugated metabolites from the bile duct into the intestine may result in conditions for enterohepatic recirculation that will permit a toxicant to maintain a potentially hazardous condition for lengthy periods. This topic will be discussed in Chapter 9.

2.1.4c. Respiratory Penetration

The respiratory system is an organ in direct contact with environmental air as an unavoidable part of living. A number of toxicants are in gaseous (CO, NO_2), vapor (benzene, CCl_4), and aerosol (lead from automobile exhaust, silica, asbestos) forms and are potential candidates for entry via the respiratory system. Opportunities for absorption are most favored through the respiratory route as the cells lining the alveoli are very thin and profusely bathed by capillaries, and the surface area of the lung is large—50–100 m^2, some 50 times the area of the skin.

At the alveoli (site of gas exchange), the membranes are exceedingly thin and have an intimate association with the vascular system. During each passage through the lung, blood cells must pass single file in immediate proximity to the site of gas exchange. The distance from vasculature to "outside" membrane is about 1.5 μm for the lung, as contrasted to approximately 30 μm for the gastrointestinal tract and over 100 μm for the skin. This enables an exceedingly rapid exchange of gases, approximately 5 sec in the case of CO_2 and 1/5 sec for O_2. A thin film of fluid wetting the alveolar walls aids in the initial absorption of toxicants from the alveolar air. However, the phospholipids of the surfactant monolayer may interact with more lipophilic compounds to slow uptake in some cases.

The sequences of respiration involving several interrelated air volumes define both the capacity of the lung and factors important to particle deposition and retention. Among the elements important in total lung capacity is the residual volume, the amount of air retained by the lung despite maximal expiratory effort. Largely due to slow release from this volume, toxicants in the respiratory air are not cleared immediately, but many expirations may be necessary to rid the lung air of residual toxicant.

Solvents and vapors. The rate of entry of vapor-phase toxicants is controlled by the alveolar ventilation rate, and toxicant is presented to the alveoli in an interrupted fashion about 20 times/min. The diffusion coefficient of the gas in the fluids of, and associated with, pulmonary membranes is an important consideration, but doses are more appropriately discussed in terms of the partial pressure of the toxicant in the inspired air. Upon inhalation of a constant tension of a toxic gas, arterial plasma tension of the gas approaches the tension of gas in the expired air. The rate of entry is then determined by blood solubility of the toxicant. If there is a high blood/gas partition coefficient, a larger amount must be dissolved in the blood to raise the partial pressure. Gases with a high blood/gas partition coefficient require a longer period to approach the same tension in the blood as in inspired air than it takes for less soluble gases. Simple diffusion accounts for the somewhat complex series of events in the lung regarding gas absorption.

Aerosols and particulates. The entry of aerosols and particulates is affected by a number of factors designed to preclude their entry. A coal miner is subject to inhalation of 6000 g of coal dust particles during his occupational lifetime, and only 100 g are found postmortem; it is therefore obvious that the protective mechanism is an effective one. The parameters of air velocity and directional air changes favor impaction of particles in the upper respiratory systems. Particle characteristics such as size, coagulation, sedimentation, electrical charge, and diffusion are important to retention, absorption, or expulsion of air-borne particles. In addition to the other lung characteristics mentioned, a mucous blanket propelled by ciliary action clears the tract of particles by directing them to the gastrointestinal system (via the glottis) or to the mouth for expectoration. This system is responsible for 80% of toxicant lung clearance. The deposition of various particle sizes in different respiratory regions is summarized in Table 2.3, where it is shown that particles larger than 2 μm do not reach the alveolus. In addition to this mechanism, phagocytosis is very active in the respiratory tract, both coupled to the directed mucosal route and via penetration through interstitial tissues of the lung and migration to the lymph, where phagocytes may remain stored for long periods in lymph nodes. Ninety percent of lung-deposited material may be cleared in less than 1 hr.

The direct penetration of air-borne toxicants at alveolar surfaces or in the upper respiratory tract is not the only action of toxicological importance. Both vapors and particulates can accumulate in upper respiratory passages to produce irritant effects. Despite the effectiveness of ciliary movement and phagocytosis, the cumulative effects of silica, asbestos, or coal dust ultimately cause important chronic fibrosis even though direct absorption is of minor importance. Thus, phagocytosis prevents acute damage but may contribute to chronic toxicity.

Table 2.3 Percent Retention of Inhaled Aerosol Particles in Various Regions of the Human Respiratory Tract (450 cm^2 tidal air)

Region	Percent retention of indicated particle sizes				
	20 μm	6 μm	2 μm	0.6 μm	0.2 μm
Mouth	15	0	0	0	0
Pharynx	8	0	0	0	0
Trachea	10	1	0	0	0
Pulmonary bronchi	12	2	0	0	0
Secondary bronchi	19	4	1	0	0
Tertiary bronchi	17	9	2	0	0
Quaternary bronchi	6	7	2	1	1
Terminal bronchioles	6	19	6	4	6
Respiratory bronchioles	0	11	5	3	4
Alveolar ducts	0	25	25	8	11
Alveolar sacs	0	5	0	0	0
Total[a]	93	83	41	16	22

[a] Remainder is expelled.

Source: Hatch and Gross, Pulmonary Deposition and Retention of Inhaled Aerosols. New York: Academic Press, 1964.

There is little evidence for active transport in the respiratory system (phenol red and disodium chromoglycate are notable exceptions), although pinocytosis may be of importance for penetration. The lung is an area of extensive metabolic activity, although detoxication mechanisms do not appear to be of major importance. It is well known that the lung is an important excretory organ for anesthetic gases. Perhaps less well known, is the fact that the lung is also an excretory route for ethanol.

2.1.5. Absorption in Some Nonmammalian Systems

Although this discussion is primarily centered on man and higher mammals, the effects of toxicants on other organisms in the environment often have a direct effect on man and require at least cursory consideration. The special cases of animals with gills, insect integument, and plant structure will be briefly discussed in relation to the absorption of toxicants.

2.1.5a. Gills

Animals equipped with this special respiratory modification are especially prone to exposure to water-dispersed toxicants. When such chemicals are highly lipid soluble and resist metabolism, the animal may accumulate concentrations in the body that are 100,000 or more times greater than in the surrounding water being passed through the gill due to partitioning into lipid membranes. Removal of an exposed animal to uncontaminated water initiates processes whereby the body burden of the toxicant may be reduced significantly within a short period of time (days).

The gill system of aquatic animals can be illustrated by the teleost fish, which has branched arches within the pharynx supported by a double row of gill filaments (Figure 2.1C) oriented such that water must pass through a narrow space between filaments. The extremely thin epithelial cells and proximity of blood channels (just large enough for the passage of one cell) offers a maximal area for diffusion. A countercurrent distribution system for movement of water around the gills ensures maximum exposure.

To illustrate the absorption of one environmental contaminant, the principal route of entry of a detergent (sodium lauryl sulfate) is across oral or respiratory membranes (80% or greater), although smaller amounts are absorbed cutaneously.

2.1.5b. Invertebrates

Although the intestinal tract of lower animals bears a superficial resemblance to vertebrates, the external covering of invertebrates is considerably modified. The integument of insects is illustrative of the differences between mammalian and invertebrate external surfaces (Figure 2.1D). The insect integument (plus the fore- and hindgut and tracheal system) is lined with a cuticle composed of three nonliving layers—epicuticle, exocuticle, and endocuticle—and the underlying epidermis, which contains the active cells. The epicuticle is a very thin layer (1–4 μm) that may have up to four sublayers. The overriding constituent of the epicuticle in regard to penetration is a lipid layer whose primary physiological function is prevention of water loss. The lipoidal nature may also enhance entry of most organic chemicals. The exocuticle is somewhat thicker (up to 10 μm), and a primary characteristic is the presence of sclerotin, a product of proteins in the exocuticle that is conjugated by action of quinones to form a somewhat impervious hardened layer. The endocuticle (and in part the exocuticle) contains chitin, a polyglucosamine that is a constituent common to many invertebrates and some plants. The endocuticle (approximately 100 μm thick) is bounded by a layer of epidermal cells that give rise to the primary constituents of the integument. A number of hairs and glands extend through the integument. An important factor for penetration may be the cuticular pore canals, which extend from the hypodermal cells to the epicuticle. These helical pores are variable in size (0.1–1.0 μm diameter) and number (15,000–1,000,000/mm^2 surface).

The mechanisms of penetration through the insect integument are controversial. One group believes that diffusion through the integument adequately accounts for penetration—lipid solubility and nonionizability favoring diffusion. Small electrolytes are also easily transported, but large ionized molecules are excluded. There appears to be a correlation between an increased number of pore canals and penetration. A second hypothesis favors the lateral movement of penetrants along the cuticle to areas favoring penetration (thin intersegmental membranes), and the extreme of this hypothesis is that toxicants diffuse laterally along the integument to ultimately enter the system via the respiratory system (tracheal canals).

A body of literature suggests that variations in the integument of insects and mammals account for selective toxicity due to differences in the rate of penetration of toxicants. Evidence has been presented that a number of insecticides are more toxic to insects than to man when applied dermally, whereas injected or oral doses give approximately equal LD_{50} values. Thus, it is frequently proposed that lower absorption through skin offers decreased toxicity for mammals compared to absorption through the highly lipoidal integument of the invertebrate. Such evidence is entirely indirect, and there are a number of exceptions to even those data. In addition, recent in vitro experiments of a direct nature (both dermal and oral) have failed to disclose any consistent difference between the penetration of insecticides among animal groups. These recent investigations suggest that penetration is much less important than detoxication mechanisms in explaining selectivity.

2.1.5c. Plants

Approximately 90% of the terrestrial biomass in the United States is composed of plants; thus, some consideration of the penetration of toxicants into these organisms seems justified. Toxicants may enter plants via leaves, stems, and to a lesser extent, roots. Uptake by leaves is the predominant route of entry of most environmental contaminants, except certain heavy metals.

The primary entry of volatile environmental pollutants is through the stomatal pores. These pores may occur on both leaf surfaces or on a single surface (usually the lower); they may close in response to various environmental and chemical cues (Figure 2.1E). When open, stomata take on atmospheric CO_2 and O_2 and transpire water vapor, in addition to readily admitting water-soluble gaseous pollutants. Thus, uptake of any gas usually correlates highly with stomatal activity.

Gaseous pollutant transfer to internal leaf surfaces occurs primarily by molecular diffusion through the stomatal pores followed by movement into the intercellular spaces of the mesophyll tissue. When gaseous materials come into contact with water-rich cell walls, they go into solution or, in the case of oxidants such as ozone, tend to react with membrane components rather than being transported. The movement of other gases into the symplast then involves transport through membranes.

The aerial plant parts are covered by a waxy, lipoidal, noncellular layer called the cuticle. This layer serves as one of the primary barriers to aboveground penetration of substances into plants. The cuticle has several components. The outer surface is covered by epicuticular waxes, which are complex mixtures of long-chain (usually C_{21}–C_{37}) alkanes, alcohols, ketones, aldehydes, esters, and fatty acids. A chemically similar waxy layer is embedded in the underlying layer. Cutin, which comprises the structural matrix of the cuticle, is a polyester of long-chain fatty acids and hydroxy fatty acids whose exact structure is unknown. Cutin behaves like a highly cross-linked, high-capacity, ion-exchange resin of a weak organic acid type. Since cutin contains both polar and nonpolar groups, it has both hydrophilic and hydrophobic properties. Between the cutin matrix and epidermal cell wall is a pectin-rich region.

Plants provide a potential trap (vegetative sink) for toxicants, especially for the gaseous ones. A continuous cover of alfalfa has been estimated to remove 0.25 ton of NO_2 or SO_2/mi_2 from air containing concentrations of these substances normally found in polluted areas. Figure 2.4 shows the rate of penetration of a number of pollutants by an alfalfa canopy. There is an excellent association between penetration of these gases and their water solubility (shown in parentheses).

A variety of chemically dissimilar polar and nonpolar compounds penetrate the leaf, primarily via the stomata and also directly through the cuticle, depending upon species and foliar maturity. The exact pathways are unknown, but there is much agreement that polar compounds follow an aqueous route, while nonpolar compounds follow a lipoidal one. Surface tension presents the biggest problem to the absorption of water-soluble compounds through the cuticle—hence the widespread use of surfactants in applying many pesticides.

The epicuticular wax is the main barrier to the penetration of nonvolatile contaminants. When epicuticular waxes were removed, an eight-fold increase in penetration was noted, whereas removal of both epicuticular and cuticular waxes increased absorption by only ninefold.

Although there is little controversy regarding the entrance of lipid-soluble compounds (diffusion through lipoidal components), the pathway for the entry of water-soluble or ionic compounds is less clearly understood. It is also apparent that compared to nonpolar substances, water-soluble ones are transported more readily through plant than animal membranes. Much evidence exists on cuticular transpiration for ready movement of some water or water vapor through the cuticle, but there is little direct evidence that xenobiotics enter by traversing the same routes in reverse. Pores and microchannels have been much acclaimed as routes of increased absorption, but there is little scientific evidence to support such claims. Specialized structures in leaves, especially the stomata,

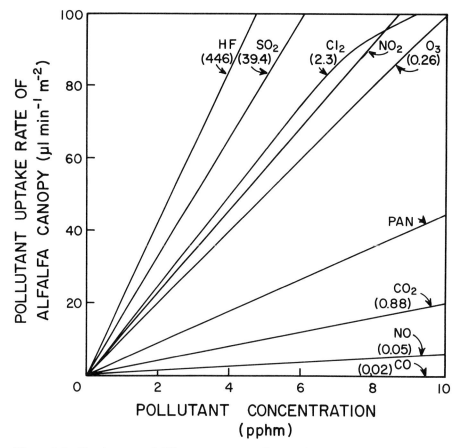

Figure 2.4 Uptake rates of different gaseous pollutants by an alfalfa canopy. Numbers in parentheses are solubility at 20°C/cc gas/cc H₂O.
SOURCE: *Modified from Hill, J. Air Pollut. Contr. Assoc. 21 (1976), 341.*

have been shown to play a role in xenobiotic penetration. Because of modifications in their cuticle layer, penetration may be facilitated into the guard cells of the stomata as compared to other epidermal cells.

Penetration through the stem varies considerably depending upon growth characteristics and age. A greatly reduced surface area (in comparison to foliage) is one obvious deterrent to uptake after exposure to xenobiotics. Movement is largely reduced due to the presence of the periderm, which replaces the epidermis. Penetration into bark is usually of little importance.

The purposeful application of herbicides to bark is aided by high volumes of solution in a highly lipid-soluble form.

A large volume of data exists on absorption of herbicides and, to a lesser extent, air pollutants into plants, but relatively little is known about absorption of other environmental chemicals. Canopy height, wind velocity, stomatal closures by pollutants, light, temperature, and season all affect the absorption of such substances.

2.2. Distribution

This section is concerned with the interactions involved in the distribution of toxicants. The toxicodynamic events involving compartmentalization and other dynamic factors are discussed in Chapter 3.

2.2.1. Distribution by Body Fluids

Body fluids are distributed between three primary compartments, only one of which, vascular fluid, is thought to have an important role in the distribution of toxicants. Human plasma amounts to about 4% of the total body weight and 53% of the total blood volume. By comparison, the interstitial tissue fluids account for 13% of body weight and intracellular fluids comprise 41%. The concentration that a toxicant may achieve in the blood following exposure will depend in part upon its apparent volume of distribution. If it is distributed only in the plasma, a high concentration could be achieved within the vascular tissue. On the other hand, the concentration would be markedly lower if the same quantity of toxicant were distributed in a larger pool including the interstitial water and/or cellular fluids.

Following entry into the circulatory system, a toxicant is distributed throughout the body and may accumulate at the site of toxic action, be transferred to a storage depot, or be transported to organs that will detoxify/intoxify or eliminate the compound. Although many toxicants have sufficient solubility in the aqueous component of blood to account for simple solution as a route of distribution,

Figure 2.5 (A–G)   Some aspects of macromolecules related to distribution of toxicants.

A.   Plasma proteins depicted according to relative amounts (*y* axis) and electrophoretic mobilities (*x* axis).
SOURCE: *Modified from Putnam, in The Proteins (Naurath, ed.), Vol. 3. New York: Academic Press, Inc., 1965.*

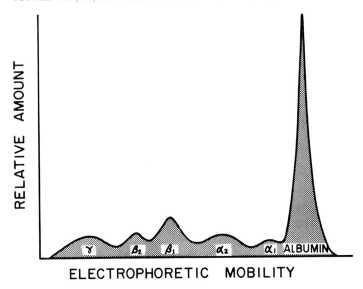

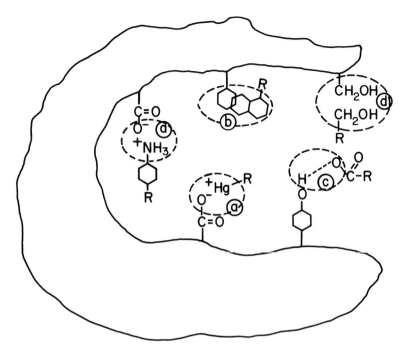

B. Schematic representation of noncovalent bonds that stabilize protein and ligand. Bonds from "protein molecule" extend into "protein pore" where ligands interact, **a.** ionic forces, **b.** hydrophobic bonding, **c.** hydrogen bonding, **d.** van der Waals forces.
SOURCE: *Modified from Afnfinson, The Molecular Basis of Evolution (1963).*

C. Scatchard plot of binding of salicylate to human serum proteins.
SOURCE: *Moran and Walker, Biochem. Pharmacol. 17 (1968), 153.*

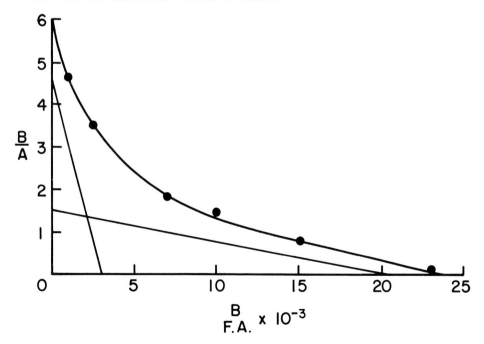

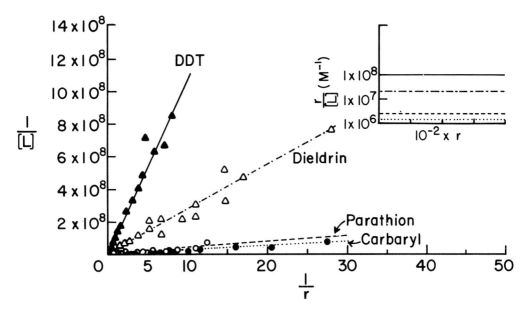

D. Double reciprocal plot of binding of rat serum lipoprotein fraction with four insecticides. Insert illustrates magnitude of differences in slopes with Scatchard plot. ▲ DDT; △ dieldrin; ○, parathion; ●, carbaryl.

SOURCE: *Skalsky and Guthrie, Pestic. Biochem. Physiol. 7 (1977), 289.*

E. Double reciprocal plot of binding of DDT to human serum fractions.

SOURCE: *Skalsky and Guthrie, Toxicol. Appl. Pharmacol. 43 (1978), 229.*

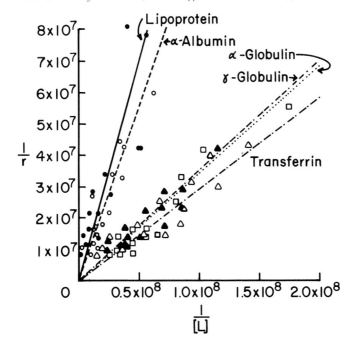

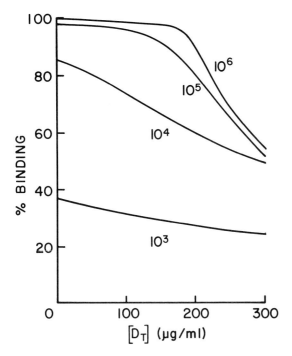

F. Effects of drug concentration (D_T) on percent binding of a drug in plasma. Each curve a different value of K.

SOURCE: *Keen, in Concepts in Biochemical Pharmacology (Brodie and Gillette, ed.), Vol. 28, Pt. 1. New York: Springer Verlag, 1971.*

G. Competitive binding between phenyl butazone and warfarin for human albumin.
SOURCE: *Solomon et al., Biochem. Pharmacol. 17 (1968), 143.*

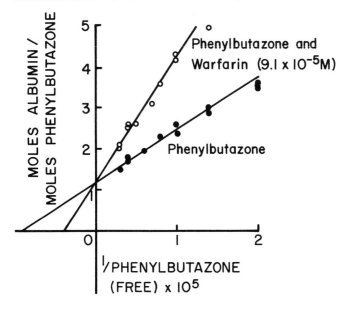

the primary distribution mechanism for toxicants appears to be in association with plasma proteins. Cellular components may also be responsible for transport of toxicants, but such transport is seldom the major route. The transport of toxicants by lymph is usually quantitatively of little importance since the intestinal blood flow is 500–700 times the intestinal lymph flow. It must be recognized, however, that both erythrocytes and lymph can play roles in the transport of xenobiotics, and in some instances to an important extent.

Studies on plasma proteins have shown the albumin to be particularly important in the binding of drugs (Figure 2.5A). Studies with toxicants have been more limited, but there is evidence that suggests a significant, perhaps even more important, role for lipoproteins.

Toxicants are often concentrated in specific tissues, either at sites of storage or directly at the site of toxic action, as in the binding of hemoglobin. If a toxicant is stored in a depot removed from the site of action (such as polychlorinated biphenyls in fat or lead in bone), no adverse effect may be manifested immediately, although a potential toxicity exists. For example, lead stored in bone is not thought to cause harm, but it has the potential for mobilization into soft tissues, whereupon toxic symptoms may appear. As the toxicant in storage depots is in equilibrium with the free toxicant in plasma, mobilization is constant, and exposure to the target organ is constant (although at a low level). Thus, the opportunity for chronic toxicity is continuous.

2.2.2. Ligand–Protein Interactions

An interesting aspect of toxicology is the apparent contradiction that although many toxicants are "unreactive" in a strictly chemical sense, they can be reversibly bound to a variety of biological constituents. In the case of most ligand–protein interactions, reversible binding is established which follows the Law of Mass Action and provides a remarkably efficient means whereby toxicants can be transported to various tissues.

The toxicant–protein interaction may be simply described according to the Law of Mass Action as

$$[T]_F + [\text{Free sites}] \underset{k_2}{\overset{k_1}{\rightleftarrows}} [T]_B$$

where $[T]_F$ and $[T]_B$ are free and bound toxicant molecules, respectively, and k_1 and k_2 are the specific rate constants for association and dissociation. It is important to stress that k_2, which governs the rate of binding to the protein, dictates the rate of toxicant release at a site of action, inaction, or storage. The ratio k_2/k_1 is identical with the dissociation constant, K_{diss}. Among a group of binding sites on proteins, those with the smallest K_{diss} values for a given toxicant will bind it most tightly. In contrast to reversible binding, some potentially carcinogenic metabolites that are formed from chlorinated hydrocarbons (such as CCl_4) are covalently bound to tissue proteins. In this case, there is no true distribution of the ligand, as k_2 is nonexistent; thus there is no opportunity for dissociation. The distinction between flow rate–limited distribution and affinity-limited distribution is discussed in Chapter 3.

Once a molecule binds to a plasma protein, it moves throughout the circulation until it dissociates, usually for attachment to another large molecule. Dissociation occurs when the affinity of another biomolecule or tissue component is greater than that of the plasma protein to which the toxicant was originally bound. Thus, forces of association must be strong enough to establish an initial interaction, but they must also be weak enough such that a change in the physical or chemical environment can lead to dissociation [binding to proteins of greater affinity (lower K_{diss} values), binding with a higher concentration of proteins of lower affinity, or changes in K_{diss} with changes in ionic strength, pH, temperature, etc.]. As long as binding is reversible, redistribution will occur whenever the concentration of one pool (i.e., blood or tissue) is diminished. Redistribution must occur when a pool is diminished in order to reestablish equilibrium.

2.2.3. Types of Binding

Proteins complex with ligands by a variety of mechanisms (Figure 2.5B), which are described below.

2.2.3a. Covalent Binding

Covalent binding may have a profound direct effect on an organism due to modification of an essential molecule, but it usually accounts for a minor portion of the total dose and is of no importance in further distribution of toxicants since such compounds cannot dissociate. As previously mentioned, when metabolites of some compounds are covalently bound to proteins, there may be no opportunity for subsequent release of the ligand apart from release upon breakdown of the protein itself.

2.2.3b. Noncovalent Binding

Noncovalent binding is of primary importance with respect to distribution because of the opportunities to dissociate after transport. In rare cases, the noncovalent bond may be so tight (K_{diss} extremely small) that a compound remains in the blood for very lengthy periods. For example, 3-hydroxy-2,4,4-triiodo-α-ethyl hydrocinnamic acid has a half-life of about 1 year with respect to its binding to plasma albumin. Types of interactions that lead to noncovalent binding include the following:

Ionic binding. Electrostatic attraction occurs between two oppositely charged ions. Proteins are capable of binding with metal ions. The degree of binding varies with the chemical nature of each compound and the net charge. Dissociation of ionic bonds usually occurs readily, but some members of the transition group of metals exhibit high association constants (low K_{diss} values) and exchange is slow. Ionic interactions may also contribute to binding of alkaloids with ionizable nitrogenous groups and other ionizable toxicants.

Hydrogen bonding. Hydrogen bonds arise when a hydrogen atom, covalently bound to one electronegative atom, is "shared" to a significant degree with a second electronegative atom. As a rule, only the most electronegative atoms (O, N, and F) form stable hydrogen bonds. Protein side chains containing hydroxyl, amino, carboxyl, imidazole, and carbamyl groups can form hydrogen bonds, as can the N and O atoms of peptide bonds themselves. Hydrogen bonding plays an important role in the structural configuration of proteins and nucleic acids.

Van der Waals forces. These are very weak forces acting between the nucleus of one atom and the electrons of another atom, i.e., between dipoles and induced dipoles. The attractive forces arise from slight distortions induced in the electron clouds surrounding each nucleus as two atoms are brought close together. The binding force is critically dependent upon the proximity of interacting atoms and diminishes rapidly with distance. However, when these forces are summed over a large number of interacting atoms that "fit" together spatially, they can play a significant role in determining specificity of toxicant–protein interactions.

Hydrophobic interactions. When two nonpolar groups come together they exclude the water between them, and this mutual repulsion of water results in a hydrophobic interaction. In the aggregate they present the least possible disruption of interactions among polar water molecules and thus can lead to stable complexes. Some authorities consider this a special case involving van der Waals forces. The minimization of thermodynamically unfavorable contact of a polar grouping with water molecules provides the major stabilizing effect in hydrophobic interactions.

2.2.4. Experimental Treatment of Interactions

2.2.4a. Method of Study

A number of methods have been employed to study ligand–protein interactions, including ultrafiltration, electrophoresis, equilibrium dialysis, solvent extraction, solvent partition, ultracentrifugation, spectrophotometry, and gel filtration or equilibrium (see Westphal[1] for a description of methods).

2.2.4b. Factors Involved

Characteristic of ligand–protein interactions is the great number of binding possibilities for attachment of a small molecule (toxicant) to a large molecule (protein). Although highly specific (high-affinity, low-capacity) binding is known to occur with a number of drugs, examples of specific binding for toxicants are limited. In most cases, low-affinity, high-capacity binding describes the interactions, and oftentimes the number of binding sites cannot be accurately determined because of the nonspecific nature of the interactions.

To understand the physiochemical and biological significance of toxicant binding to a protein, several factors must be considered. The number of ligand molecules bound per protein molecule, $\bar{\nu}$, and the maximum number of binding sites, n, are important considerations as they comprise the definitive binding capacity of the protein. Another consideration is the binding affinity, $K_{binding}$ (or $1/K_{diss}$). If the protein has but one binding site for the toxicant, a single value of

---

[1] Westphal, U. Steroid–Protein Interactions. New York: Springer, 1971.

K_{diss} (or $K_{binding}$) describes the strength of the interaction. More usually, the value of the binding constant will vary when more than one binding site is present, each site having its intrinsic association constant, $K_1, K_2, \cdots, K_n$. Rarely is the situation found where $K_1 = K_2 = \cdots = K_n$, wherein a single value would suffice for the affinity constant at all sites. This is especially true in the case of those toxicants for which van der Waals forces and hydrophobic binding appear to contribute to binding of a nonspecific, low-affinity nature. Of course, the chemical nature of the binding site is of critical importance in determining the binding characteristics. The environment of the protein, the three-dimensional molecular structure of the binding site, the general location in the overall protein molecule, cooperativity, and allosteric effects are all factors that influence binding. Studies with toxicants, and even more extensive investigations with drugs, have not generally provided an adequate elucidation of these factors; i.e., binding is usually too complex to be accurately described by any one set of equations.

2.2.4c. Analysis of Data

Methods for analyzing binding phenomena are legion, and the examples given here will be those of a less complex nature. Toxicant–protein complexes that are held together by relatively weak bonds (energies of the order of hydrogen bonds or less) readily associate and dissociate at physiological temperature, and a state of thermodynamic equilibrium can be readily attained. The Law of Mass Action can be applied as follows:

$$K_{binding} = \frac{[TP]}{[T][P]} = \frac{1}{K_{diss}}$$

where $K_{binding}$ is the equilibrium constant for association, [TP] is the concentration of toxicant–protein complex, [T] is the concentration of free toxicant, and [P] is the concentration of total protein. This equation does not describe the binding sites nor binding affinity. To incorporate these parameters and estimate the extent of binding, double reciprocal plots (1/[TP] versus 1/[T]) may be utilized to test the specificity of binding; in these plots regression lines passing through the origin imply infinite binding. In the case of infinite binding, calculation of an affinity constant becomes questionable.

The two observed groups of toxicant–protein binding may be defined as (a) specific, high-affinity, low-capacity, and (b) nonspecific, low-affinity, high-capacity. The term high affinity implies an affinity constant, ($K_{binding}$) of the order $10^8 \, M^{-1}$ or greater, while low affinity implies a $K_{binding}$ of the order of $10^4 \, M^{-1}$ or less. Nonspecific, low-affinity binding appears to be most characteristic of binding of nonpolar compounds.

Where high-affinity binding is manifest, the method of Scatchard is perferable for describing the action in which the equation

$$\bar{\nu} = \frac{nK\,[A]}{1 + K[A]}$$

is rearranged for purposes of graphing to

$$\frac{\bar{\nu}}{[A]} = K(n - \bar{\nu})$$

where $\bar{\nu}$ is the moles of ligand bound per mole of protein, [A] is the concentration of free ligand, K is the intrinsic affinity constant, and n is the number of sites exhibiting such affinity. When $\bar{\nu}/[A]$ is plotted against $\bar{\nu}$, a straight line is obtained (provided the protein has only one class of binding sites), the slope being $-K$ and the intercept on the $\bar{\nu}$ axis being n. With more than one class of sites, a curve is obtained from which the constants may be derived. This is illustrated for binding of salicylate to human serum protein (Figure 2.5C), for which the data show not one but two species of binding sites: one with a low capacity but high affinity, the other with approximately three times the capacity but with low affinity. Computer programs usually solve such data by determining one line for the specific binding and one line for nonspecific binding, the latter being an average of many possible solutions.

Figure 2.5D shows double reciprocal plots of the binding of rat plasma lipoprotein with four insecticides for which the intercepts were found to intersect at the origin, implying "infinite" binding. The insert shows the low-affinity, "unsaturable" nature of binding of such highly lipophilic, nonionized toxicants, and hydrophobic interaction is implied.

Where hydrophobic binding of highly lipid toxicants occurs, as shown in Figure 2.5D (probably true for many environmental contaminants), binding is probably not limited to a single plasma protein. From the experimental data illustrated in Figure 2.5E, the binding of DDT to five human plasma proteins was determined, and it was found that although binding was strongest for proteins of the albumin and lipoprotein fractions, binding to any of three other proteins could adequately explain transport of DDT in the blood. Similar results were found for dieldrin, parathion, and carbaryl.

Protein-binding data are frequently expressed in terms of percent of ligand bound. Although useful, the limitations should be recognized, for as ligand concentration is lowered, the percentage of it binding increases, as shown in Figure 2.5F. It can be seen that when a compound has a high affinity for a protein (albumin in this case), percent binding falls sharply when the total ligand concentration $[D_t]$ exceeds a certain value.

2.2.4d. Competitive Binding

If a toxicant or drug is administered after binding sites on a protein are occupied by another, competition for the site occurs, and toxic effects may be noted due to a higher concentration of free toxicant. A number of fatty acids and derivatives, as well as the drug phenylbutazone, bind to the same site as the anticoagulant warfarin. Figure 2.5G illustrates the situation in which phenylbutazone displaces warfarin from its binding site of albumin. The increased anticoagulant effect observed in vivo when the compounds are administered concurrently may be attributable to an increase of free warfarin at its cell receptor site. To further illustrate, Hg^{2+} has a greater affinity for metallothionein than has Cd^{2+} and replaces Cd from the protein in vitro.

Competition for the same site on plasma proteins may have especially important consequences when one of the potentially toxic ligands has a very high affinity. If compound A has low fractional binding (for example, 30%) and compound B displaces 10% of A from the protein, the net increase of free A is from 70% to 73%, a negligible increase. However, if A were 98% bound and 10% is displaced, the amount of free A increases from 2% to 12%, a sixfold increase in free toxicant, which could result in a severe reaction.

A change in binding may also occur when a second ligand produces an allosteric effect resulting in altered affinity (binding or stimulation) of the protein for the originally bound compound (noncompetitive binding). Competitive binding for very nonpolar compounds with infinite binding sites (insert of Figure 2.5D) would be unlikely to occur at physiological concentrations.

2.2.4e. Other Factors Affecting Distribution

Among the factors that affect distribution, apart from binding to blood macromolecules per se, are the route of administration, rate of metabolism, polarity of the parent toxicant or metabolic products, and rate of excretion.

Gastrointestinal absorption and intraperitoneal administration provide immediate passage of a compound to the liver, whereas dermal or respiratory routes provide at least one passage through the systemic circulation prior to reaching the liver. The metabolism of most toxicants results in products that are more polar and thus more readily excreted (than the parent molecule). Therefore, the rate of metabolism is a critical determinant in the distribution of a compound since those compounds that are readily metabolized are usually readily excreted, and thus are proportionally less prone to accumulate in the tissues. The same principle holds for polarity, since the greater the polarity the more readily a xenobiotic may be excreted. For a more detailed discussion of these factors, especially their interrelations, see Chapter 9.

In summary, the binding of drugs to plasma proteins is of considerable interest to toxicologists and is of key importance in transport. Many organic and inorganic compounds of low molecular weight appear to bind to lipoproteins, albumins, and other plasma proteins. Ionic, hydrophobic, hydrogen bonding, and van der Waals interactions are implicated in such binding. It is generally accepted that the fraction of toxicant that is bound does not possess toxicological action per se. Many toxicants and endogenous compounds appear to compete for the same binding site, and thus one compound may alter the unbound fraction of another by displacement, thereby increasing toxic effects.

Suggested Reading

General

Brodie, B. B., Gillette, J. R., Ackerman, H. S. (Eds.). Handbook of Experimental Pharmacology Vol. 28, Part 1, Concepts in Biochemical Pharmacology. Berlin: Springer, 1971.

Casarett, L. J., Doull, J. (Eds.). Toxicology: The Basic Science of Poisons. New York: Macmillan, 1975.

Goldstein, A., Aranow, L., Kalman, S. M. Principles of Drug Action. New York: Wiley-Health, 1974.

Hayes, W. J., Toxicology of Pesticides. Baltimore: Williams & Wilkins, 1975.

Absorption

Brooks, G. T., Penetration and distribution of insecticides. In Wilkinson, C. F. (Ed.). Insecticide Biochemistry and Physiology. New York: Plenum Press, 1976, pp. 3–58.

Bukov, M. J. Herbicide entry into plants. In Audus, I. J. (Ed.). Herbicides: Physiology, Biochemistry, and Ecology. New York: Academic Press, 1976, pp. 335–364.

Eisenberg, M., McLaughlin, S. M. Lipid bilayers as models for biological membranes. BioSciences 26 (1976), 436.

Hull, H. M. Leaf structure as related to absorption of pesticides and other compounds. Residue Rev. 31 (1970), 1.

Mudd, J. B., Kozlowski, T. T. (Eds.). Plant Responses to Air Pollution. New York: Academic Press, 1975.

Lee, D. H. K., Falk, H. L. Murphy, S. D. (Eds.). Handbook of Physiology, Section 9, Reaction to Environmental Agents. Bethesda, Md.: American Physiological Society 1977. [See chapters on skin (p. 299), gastrointestinal tract (p. 349), and respiration (p. 213).]

Weissmann, G., Claiborne, R. (Eds.). Cell Membranes: Biochemistry, Cell Biology, and Pathology. New York: H. P. Publishing 1975.

Distribution

Rose, M. S. Reversible binding of toxic compounds to macromolecules, Br. Med. Bull. 25 (1967), 227.

Westphal, U. Steroid–Protein Interactions. New York: Springer, 1971.

Daniel B. Tuey

3

Toxicokinetics

3.1. Introduction

Pharmacokinetics deals with the movement of chemicals in biological systems. Its goal is to quantitate the dynamic time course of chemical absorption, distribution, biotransformation, and elimination processes in living organisms. *Pharmacodynamics* deals with the biochemical and physiological effects of chemicals and their mechanisms of action. Thus, while pharmacokinetics is primarily concerned with movement, pharmacodynamics is more generally concerned with the underlying forces and their relationship to movement. The purpose of this chapter is to introduce some pharmacokinetic concepts and principles and to demonstrate their utility for elucidating how, why, and to what extent kinetic events can affect the disposition of toxicants in the body.

Many of the pharmacokinetic methodologies and principles used by pharmacologists are directly applicable to the work of toxicologists. Both fields are concerned with the time course and tissue or organ specificity of chemical agents. However, while the pharmacologist is mainly interested in establishing and maintaining therapeutically effective levels of medicinal agents in the body, the toxicologist is concerned with avoiding toxicity (for example, by maneuvering processes governing the accumulation of chemicals in the body in favor of elimination) and assessing whether and what safe levels exist. Pesticide and environmental toxicologists must in addition be cognizant of species specificity and susceptibility and contend with chronic exposures to low or unknown levels and mixtures of xenobiotic agents. The terms *toxicokinetics* and *toxicodynamics* are used to emphasize the special concerns of the toxicologist.

An important and most promising area for new developments in and applications of toxicokinetics is that dealing with nonlinear phenomena. Toxicities often occur only after the saturation of capacity-limited elimination pathways, or as a result of enzyme-mediated metabolic activation–deactivation reactions that produce reactive intermediates. A toxic response can also cause altered kinetics. However, the treatment of such effects is beyond the scope of this chapter. Since the aim here is to motivate a desire to seek out more comprehensive treatments, only a few of the simplest and most straightforward toxicokinetic concepts are introduced. Linear kinetics are considered throughout, and it is assumed that the toxic agent is either the parent compound or a linear function of it. Toxicodynamic mechanisms are ignored. Although many of the "sticky" mathematical details are deftly skirted, the presentation is rigorous. The reader should think of, and attempt to interpret, each equation encountered as a precise symbolic statement of the assumptions made and the consequences that follow.

3.2. Basic Concepts

3.2.1. Exponential Growth and Decay

In studying the disposition of chemicals in biological systems one frequently observes variables that exhibit *first-order kinetics;* that is, the rate of change of a variable over time appears to be proportional to its instantaneous magnitude. Symbolically, if y is the magnitude of a variable and dy/dt is the instantaneous rate of change in its magnitude at any time t, a mathematical description of this observation is provided by the linear differential equation

$$- \frac{dy}{dt} = ky \tag{3.1}$$

where k is a constant of proportionality. The minus sign corresponds to a decaying y; the sign would be positive if the process were growing. Equation (3.1) states in precise mathematical terms that the larger the magnitude of y, the faster it will change. The parameter k is called a *rate constant* because it has the dimensions of reciprocal time. It should be clear that it is the proportionality between dy/dt and y that is constant, not the rate of change.

If y_0 is the magnitude of y at some instant in time t_0, the integrated form of Equation (3.1) is the exponential equation

$$y(t) = y_0 e^{-kt}, \qquad t \geq t_0. \tag{3.2}$$

Equation (3.2) expresses y explicitly as a function of time (Figure 3.1a). Thus the magnitude of y can be calculated at any point in time after t_0, provided that the values of y_0 and k are known.

Taking the logarithm of both sides transforms Equation (3.2) into a linear one,

$$\ln y(t) = \ln y_0 - kt \tag{3.3}$$

using natural logarithms, or

$$\log y(t) = \log y_0 - (0.434)kt \tag{3.4}$$

using base 10 common logarithms. If $\log y$ were plotted as a function of time it would appear as shown in Figure 3.1b, a straight line having intercept $\log y_0$

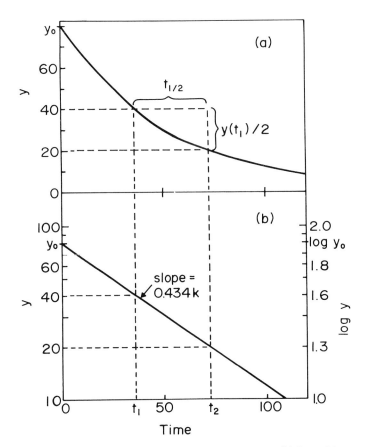

Figure 3.1 Exponential decay: (a) $y(t)$ versus t; (b) $\log y(t)$ versus t.

and slope $-(0.434)k$. A convenient method of characterizing the rate of decay of y is by means of its half-life $t_{1/2}$. If t_1 and t_2 are two distinct time points such that the magnitude of y at time t_2, $y(t_2)$, is one-half its magnitude at time t_1, $y(t_1)$, then, from Equation (3.2),

$$\frac{y(t_2)}{y(t_1)} = \frac{1}{2} = e^{-k(t_2 - t_1)} \tag{3.5}$$

and the logarithm of this result yields

$$t_2 - t_1 = \frac{\ln 2}{k} = \frac{\log 2}{0.434k} = \frac{0.693}{k} = t_{1/2}. \tag{3.6}$$

Note that while the time point t_1 can be selected arbitrarily and may, but need not, correspond to y_0, this choice then determines the time t_2. The interval between these two time points is the half-life, which, according to Equation (3.6), is a constant whose value depends only on the rate constant k.

To summarize, exponential changes correspond to first-order kinetics that can be described by linear differential equations and characterized by half-lives.

3.2.2. Curve Fitting

The fitting of curves to experimental data is a standard procedure in the study of toxicant disposition kinetics. For example, if serial measurements of the amount or concentration of a toxicant in the body were plotted as a function of time on semilog graph paper and appeared to fall on a straight line, the analysis described in the previous section could be applied directly. Thus it could be inferred that the process that generated the experimental results is described by Equation (3.1). The toxicant's disposition kinetics could be further characterized by graphically determining its half-life in the body. In Section 3.3 it will be seen that some additional inferences can be made with the aid of a compartmental model.

If it is apparent that a semilog plot of the experimental data does not approximate a straight line and it is unlikely that the discrepancy is the result of experimental error and biological variability, one might then attempt to fit a biexponential function to the data, or even a multiexponential function. A typical biexponential function is given by

$$y(t) = Ae^{-\alpha t} + Be^{-\beta t} \tag{3.7}$$

where A, α, B, and β are constants to be determined from the experimental data. Provided that these experimental constants can be determined, similar analyses could be applied to help characterize the toxicant's biexponential disposition kinetics.

The method of residuals is a commonly used technique for resolving multiexponential functions such as Equation (3.7) into their individual components. The method consists of sequentially feathering, or peeling off, successive exponential terms. Generally the successive exponents must differ in magnitude from one another by at least a factor of 3 in order for this graphic technique to succeed, and in practice the procedure rarely works for more than two or three exponential terms. More often it is used to obtain initial estimates for use in a more refined parameter estimation method such as iterative nonlinear least squares regression. Standard computer programs exist for performing this parameter estimation, although one should be aware that meaningful results are by no means guaranteed due to the inherently nonlinear nature of exponential functions.

The biphasic decay described by Equation (3.7) can be characterized at early times by its initial half-life, equal to $0.693/\alpha$, and at later times by its terminal half-life, equal to $0.693/\beta$. However, without additional information there is no way of knowing whether a third exponential term might have shown up if data had been obtained at earlier or later time points, or whether more precise measurements might have revealed that the apparent biphasic decay components are actually combinations of other exponential terms. This is because, unlike a physical process such as radioactive decay, a toxicant's disposition kinetics in a biological system is in general the result of many complex, interacting phenomena. It is therefore important to keep in mind that while biological half-lives and mathematical models are useful concepts for characterizing curves fit to data from physicochemical phenomena, their uniqueness is by no means assured.

3.2.3. Pharmacokinetic Models

A quantitative description and evaluation of a toxicant's biological fate is often greatly facilitated by representing the body as a system of interconnected compartments. In the language of pharmacokinetics, the term *compartment* refers to all those tissues, organs, and fluids within the body that are kinetically indistinguishable from each other. For example, a compartment might refer to a particular cluster of cells within a specific organ, or to the blood, extracellular water, and all well-perfused tissues taken together. What constitutes a compartment will depend on the properties of the chemical being studied, i.e., its molecular size, lipophilicity, binding affinity, etc., as well as how closely and accurately the biological system is or can be monitored.

A *pharmacokinetic model* is simply a functional representation that possesses the ability to describe the movement of a chemical over time in a real biological system. Several model analogies are depicted in Figure 3.2: an animal model used in lieu of human subjects (Figure 3.2a), a hydraulic model (Figure 3.2b), a symbolic compartmental model (Figure 3.2c), and a differential equation model (Figure 3.2d). If the concentration of a toxicant in serial blood samples from the animal model declines exponentially over time, since the hydraulic, com-

Figure 3.2 Equivalent pharmacokinetic models: (a) animal model, curve fit to serial blood sample data; (b) hydraulic model, $c(t)$ is the concentration of solute; (c) symbolic compartmental model, k is a first-order rate constant; and (d) differential equation model.

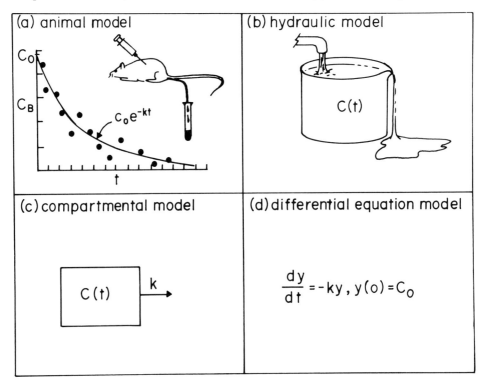

partmental, and mathematical analogies can all be made to describe the same exponential function, all of these models are pharmacokinetically equivalent.

Toxicokinetic analysis is concerned with deriving a formal compartmental model interpretation of toxicant disposition time-course data; toxicokinetic synthesis attempts to formulate from physicobiochemical concepts a compartmental model that will describe the experimental observations.

3.3. Toxicokinetic Analysis

3.3.1. Toxicokinetic Analysis Models

Toxicokinetic analysis models depend on the ability to fit curves to experimental data that generally consist of serial blood and/or excreta samples. As pointed out earlier, the size and number of compartments derived from such data are highly dependent on the specific disposition characteristics of the particular toxicant being studied, and generally will not correspond directly to any clearly defined real anatomical body tissue. However, it is often both possible and sufficient, for toxicokinetic analysis purposes, to interpret the derived compartments and model parameters as being representative of functionally homogeneous tissue groups possessing common characteristics insofar as toxicant disposition is concerned. For example, a three-compartment model of the body might consist of a central compartment representing the blood and well-perfused body tissues, a peripheral compartment representing the poorly perfused tissues, and a third compartment for a tissue or organ of special interest. In practice, one- and two-compartment analysis models are by far the most common.

3.3.2. One-Compartment Model

3.3.2a. First-Order Elimination

The simplest compartmental model depicts the body as a single homogeneous unit within which a chemical toxicant is uniformly distributed at all times. If toxicant elimination approximates first-order kinetics, then its rate of loss from the body is described by

$$\frac{dX}{dt} = -k_e X, \qquad X(0) = X_0 \tag{3.8}$$

where X is the amount in the body at time t, k_e is the rate constant for first-order elimination, and X_0 is the initial amount in the body. This equation was introduced as Equation (3.1), where the symbol y was used in place of X.

In compartmental analysis k_e is often referred to as an *apparent first-order elimination* rate constant, to emphasize that the underlying processes may in reality only approximate first-order kinetics. For example, the toxicant might actually be eliminated by active biliary secretion for which zero-order saturation kinetics would be observed under suitable conditions.

If the amount of chemical in the body is negligible prior to the rapid introduction of a known amount D, the total amount of chemical initially in the body will be approximately

$$X(0) = D. \tag{3.9}$$

Therefore, solving Equation (3.8) by integration subject to the initial condition given in Equation (3.9) gives the result

$$X(t) = De^{-k_e t} \tag{3.10}$$

which describes the amount remaining in the body at any time t thereafter (Figure 3.3a).

The body is obviously not a single homogeneous unit, and in actuality a chemical will be distributed throughout the body at concentrations that are different for each tissue. Often, however, a dynamic distribution equilibrium will be maintained between the tissues so that tissue/blood concentration ratios are approximately constant. Under these circumstances the total amount of chemical in the body will be proportional to its concentration in blood,

$$X = VC \tag{3.11}$$

where V is a constant of proportionality and C is the concentration in blood or plasma. Since V happens to have the units of volume, it is referred to as the *apparent volume* of distribution. However, it is important to remember that V is in reality simply a convenient proportionality constant. If the initial blood con-

Figure 3.3 One compartment model with first-order elimination and (a) instantaneous absorption; (b) first-order absorption; (c) constant input. D is the dose or dose rate, f is the fraction absorbed, k_a and k_e are rate constants, and X_a, X, and X_e are amounts.

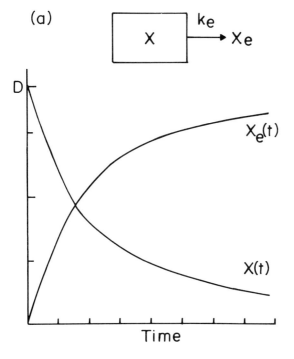

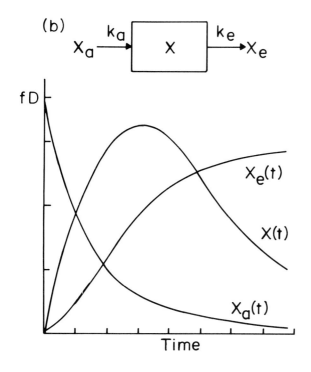

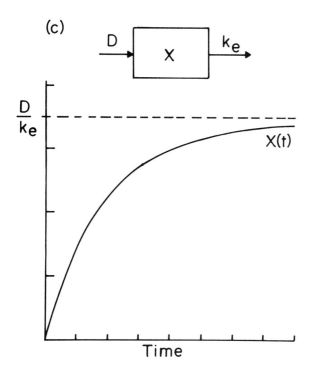

centration C_0 is known, this apparent distribution volume can be estimated from Equation (3.11) as

$$V = \frac{D}{C_0}.$$ (3.12)

Combining Equations (3.10) and (3.11) and solving for C gives the concentration of toxicant in the blood as a function of time,

$$C(t) = \frac{D}{V} e^{-k_e t}.$$ (3.13)

Taking logarithms transforms this equation into a linear one:

$$\log C(t) = \log \left(\frac{D}{V}\right) - (0.434)k_e t$$ (3.14)

which can be used as described in Section 3.2.1 to estimate, from serial blood or plasma samples, the rate constant k_e and the half-life $t_{1/2}$ for toxicant elimination from the body.

An alternative method of assessing a toxicant's disposition kinetics is to monitor its appearance in excreta. Since the elimination of toxicant is assumed to be first order, its rate of appearance in excreta will be proportional to the instantaneous amount in the body,

$$\frac{dX_e}{dt} = k_e X, \qquad X_e(0) = 0$$ (3.15)

where k_e is again the apparent first-order elimination rate constant and X_e, the amount in excreta, is initially zero. Since Equation (3.10) gives the amount of chemical in the body as an explicit function of time, substituting for X in Equation (3.15) and integrating gives the cumulative amount excreted as a function of time:

$$X_e(t) = D(1 - e^{-k_e t})$$ (3.16)

shown in Figure 3.3A. This equation can also be logarithmically transformed into a more convenient form for estimating k_e and $t_{1/2}$:

$$\log \left[\frac{D - X_e(t)}{D}\right] = -(0.434)k_e t.$$ (3.17)

3.3.2b. First-Order Absorption

In the previous discussion, toxicant intake was assumed to be essentially instantaneous compared to distribution and elimination. If intake more closely approximates a first-order absorption process, the rate of change in the amount of chemical in a one-compartment model of the body with first-order elimination, Equation (3.8), becomes

$$\frac{dX}{dt} = -k_e X + k_a X_a \tag{3.18}$$

where k_e and X are as defined previously, k_a is the *apparent first-order absorption rate constant*, and X_a is the amount of chemical at the absorption site. The rate of loss of chemical from the absorption site is given by

$$\frac{dX_a}{dt} = -k_a X_a. \tag{3.19}$$

The solution to Equation (3.19), assuming $X_a(0) = fD$, where f is the fraction of the dose D that is actually absorbed, is

$$X_a(t) = fDe^{-k_a t}. \tag{3.20}$$

Substituting Equation (3.20) into Equation (3.18) and solving gives

$$X(t) = \frac{fDk_a}{k_a - k_e} (e^{-k_e t} - e^{-k_a t}) + X_0 e^{-k_e t} \tag{3.21}$$

where X_0 is the initial amount of chemical already in the body. Substituting Equation (3.21) into Equation (3.15) and integrating gives the cumulative amount excreted:

$$X_e(t) = fD\left[1 - \left(\frac{k_a e^{-k_e t} - k_e e^{-k_a t}}{k_a - k_e}\right)\right] + X_0\left(1 - e^{-k_e t}\right). \tag{3.22}$$

The first term in the last two equations is the contribution due to D, while the second term is due to the nonzero initial amount X_0 in the body. Typical plots of $X_a(t)$, $X(t)$, and $X_e(t)$ versus time are shown in Figure 3.3B.

If X_0 is much less than fD and the rate of absorption is fast compared to the rate of elimination, then after a short period of time the term $e^{-k_a t}$ will be negligible and Equation (3.21) will closely approximate

$$X(t) = fDe^{-k_e t}. \tag{3.23}$$

This result is essentially identical to Equation (3.10), previously obtained assuming instantaneous absorption and $X_0 = 0$. The same analysis applies to $X_e(t)$.

3.3.2c. Constant Input

If a chemical is ingested chronically, such as a contaminant in food, and is slowly eliminated from the body, the dose rate can often be treated as though it were a constant input. In this case the differential equation describing the rate of change in the amount of toxicant in the body, again assuming a one-compartment model with first-order elimination, is

$$\frac{dX}{dt} = -k_e X + D, \qquad X(0) = X_0 \tag{3.24}$$

where k_e, X, and X_0 are as previously defined, and now D is a constant-input dose rate expressed as an amount per unit time. Letting $X_0 = 0$, the solution to this equation is

$$X(t) = \frac{D}{k_e} (1 - e^{k_e t}) \tag{3.25}$$

which describes the accumulation of toxicant in the body with time as depicted in Figure 3.3C.

After a period of time exceeding five or six half-lives, the exponential term in Equation (3.25) will be negligible, and thus the amount in the body will essentially be constant. Using Equation (3.11) to express this *steady-state* condition in terms of blood concentration gives

$$C_{ss} - \frac{D}{Vk_e} \tag{3.26}$$

where C_{ss} is the steady-state concentration of chemical in the body. It is apparent that this steady-state or *plateau level* will be directly proportional to the dose rate, and that when this condition is attained, elimination from the body exactly balances input. Equation (3.26) also provides a convenient relationship at steady state for determining the apparent volume of distribution if k_e, C_{ss}, and D are known.

3.3.3. Two-Compartment Model

If a chemical does not distribute and equilibrate throughout the body rapidly, a two-compartment model may provide a better description of toxicant disposition kinetics. Typically, the main or central compartment is assumed to represent the blood and highly perfused organs and tissues, such as the liver and kidney, that are in rapid distribution equilibrium with the blood, while the second or peripheral compartment corresponds to poorly perfused tissues, such as the muscle, fat, and lean tissues. As noted earlier, in practice, whether a particular tissue is associated with the central or peripheral compartment will depend on the individual characteristics of the compound being modeled. In the following discussion it is assumed that the elimination and intercompartment transfer rates all obey first-order kinetics and that elimination occurs only from the central compartment.

The model just described is depicted in Figure 3.4 and is called a *two-compartment open pharmacokinetic model*. The differential equations describing the rate of change in the amount of chemical in the central and peripheral compartments are

$$\frac{dX_c}{dt} = -(k_{10} + k_{12})X_c + k_{21}X_p, \qquad X_c(0) = X_0, \tag{3.27}$$

$$\frac{dX_p}{dt} = k_{12}X_c - k_{21}X_p, \qquad X_p(0) = 0 \tag{3.28}$$

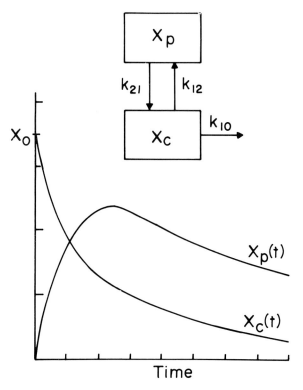

Figure 3.4 Two compartment model: k_{12}, k_{21}, and k_{10} are first-order rate constants; X_0 is the initial amount, X_c is the amount in the central compartment, and X_p is the amount in the peripheral compartment.

where X_c and X_p are the amount of toxicant in the central and peripheral compartments, respectively, k_{12} and k_{21} are the apparent first-order intercompartment transfer rate constants, k_{10} is the apparent first-order elimination rate constant, and the initial conditions $X_c(0)$ and $X_p(0)$ are assumed to be as specified.

The solution to these simultaneous equations is

$$X_c(t) = X_0 \left[\left(\frac{\alpha - k_{21}}{\alpha - \beta} \right) e^{-\alpha t} + \left(\frac{k_{21} - \beta}{\alpha - \beta} \right) e^{-\beta t} \right] \tag{3.29}$$

$$X_p(t) = \frac{k_{12} X_0}{\alpha - \beta} \left(e^{-\alpha t} - e^{-\beta t} \right) \tag{3.30}$$

where α and β are given by

$$\begin{bmatrix} \alpha \\ \beta \end{bmatrix} = \frac{1}{2} \left[(k_{12} + k_{21} + k_{10}) \pm \sqrt{(k_{12} + k_{21} + k_{10})^2 - 4k_{21}k_{10}} \right] \tag{3.31}$$

and are called the *apparent first-order decay rate constants*. Thus, the pharmacokinetics of a two-compartment model describe a biexponential decay in the amount of toxicant in the body. Typical curves are shown in Figure 3.4.

Analogous to a one-compartment model, since a distribution equilibrium is assumed to exist within each compartment, Equation (3.29) can be expressed in terms of blood concentration:

$$C(t) = Ae^{-\alpha t} + Be^{-\beta t} \tag{3.32}$$

where

$$A = \frac{X_0}{V_c}\left(\frac{\alpha - k_{21}}{\alpha - \beta}\right), \qquad B = \frac{X_0}{V_c}\left(\frac{k_{21} - \beta}{\alpha - \beta}\right) \tag{3.33}$$

and V_c is the apparent volume of the central compartment. The use of excretion data to assess the pharmacokinetics of a chemical that exhibits two-compartment model characteristics is also analogous to the procedures described for a one-compartment model.

By convention, $\alpha > \beta$, so that the term $Ae^{-\alpha t}$ will approach zero faster than $Be^{-\beta t}$, at which time Equation (3.32) reduces to

$$C(t) = Be^{-\beta t}. \tag{3.34}$$

This equation describes the *postdistributive phase*, and β is called the *disposition rate constant*. Thus, analogous to a one-compartment model, the terminal half-life for a two-compartment model is given by

$$t_{1/2} = 0.693/\beta \tag{3.35}$$

and is referred to as the *biological half-life* of the toxicant. It is important to note that the biological half-life is not simply a function of the elimination rate k_{10}, but depends, as Equation (3.31) shows, on the intercompartment transfer rate constants k_{12} and k_{21} as well.

According to Equation (3.32), a plot of the logarithm of blood concentration versus time will yield a biphasic decay from which the constants A, B, α, and β can be estimated either graphically or by nonlinear regression analysis. Once these experimental constants have been determined the pharmacokinetic parameters k_{12}, k_{21}, k_{10}, and V_c can be calculated from relationships that result from the solution to Equations (3.27) and (3.28). The numerical values of these parameters can aid in assessing the relative importance of tissue distribution and elimination to the disposition of the toxicant.

3.3.4. Chronic Ingestion

It was shown in Section 3.3.2c. that when the ingestion of a chemical approximates a constant dose rate the amount in the body will accumulate up to a steady-state plateau level. The time to reach this steady state will depend on the elimination rate, while the amount of toxicant in the body at plateau will depend on both the dose and the elimination rate. Accumulation can also occur during chronic daily or even intermittant ingestion, depending on the toxicant's disposition kinetics. For example, the amount in the body following n equal

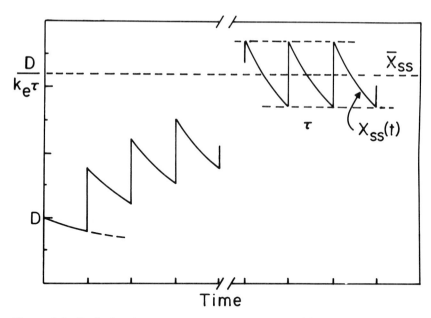

Figure 3.5 Body burden in a one compartment model receiving repeated doses of a toxicant: D is the amount of each dose, k_e is the first-order elimination rate constant, τ is the time between doses, $X_{ss}(t)$ is the amount in the body at plateau, and $\bar{X}_{ss}$ is the average body burden at plateau.

doses of a toxicant whose single-dose kinetics are as described in Section 3.3.2.a is

$$X_n(t) = D(e^{-k_e((n-1)\tau+t)} + e^{-k_e((n-2)\tau+t)}$$
$$+ \cdots + e^{-k_e(\tau+t)} + k^{-k_e t}) \tag{3.36}$$

where t and $X_n(t)$ are the time and the amount after dose n, and τ is the interval between doses. The first exponential term in Equation (3.36) is the residue from the first dose, the second term is the residue from the second dose, and so on. Rearrangement of Equation (3.36) results in

$$X_n(t) = D\left(\frac{1 - e^{-nk_e\tau}}{1 - e^{-k_e\tau}}\right) e^{-k_e t}. \tag{3.37}$$

A representative plot of this equation is shown in Figure 3.5. At steady state the amount in the body, $X_{ss}(t)$, will fluctuate between successive doses according to

$$X_{ss}(t) = \frac{De^{-k_e t}}{1 - e^{-k_e\tau}}. \tag{3.38}$$

The maximum amount in the body at steady state will occur immediately after each dose, while the minimum will occur at the end of each dose interval. The average amount at steady state is given by

$$\overline{X}_{ss} = \frac{1}{\tau} \int_0^{\tau} X_{ss}(t) \, dt \tag{3.39}$$

which, upon substitution of Equation (3.38) and integration, yields

$$\overline{X}_{ss} = \frac{D}{k_e \tau} = \frac{(1.44)t_{1/2}D}{\tau} \tag{3.40}$$

where k_e has been replaced by the half-life according to Equation (3.6). Equation (3.40) shows clearly that the average amount of toxicant in the body will accumulate to a steady-state level that can be much higher than the chronic ingestion level if the half-life for elimination is long.

Similar analyses apply when toxicant intake is first order, and also for multicompartmental models of toxicant disposition in the body, in which additional distribution effects come into play. Thus, understanding the kinetic fate of a toxicant in the body takes on added importance when ingestion is chronic. It should also be remembered that an ideal situation has been described above; aging, stress, and toxicities that arise during chronic ingestion can alter physiological function and change the pharmacokinetics of a toxicant during the time course of the exposure.

3.4. Toxicokinetic Synthesis

3.4.1. Physiological Compartmental Models

Although compartmental analysis models are convenient to use and provide useful descriptions of the overall time course of toxicant disposition, the practical limitations of curve fitting to experimental data generally restrict such models to one- or two-compartment descriptions of the body. Alternatively, it is often possible to synthesize a compartmental model from physiological principles and thereby circumvent the inherent limitations of curve-fitting analysis.

A physiological compartmental model is one that is constructed using physical and biochemical parameters such as blood flow rates, tissue and organ sizes, binding, and metabolic rates. Even though they are generally more complex and require the specification of many more parameters than are needed for analysis models, physiological compartmental models are still in many ways simplified representations of real biological systems. In addition, the accurate determination of physical and biochemical parameters is often both difficult and variable. However, the physiological framework provides several advantages: the physical definition of compartments and transfer rates facilitates the incorporation of existing knowledge about the quantitative behavior of biological systems into the model; physiological changes with time during chronic exposure to a chemical, such as those due to physical growth, or induction of metabolism and excretion rates, can be introduced naturally; and, most important, a reasonable basis exists for extrapolating the pharmacokinetics of a chemical beyond the original data base, so that attempts can be made to predict the disposition of a chemical following various types and patterns of exposure, in the same as well as in other animal species.

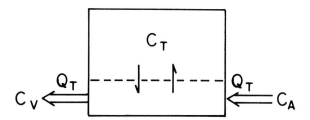

Figure 3.6 Schematic representation of a physiological compartment. Dashed line separates intracellular and extracellular regions; C is the toxicant concentration in tissue (C_T), arterial blood (C_A), and venous blood (C_V); Q_T is the blood or plasma flow rate. For a flow-limited compartment membrane permeabilities are large compared to the perfusion rate.

In this brief introduction to physiological compartmental models the concepts of mass balance and flow-limited transport are introduced; examples are then given of their use in the formulation of compartmental models to predict, the disposition of some environmental chemical pollutants in laboratory animals.

3.4.2. Mass Balance and Flow-Limited Transport

The blood serves to distribute a toxicant from its site of absorption to the other parts of the body. In the normal sequence of events, a chemical entering the blood stream will often distribute within the blood pool with sufficient rapidity such that its blood concentration can be considered to be essentially uniform. Figure 3.6 is a schematic representation of a typical physiological compartment, which may be an organ, a tissue, or a group of tissues that are sufficiently uniform in their properties. The chemical enters and leaves the compartment with the blood flow and diffuses or is transported between blood and tissue. The chemical may also undergo a variety of physical interactions, such as binding to blood and tissue macromolecules, and the result is that a partitioning will occur between tissue (T) and blood (B) depending on the chemical's particular affinity for each medium. At equilibrium, this partitioning (R) can be expressed as a tissue/blood concentration ratio

$$R_T = \frac{C_T}{C_B}\bigg]_{eq} . \tag{3.41}$$

Diffusion or transport directly between adjacent compartments, enzymatic transformations, and excretion may also occur. The net result of all of these changes is expressed by a *mass balance* differential equation, which is simply a mathematical statement of the conservation of mass. In words,

[Rate of change in the amount of chemical in the compartment]
   = [Rate of influx with blood] − [Rate of efflux with blood]
     + [Rate of diffusion or other transport in]
       − [Rate of diffusion or other transport out]
    + [Rate of formation] − [Rate of conversion]
    + [Rate of absorption or injection] − [Rate of excretion].   (3.42)

Frequently this mass balance equation can be greatly simplified since many of the terms may not apply to a particular compartment. For example, the rate of mass change in a compartment due to transport of chemical by blood flow alone is given by the balance equation

$$V_T \frac{dC_T}{dt} = Q_T C_A - Q_T C_V \tag{3.43}$$

where V_T is the (constant) volume of the compartment, Q_T is the blood flow rate, and C_T, C_A, and C_V are the concentrations of chemical in tissue, arterial blood, and venous blood, respectively. If exchange of the chemical between the blood and tissue regions is rapid, the concentration of the chemical in the venous blood leaving this compartment will essentially be in equilibrium with the tissue concentration. In this *flow-limited* case, Equation (3.43) can be simplified using Equation (3.41), which yields

$$V_T \frac{dC_T}{dt} = Q_T \left(C_A - \frac{C_T}{R_T} \right) . \tag{3.44}$$

When the movement of a toxicant in the body is flow limited, the rate and amount of blood flow to the various tissues and organs will determine the initial distribution, while the tissue masses and their affinity for the toxicant will determine the final distribution.

3.4.3. Polychlorinated Biphenyls: An Example

Studies involving the use of physiological pharmacokinetic models as an aid to extrapolating and assessing the significance of chemical disposition and toxicity data from one animal species to another have been initiated for the polychlorinated biphenyls (PCBs). Much of the recent interest in these compounds exists because they are representatives of a major class of environmental contaminants, the halogenated hydrocarbons, as well as being ubiquitous environmental pollutants in themselves. There are 210 possible PCBs, all having the same biphenyl carbon skeleton and differing only in the number and position of the chlorine atoms. Because it would be an enormous task to study the individual disposition of every PCB, the pharmacokinetics of five differently chlorinated biphenyl compounds was examined: 4-monochlorobiphenyl (1CB), 4,4'-dichlorobiphenyl (2CB), 3,3',5,5'-tetrachlorobiphenyl (4CB), 2,2',4,5,5'-pentachlorobiphenyl (5CB), and 2,2',4,4',5,5'-hexachlorobiphenyl (6CB).

Preliminary laboratory experiments suggested that a flow-limited compartmental model could be used to predict the pharmacokinetics of these PCBs in the rat. Figure 3.7 is a schematic diagram of the model. The liver, muscle, skin, and adipose tissue masses were each represented as a compartment in which PCB entered with the arterial blood flow at one concentration and left with the venous blood flow at another concentration. For flow-limited transport the concentration in venous blood depends on the tissue/blood partition ratio of the tissue it flows through. Metabolism was assumed to be a first-order process that occurred only in the liver. Metabolized PCB was distributed to the other tissues with the blood flow and was also excreted with the bile. The excreted

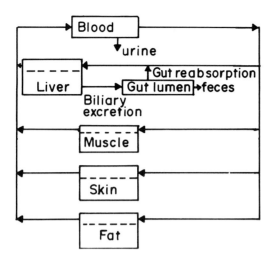

Figure 3.7 Flow diagram for a pharmacokinetic model of PCB disposition in the rat.
SOURCE: *Lutz et al., Drug Metab. Dispos. 5 (1977), 386.* © 1977 *American Society for Pharmacology and Experimental Therapeutics.*

metabolites were partially reabsorbed as material moved down the intestines by bulk flow. PCB metabolites were eventually eliminated from the body with the feces, and also by excretion in urine.

Mass balance differential equations were written to describe the rate of change of PCB in each compartment; a second set of equations was similarly written for PCB metabolites. For example, the mass balance equation for PCB in the liver compartment is

$$V_L \frac{dC_L}{dt} = Q_L C_B - Q_L \left(\frac{C_L}{R_L}\right) - k_m \left(\frac{C_L}{R_L}\right) \tag{3.45}$$

where V_L is the volume of the liver, C_B and C_L are the PCB concentrations in the blood and liver tissues, respectively, Q_L is the average blood flow rate to the liver, R_L is the liver/blood equilibrium distribution ratio, and k_m is the apparent first-order metabolic rate constant. The mass balance equation for PCB metabolites in the liver is

$$V_L \frac{dC'_L}{dt} = Q_L C'_B - Q_L \left(\frac{C'_L}{R'_L}\right) + k_m \left(\frac{C_L}{R_L}\right) - k_b \left(\frac{C'_L}{R'_L}\right) + k_G V_G C'_G \tag{3.46}$$

where k_b and k_G are the apparent first-order rate constants for biliary clearance and gut reabsorption, respectively, V_G is the volume of the gut lumen compartment, and all other terms are as previously defined, with primes denoting metabolites. The complete mathematical description of the model, including the rate of accumulation of metabolites in urine and in feces, consisted of 13 simultaneous differential equations with the appropriate parameters and initial conditions specified for each PCB.

Although knowledge of a considerable number of parameters was required, the physiological framework of the model permitted many of the necessary parameter values to be obtained from the literature; where necessary, they were determined experimentally in the laboratory. Table 3.1 gives the parameter values used for each of the five PCBs studied. In principle, the explicit analytical solution to the model equations could be determined; in practice it is easier to solve the equations numerically on a computer.

Computer simulations using the model equations to predict the tissue distribution and excretion of these PCBs as a function of time were quite accurate for the slowly metabolized compounds. An example is shown in Figure 3.8 for 6CB disposition in the rat, where the lines are the computer simulation results. The lines were not curve fit to the data points, which were obtained from actual laboratory experiments following a single iv dose of 6CB. It can be seen that the physiological compartmental model gave good predictions of the disposition of this compound in this animal species. Model predictions were best for those compounds whose in vivo metabolic rates could be most accurately estimated, which were for the most slowly metabolized PCBs. Fortunately, the more readily metabolized PCBs are also the least persistent in the environment, and consequently are of less concern.

Table 3.1   PCB[a] Model Parameters for a 250-g Rat

Compartment	Volume (ml)	Parent tissue blood ratios				
		1CB	2CB	4CB	5CB	6CB
Blood	22.5	1	1	1	1	1
Gut lumen	14	1	1	1	1	1
Muscle	125	1	2	1	1	4
Liver	10	1	3	6	6	12
Skin	40	10	10	7	7	30
Fat	17.5	30	70	220	70	400

Compartment	Blood flow (ml/hr)	Metabolite tissue blood ratios				
		1CB	2CB	4CB	5CB	6CB
Blood	—	1	1	1	1	1
Gut lumen	—	1	1	1	1	1
Muscle	450	0.14	0.40	0.10	0.10	0.30
Liver	960	2	5	2	2	4
Skin	30	0.25	0.30	0.30	0.10	2
Fat	24	0.40	0.60	0.50	0.40	2

Kinetic parameters	1CB	2CB	4CB	5CB	6CB
Metabolism rate k_m (ml/hr)	600	120	14.2	23.4	2.7
Kidney clearance k_k (ml/hr)	12	8	0.7	2	1.8
Biliary clearance k_b (ml/hr)	12	21	12.1	18	18
Gut reabsorption k_G (hr^{-1})	0.0096	0.0096	0.01	0.0096	0.0096
Fecal transport k_f (hr^{-1})	0.048	0.048	0.05	0.048	0.048

Source: Data from Lutz et al., *Drug Metab. Dispos.* 5 (1977), 386; and Tuey and Matthews, *Drug Metab. Dispos.* 5 (1977), 444.

[a] 1CB, 4-monochlorobiphenyl; 2CB, 4,4'-dichlorobiphenyl; 4CB, 3,3',5,5'-tetrachlorobiphenyl; 5CB, 2,2',4,5,5'-pentachlorobiphenyl; 6CB, 2,2',4,4',5,5'-hexachlorobiphenyl.

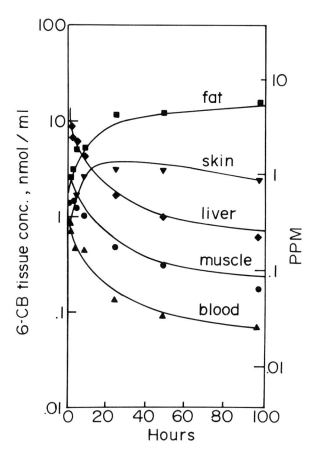

Figure 3.8 6CB tissue concentrations in the rat after a single 0.6 mg/kg iv dose. Points represent mean ($n = 3$) experimental data; lines are the model computed predictions.
SOURCE: *Lutz et al., Drug Metab. Dispos. 5 (1977), 386.* © *1977 American Society for Pharmacology and Experimental Therapeutics.*

Initial attempts at using this model as a means for extrapolating toxicant disposition kinetics from one animal species to another were also successful, again most favorably for those PCBs whose rates of metabolism could be most accurately determined. The model described above for a 250-g rat was scaled using physiological parameter values appropriate for a 38-g mouse, and computer simulations were again performed. An example of the results obtained in the mouse for the predicted disposition of the same 6CB compound is shown in Figure 3.9. The lines shown in this figure were generated by computer using the scaled model and, as for the rat, are not curve fits of the mouse experimental data points.

3.4.4. Hexabromobiphenyl: An Example

As a second example of toxicokinetic synthesis techniques, a physiological compartmental model for the disposition of 2,2′,4,4′,5,5′-hexabromobiphenyl (PBB) will be described. This brominated biphenyl compound is the major constituent (54–68%) of Firemaster BP-6, the fire retardant chemical that accidentally con-

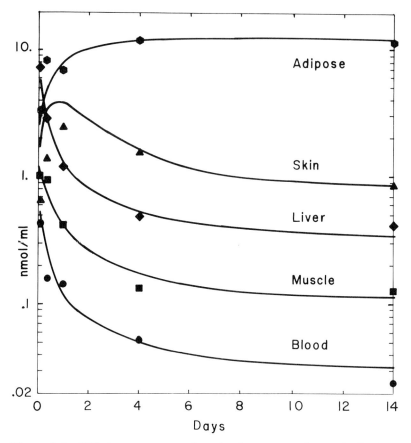

Figure 3.9 6CB tissue concentrations in the mouse after a single 0.6 mg/kg iv dose. Points represent mean ($n = 3$) experimental data; lines are the scaled model predictions. SOURCE: *Tuey and Matthews, Toxicol. Appl. Pharmacol. 41 (1977), 158.*

taminated livestock feed and subsequently much of the livestock, animal produce, and human population of Michigan in 1973 and 1974. Figure 3.10 is a flow diagram for the disposition of PBB in the rat. Preliminary experimental data indicated that metabolism was negligible. Distribution to tissues was similar to that of the PCBs, and was again assumed to be by flow-limited transport. An iv dose of PBB was eliminated slowly and primarily in the bile. Urine was a negligible route of elimination.

In order to account for the rate of both oral and iv doses, the gut was described in more detail than was necessary for the PCB model. Bile duct cannulations were performed on animals for 1 hr prior to sacrifice 24 hr after a single iv dose, and the amount of PBB-derived material excreted was used in conjunction with the concentration in liver tissue to estimate a first-order biliary excretion rate constant k_b. Mass transfer of PBB between intestinal tissue and its lumenal contents was assumed to occur by passive bidirectional diffusion. A permeability constant k_G, was estimated from the results observed for orally administered doses of PBB, which were assumed to be absorbed primarily from the intestines.

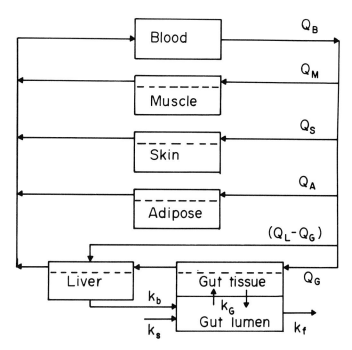

Figure 3.10 Flow diagram for a pharmacokinetic model of PBB disposition in the rat. Q_T, $T = B, M, S, A, L, G$, are blood flow rates; k_b, biliary excretion rate; k_G, permeability constant; k_S, stomach transport rate; k_f, fecal transport rate.
SOURCE: *Tuey and Matthews, Toxicol. Appl. Pharmacol. 45 (1978), 337.*

The small and large intestines were combined and modeled as a single gut tissue having a distant lumen compartment. A transport time $1/k_S$, was estimated for material passing from the stomach into the small intestine, while the average residence time of intestinal contents $1/k_f$, was determined from the experimental data. The mass balance equations for the liver, intestines, and lumen were

Liver:

$$V_L \frac{dC_L}{dt} = (Q_L - Q_G)C_B + Q_G\left(\frac{C_G}{R_G}\right) - Q_L\left(\frac{C_L}{R_L}\right) - k_b C_L \qquad (3.47)$$

Intestinal tissue:

$$V_G \frac{dC_G}{dt} = Q_G\left(C_B - \frac{C_G}{R_G}\right) + k_G(V_{GL}C_{GL} - V_G C_G) \qquad (3.48)$$

Intestinal lumen:

$$V_G \frac{dC_{GL}}{dt} = k_G(V_G C_G - V_{GL}C_{GL}) + k_b C_L + k_S M_S - k_f V_{GL}C_{GL} \qquad (3.49)$$

where M_S is the amount of PBB in the stomach. For multiple oral doses the amount in the stomach compartment was described by

$$\frac{dM_S}{dt} = -k_S M_S + Dg(t) \tag{3.50}$$

where D is the daily dose and $g(t)$ is a normalized injection function. An iv dose was simulated by introducing $Dg(t)$ directly into the blood compartment.

Since fat is the major long-term storage site of lipophilic xenobiotics, changes in the amount of this tissue can significantly alter distribution and excretion. Rat body weights increased from 250 g to over 400 g during the 42-day study, and a significant fraction of this weight increase occurred in adipose tissue. In order to account for this change, the volume of the adipose tissue compartment was computed from equations that were fit to experimental data of the change in body weight and fat fraction as a function of time:

$$V_A(t) = W_0(1 + 0.0007t)[0.07 + 0.04(1 - e^{-0.003t})] \tag{3.51}$$

where W_0 is the initial body weight in grams and t is time in hours. The mass balance equation for PBB in the growing adipose tissue compartment was

$$V_A(t)\frac{dC_A}{dt} = Q_A\left(C_B - \frac{C_A}{R_A}\right) - C_A\frac{dV_A}{dt}. \tag{3.52}$$

These growth equations were originally developed to describe the long-term disposition of 6CB.

Mass balance equations describing PBB in the blood, muscle, and skin compartments were identical to those for the PCB model with no excretion in urine and completed the mathematical description of the PBB disposition model. Computer simulations were performed, and the predicted and experimental results following a single 1.0 mg/kg iv dose are shown in Figure 3.11. As for the PCB results, the lines shown here are the PBB time courses predicted by the model and were not curve fitted to the experimental data points.

It is instructive to describe some of the inferences that can be drawn from the model predictions. Less than 7% of the dose was excreted after 42 days, and the daily excretion rate after 7 days was less than 0.2%/day. The model predicted the cumulative excretion of PBB in bile after 4 hr to be 0.65%, compared to $0.5 \pm 0.14\%$ measured experimentally in bile duct cannulated animals. The predicted cumulative excretion in bile after 7 days was 5.07% of the dose. Since total excretion in feces at this time was only 3.28% of the dose, approximately 35% of the biliary excretion of PBB was reabsorbed through the intestinal wall. The model showed that, similar to the PCBs, even though lean muscle tissue is poorly perfused and has a low affinity for PBB, it was initially the major storage compartment because of its large volume. Only later did the higher affinity adipose and skin compartments become the major storage sites. As observed for the higher chlorinated PCBs, the equilibrium PBB fat/blood distribution ratio was much higher than that for any of the other tissues sampled. Adipose tissue growth had an additional marked effect on long-term disposition kinetics. Fat volume increased on the average by more than 250% during the study, and the model showed that while the concentration of PBB in adipose tissue peaked at 11.84 nmoles/ml around 4 days and subsequently declined slowly, the total amount of PBB in this tissue was still rising at 42 days (Figure 3.11). Thus it

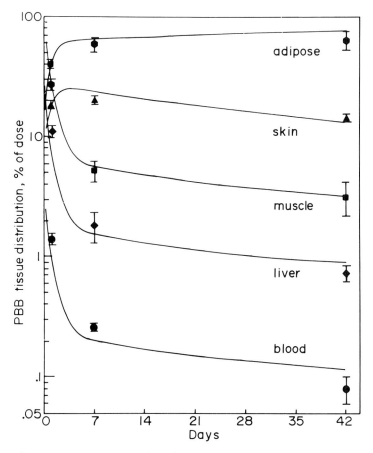

Figure 3.11 PBB tissue distributions in the rat after a single 1.0 mg/kg iv dose. Points and bars represent mean ± SD (n = 3) experimental data; lines are the model computed predictions.

SOURCE: *Tuey and Matthews, Toxicol. Appl. Pharmacol. 45 (1978), 337.*

could be demonstrated that dilution and redistribution due to the increasing fat volume was the major factor responsible for the declining PBB tissue concentrations observed after 7 days, not excretion.

Figure 3.12 shows the cumulative excretion of PBB in feces during and after four oral doses, plotted as a percentage of the doses given versus time. Similar to the iv results, about 2% of each oral dose was excreted in bile during the following 24-hr period. The tissue levels predicted by the model during the 7-day multiple oral dose study were in reasonable agreement with the PBB concentrations found in samples taken at 1 and 7 days (Figure 3.13).

According to the model, net diffusion of PBB through the intestinal wall following an iv dose favored reabsorption, and thus tended to reduce the amount eliminated in feces. Similarly, at all times following each oral dose the model showed that PBB concentration would be higher in the lumen than in intestinal tissue, so that net absorption would prevail. While about 2% of an iv dose was excreted in feces during the first 24 hr, approximately 12% of each oral

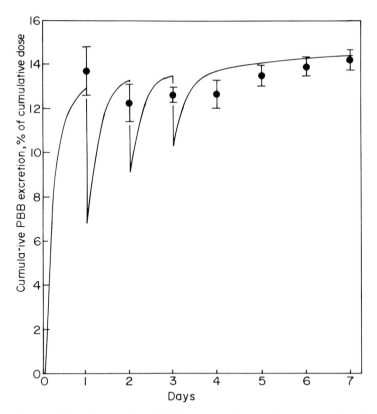

Figure 3.12 Cumulative PBB fecal excretion by the rat as a function of time and doses given at the daily rate of 1.0 mg/kg po for 4 days. Points and bars represent mean ± SD (*n* = 3) experimental data; lines are the model computed predictions.

dose was excreted during a similar time period. Biliary excretion accounted for only about 2% of the dose by either route after 24 hr. Consequently, enterohepatic recycling was probably insignificant and at least 10% of each oral dose was excreted unabsorbed. Since the absorbed portions of the oral doses eventually exhibited tissue distribution and excretion kinetics similar to those observed after an iv dose, differences in the fate of orally versus iv administered PBB were apparently due simply to diffusion through the intestinal wall.

In summary, this physiological compartmental model accomplished the following: (a) it gave reasonable predictions of the amounts and concentrations of PBB in all of the major tissues following both iv and multiple oral doses; (b) it demonstrated the time sequence of the relative significance of the different tissues to PBB disposition in the body; (c) it facilitated the incorporation of animal growth and demonstrated the importance of accounting for this phenomenon in chronic studies involving lipophilic compounds; and (d) it demonstrated how diffusion through the intestinal wall could account for iv verus oral dose PBB disposition. It is apparent that, at least for this compound, the benefits of pharmacokinetic synthesis amply justify the effort expended.

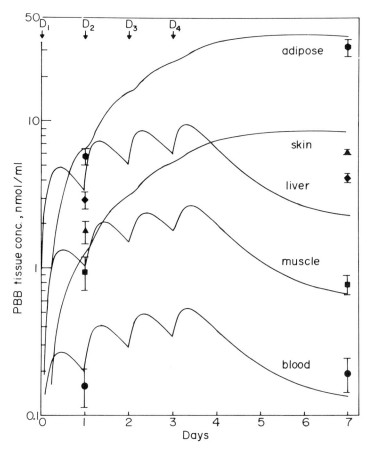

Figure 3.13 PBB tissue concentrations in the rat. Doses were given at the daily rate of 1.0 mg/kg po for 4 days. D_i, dose number. Points and bars represent mean $\pm$ SD ($n = 3$) experimental data; lines are the model computed predictions.

Suggested Reading

Bischoff, K. B., Brown, R. G. Drug distribution in mammals. Chem. Engr. Progr. Symp. Ser. 66 (1966), 33.

Bischoff, K. B., Dedrick, R. L., Zaharko, D. S., Longstreth, J. A. Methotrexate pharmacokinetics. J. Pharm. Sci. 60 (1971), 1128.

Borchard, R. E., Welborn, M. E., Wiekhorst, W. B., Wilson, D. W., Hansen, L. G. Pharmacokinetics of polychlorinated biphenyl components in swine and sheep after a single oral dose. J. Pharm. Sci. 64 (1975), 1294.

Chen, C. N., Andrade, J. R. Pharmacokinetic model for simultaneous determination of drug levels in organs and tissues. J. Pharm. Sci. 65 (1976), 717.

Dedrick, R. L. Animal scale-up. J. Pharmacokinet. Biopharm. 1 (1973), 435.

Dedrick, R. L., Forrester, D. D., Cannon, J. N., El Dareer, S. M., Mellett, L. B. Pharmacokinetics of 1-β-D-arabinofuranosylcytosine (Ara-C) deamination in several species. Biochem. Pharmacol. 22 (1973), 2405.

Garrettson, L. K., Curley, A. Dieldrin—Studies in a poisoned child. Arch. Environ. Health 19 (1969), 814.

Gibaldi, M., Perrier, D. Pharmacokinetics. New York: Marcel Dekker, 1975.

Nelson, E. Kinetics of drug absorption, distribution, metabolism, and excretion. J. Pharm. Sci. 50 (1961), 181.

Riegelman, S., Loo, J. C. K., Rowland, M. Shortcomings in pharmacokinetic analysis by conceiving the body to exhibit properties of a single compartment. J. Pharm. Sci. 57 (1968), 117.

Rose, J. Q., Ramsey, J. C., Wentzler, T. H., Hummel, R. A., Gehring, P. J. The fate of 2,3,7,8-tetrachlorodibenzo-p-dioxin following single and repeated oral doses to the rat. Toxicol. Appl. Pharmacol. 36 (1976), 209.

Teorell, T. Kinetics of distribution of substances administered to the body I. The extravascular modes of administration. Arch. Int. Pharmacodyn. Ther. 57 (1937), 205.

Teorell, T. Kinetics of distribution of substances administered to the body II. The intravascular modes of administration. Arch. Int. Pharmacodyn. Ther. 57 (1937), 226.

Westlake, W. J. Problems associated with analysis of pharmacokinetic models. J. Pharm. Sci. 60 (1971), 882.

Ernest Hodgson and
Walter C. Dauterman

4

Metabolism of Toxicants
Phase I Reactions

4.1. Introduction

The majority of xenobiotics that enter the body tissues are lipophilic, a property that enables them to penetrate lipid membranes and to be transported by lipoproteins in the body fluids. The metabolism of xenobiotics, carried out by a complex of relatively nonspecific enzymes, is usually held to consist of two phases. During phase I, a polar reactive group is introduced into the molecule; although this serves to increase the water solubility, the most important effect is to render the xenobiotic a suitable substrate for phase II reactions. In phase II, the altered compounds combine with an endogenous substrate to produce a water-soluble conjugation product that is readily excreted.

Although this sequence of events is generally a detoxication mechanism, in some cases the intermediates or final products are more toxic than the parent compound, and the sequence is termed an intoxication mechanism.

4.2. Microsomal Mixed-Function Oxidations

Microsomal mixed-function oxidation reactions are catalyzed by a nonspecific multienzyme system located in the endoplasmic reticulum of the cell. This system, which has cytochrome P-450 as the terminal oxidase, has been studied in many tissues and organisms.

4.2.1. Microsomes and Mixed-Function Oxidation:
· General Background

Microsomes are derived from the endoplasmic reticulum of the cell as a result of homogenization and are isolated by ultracentrifugation of the postmitochondrial supernatant fraction. The endoplasmic reticulum is a continuous anastomosing network of lipoprotein membranes extending from plasma membrane to nucleus and mitochondria, while the microsomal fraction derived from it consists of membranous vesicles contaminated with free ribosomes and fragments of mitochondria, nuclei, Golgi apparatus, etc. In the hepatocyte the surface area of the endoplasmic reticulum is 37 times that of the plasma membrane and 8.5 times that of the outer mitochondrial membrane.

The endoplasmic reticulum and, consequently, the microsomal vesicles, consist of two types, rough and smooth, the former having the outer surface studded with ribosomes, which the latter characteristically lack. Although both rough and smooth microsomes have all the components of the mixed-function oxidase system, the specific oxidative activity of the smooth fraction is usually higher.

Microsomes have been prepared by several methods, including column chromatography and precipitation by $CaCl_2$, but the method of choice remains homogenization followed by differential centrifugation. Typically, homogenization by one of several methods is followed by high-speed centrifugation at about 10,000 g for 10–15 min to remove mitochondria and heavier constituents such as whole cells, nuclei, etc. A microsomal pellet is then sedimented by ultracentrifugation of the post mitochondrial supernatant at about 100,000 g for 30–120 min. The microsomal pellet is then resuspended in a reaction medium suitable for the measurement of oxidative reactions for spectral examination. The microsomal fraction has been separated into rough and smooth microsomes by a two-step density gradient centrifugation, and both rough and smooth fractions can be further separated into fractions of different densities by careful selection of an appropriate gradient.

The optimum conditions for preparation may vary somewhat from tissue to tissue and from organism to organism, and a necessary preliminary to the investigation of microsomal oxidations is a careful comparison of homogenization techniques, of the optimum kind, pH and ionic strength of the homogenizing buffer, and centrifugation speeds and times. Subsequently, the same characteristics of the reaction medium should also be investigated since they may be different than those of the homogenization medium.

Mixed-function oxidations are those oxidations in which one atom of molecular oxygen is reduced to water while the other is incorporated into the substrate. The term "monooxygenases" has also been used for enzymes that catalyze the incorporation of one atom of molecular oxygen into the substrate; although this appears to be a logical name, the term of choice is still mixed-function oxidase.

Since the electrons involved in the reduction of cytochrome P-450 are derived from NADPH the overall reaction can be written as follows (where RH is the substrate):

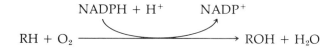

$$\text{RH} + O_2 \xrightarrow{\quad NADPH + H^+ \qquad NADP^+ \quad} \text{ROH} + H_2O$$

or, alternatively,

$$\text{RH} + O_2 \xrightarrow{\quad \text{Reduced} \atop \text{cytochrome P-450} \qquad \text{Oxidized} \atop \text{cytochrome P-450} \quad} \text{ROH} + H_2O$$

4.2.2. Constituent Enzymes of the Mixed-Function Oxidase System and the Cytochrome P-450 Reaction Mechanism

Cytochrome P-450, the carbon monoxide–binding pigment of microsomes, is a hemoprotein of the b cytochrome type. Unlike most cytochromes it is named, not from the absorption maximum of the reduced form in the visible region, but rather from the unique wavelength of the absorption maximum of the carbon monoxide derivative of the reduced form, namely 450 nm (Figure 4.1B).

The role of cytochrome P-450 as the terminal oxidase in mixed-function oxidase reactions is supported by considerable evidence, including the following:

1. The initial proof was derived from the demonstration of the light reversibility of the carbon monoxide complex, which confirmed its role in the C-21 hydroxylation of 17α-hydroxyprogesterone by adrenal gland microsomes.
2. The carbon monoxide sensitivity of microsomal mixed-function oxidase reactions, when allied with the fact that cytochrome P-450 is the only carbon monoxide–binding pigment in the microsomes, affords significant support.
3. Degradation of cytochrome P-450 to cytochrome P-420 causes a roughly proportionate loss of activity.
4. Induction of cytochrome P-450 by such inducers as phenobarbital causes an increase in activity.
5. Spectral perturbations of a particular type (to be discussed below), which can be measured as difference spectra, are brought about by almost all substrates.
6. Direct proof has been afforded, in recent years, by the demonstration that mixed-function oxidase systems, reconstituted from apparently homogenous cytochrome P-450, NADPH–cytochrome P-450 reductase, and phosphatidylcholine, can catalyze mixed-function oxidation reactions.

Cytochrome P-450, like other hemoproteins, has a characteristic absorption in the visible region. Addition of many organic and some inorganic ligands results in a perturbation of this spectrum. Since the particulate nature of microsomes gives rise to light scattering, and light scattering is a function of wavelength, such changes in the absolute spectrum are seen as fluctuations along a sloping baseline—an undesirable situation for quantitative measurements. In difference spectroscopy, light-scattering, nonspecific absorption and the absolute spectrum of the microsomal cytochromes are balanced out by placing microsomes in both cuvettes of a split-beam spectrophotometer; then only the difference caused by the addition of a ligand to the microsomes in the sample cuvette is seen as a difference spectrum (Figure 4.1A). Although the detection and measurement of such spectra requires a high-resolution instrument which must be used with considerable care, they have been of tremendous use in the characterization of cytochrome P-450.

The most important difference spectra of oxidized cytochrome P-450 are type I, with an absorption maximum at 385–390 nm and a minimum around 420 nm, and type II, with a peak at 420–435 nm and a trough at 390–410 nm (Figure 4.1C).

Type I ligands are found in many different chemical classes and include many drugs, environmental compounds, insecticides, etc. They appear to be generally

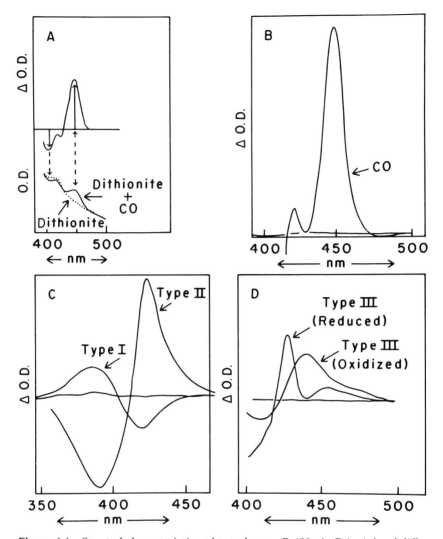

Figure 4.1 Spectral characteristics of cytochrome P-450. **A.** Principle of difference spectroscopy. **B.** Carbon monoxide-reduced cytochrome P-450 difference spectrum. **C.** Type I and Type II difference spectra with oxidized cytochrome P-450. **D.** Type III difference spectra with oxidized and reduced cytochrome P-450.

unsuitable on chemical grounds as ligands for the heme iron and are believed to bind at a hydrophobic site in the protein in close enough proximity to the heme iron to allow both perturbation of the absorption spectrum and interaction with the activated oxygen. Although the vast majority of type I ligands are substrates, it has not been possible to demonstrate a quantitative relationship between K_s (concentration required for half-maximal spectral development) and K_m (Michaelis constant).

Type II ligands, on the other hand, interact directly with the heme iron of cytochrome P-450 and are associated with organic compounds having nitrogen atoms with sp^2 or sp^3 nonbonded electrons that are sterically accessible. Such ligands are frequently inhibitors of mixed-function oxidase activity. The so-called reverse type I (or modified type II) difference spectrum caused by certain steroids and alcohols may be due to the displacement of an endogenous ligand or possibly to oxygen acting in a similar way to the nitrogen described above, i.e., as a nucleophile interacting at the sixth ligand position of the heme iron.

The most important difference spectra of reduced cytochrome P-450 are the well-known carbon monoxide spectrum, with its maximum at or about 450 nm, and the type III spectrum, with two pH-dependent peaks at approximately 430 and 455 nm (Figure 4.1D). Due to the pH dependency of the peaks, a pH equilibrium point can be determined, i.e., the pH at which the peaks are of equal size. This value has been of some use in the characterization of different cytochrome P-450s. The best known and most investigated type III ligand for cytochrome P-450 is ethyl isocyanide. This is an unstable interaction, however, since the ligand can be readily displaced. Compounds such as the methylenedioxyphenyl synergists and SKF-525A form stable type III complexes that appear to involve covalent binding and to be related to the mechanism by which they inhibit mixed-function oxidation reactions.

Reducing equivalents are transferred from NADPH to cytochrome P-450 by a flavoprotein enzyme known as NADPH–cytochrome P-450 reductase. The evidence that this enzyme is involved in microsomal mixed-function oxidation was originally derived from the observations that cytochrome c, which can function as an artificial electron acceptor for the enzyme, is an inhibitor of such oxidations. Furthermore, phenobarbital, a known inducer of enzymes, particularly cytochrome P-450 and mixed-function oxidase activity, also causes a parallel induction of the reductase. More direct evidence has become available recently since it has been shown that NADPH–cytochrome P-450 reductase is an essential component in mixed-function oxidase systems reconstituted from solubilized and purified components. Antibodies prepared from the purified reductase have been shown to be inhibitors of microsomal mixed-function oxidase activity.

The reductase has been purified from both insect and mammalian sources. It is a flavoprotein of approximately 80,000 daltons that contains one mole each of flavin mononucleotide (FMN) and flavin adenine dinucleotide (FAD) per mole of enzyme.

The only other component necessary for activity in reconstituted systems is a phospholipid, phosphatidylcholine. This substance is not directly involved in electron transfer but appears to be involved in the coupling of the reductase and the cytochrome and in the binding of the substrate to the cytochrome.

The mechanism of cytochrome P-450 function has not been established unequivocally; however, the generally recognized steps are summarized in Figure 4.2. The initial step consists of the binding of substrate to oxidized cytochrome P-450 followed by a one-electron reduction catalyzed by the NADPH–cytochrome P-450 reductase to form a reduced cytochrome–substrate complex. This complex can interact with carbon monoxide to form the CO–complex, which gives rise to the well-known difference spectrum with a peak at 450 nm.

The next several steps are less well understood. They involve an initial interaction with molecular oxygen to form a ternary oxygenated complex. This ternary complex accepts a second electron, resulting in the further formation of one or more poorly understood complexes. One of these, however, is probably

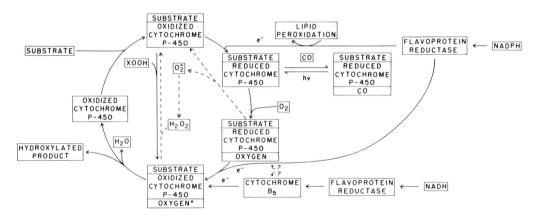

Figure 4.2 Reaction mechanism of the cytochrome P-450-dependent microsomal mixed-function oxidase system.

the equivalent of the peroxide anion derivative of the substrate-bound hemoprotein (Figure 4.2). Under some circumstances this complex may break down to yield hydrogen peroxide and the substrate–oxidized cytochrome complex. After the transfer of one atom of oxygen to the substrate and the other to form water, dismutation reactions occur that lead to the formation of the hydroxylated product, water and the oxidized cytochrome.

The possibility that the second electron is derived from NADH via cytochrome b_5 has been the subject of argument for some time and is still to be completely resolved. It is clear, however, that this pathway is not essential for all mixed-function oxidase reactions since many occur in systems reconstituted from NADPH, O_2, phosphatidylcholine, NADPH–cytochrome P-450 reductase, and cytochrome P-450. Nevertheless, evidence is available that this pathway can occur under some circumstances and that it may facilitate oxidative activity in the intact endoplasmic reticulum.

It has also been suggested that the oxygenated complex may decompose to yield the substrate–oxidized cytochrome complex and superoxide anion. If this is the case, it is of importance in such manifestations of superoxide anion toxicity as lipid peroxidation.

4.2.3. Distribution of Cytochrome P-450

In vertebrates, the liver is the richest source of cytochrome P-450 and is most active in the mixed-function oxidation of xenobiotics. Cytochrome P-450 and the other components of the mixed-function oxidase system are also found in skin, lung, and gastrointestinal tract, presumably reflecting the evolution of defense mechanisms at portals of entry. In addition to these organs, cytochrome P-450 has been demonstrated in kidney, adrenal cortex and medulla, placenta, testes, ovaries, fetal and embryonic liver, corpus luteum, aorta, and blood platelets. Although not demonstrated in the nervous system, its presence has been inferred from the presence of mixed-function oxidase activity toward xenobiotics. In man, cytochrome P-450 has been demonstrated in fetal and adult liver, placenta, kidney, testes, fetal and adult adrenal gland, skin, blood platelets, and lymphocytes.

In insects, cytochrome P-450 has been demonstrated in midgut, fatbody, and Malphigian tubes, with the midgut generally being the site of greatest concentration.

Although cytochrome P-450 is found in many tissues and organs, its function does not appear to be the same in each case. The liver cytochrome carries out a large number of xenobiotic oxidations as well as the oxidation of some endogenous steroids and bile pigments. The cytochrome P-450 of the lung also appears to be concerned primarily with xenobiotic oxidation, although the range of substrates tested has been more limited than in the case of the liver. Skin and small intestine also carry out xenobiotic oxidations, but only aryl hydrocarbon hydroxylation activity has been studied to any extent. In the uninduced mother, the placental microsomes display little or no ability to oxidize foreign compounds, appearing to function as a steroid hormone–metabolizing system. On induction, for example, in the cigarette-smoking human mother, aryl hydrocarbon hydroxylase activity is readily apparent.

The cytochrome P-450 of the kidney is active in the ω-oxidation of fatty acids such as lauric acid and, although it binds some xenobiotics, is relatively inactive in xenobiotic oxidation. Mitochondrial cytochromes, such as those of the placenta and adrenal cortex, are active in the oxidation of steroid hormones rather than xenobiotics.

Distribution of cytochrome P-450 within the cell has been studied primarily in the mammalian liver, where it is present in greatest quantity in the smooth endoplasmic reticulum and in smaller, but still appreciable, quantities in the rough endoplasmic reticulum. Other cell membranes may also possess cytochrome P-450, but the results are less certain due to cross contamination between centrifugal fractions. However, the nuclear membrane has been reported to contain cytochrome P-450 and to have detectable aryl hydrocarbon hydroxylase activity, an observation of great importance in studies of the activation of chemical carcinogens. Traces of cytochrome P-450 have been reported in lysosomes and Golgi apparatus, while its presence is virtually undetectable in hepatic mitochondria and plasma membranes. As the discussion of the multiplicity of cytochrome P-450 will indicate, recent evidence indicates that fractions of smooth microsomes of different densities contain qualitatively different cytochromes P-450.

In certain tissues, such as the adrenal cortex and placenta, there are mitochondrial cytochromes P-450 that appear to have specialized functions in steroid hormone metabolism. In other tissues the cytochrome is predominantly microsomal.

4.2.4. Multiplicity of Cytochrome P-450 and Purification and Reconstitution of Mixed-Function Oxidase Systems

Even before appreciable purification of cytochrome P-450 had been accomplished, it was already apparent from indirect evidence that mammalian liver cells contained more than one cytochrome P-450. The more recent direct evidence on the multiplicity of cytochrome P-450 is of two types: (a) following solubilization of microsomal preparations, the separation and purification of cytochromes P-450, which can be distinguished from one another by chromatographic behavior, immunological specificity, and/or substrate specificity after reconstitution; and (b) separation of distinct polypeptides by polyacrylamide gel electrophoresis, following treatment with sodium dodecyl sulfate, which can be related to distinct cytochromes P-450 present in the original microsomes.

Although each of the methods used to identify the cytochrome P-450–derived polypeptides are open to criticism, their combined use appears to be definitive.

Earlier indirect evidence bearing on the multiplicity of cytochrome P-450 may be summarized as follows:

1. Induction by polycyclic hydrocarbons such as 3-methylcholanthrene caused a shift in the λ_{max} of the carbon monoxide spectrum of hepatic microsomes and a shift in the pH equilibrium point of the ethyl isocyanide spectrum. A change in substrate specificity, manifested as an increase in aryl hydrocarbon hydroxylase activity, was also apparent. Induction by phenobarbital, initially thought to cause only a quantitative increase in cytochrome P-450, was later shown to cause more subtle changes in substrate specificity.

2. Turnover experiments, carried out by labeling the heme moiety via labeled $\triangle$-aminolevulinic acid, indicated the presence of at least two populations, one turning over rapidly and the other more slowly.

3. Kinetic experiments, both with substrates and inhibitors, frequently gave complex results that could be explained by inferring the presence of more than one cytochrome P-450 with differing affinities either for substrate or inhibitor or both. These findings were, however, less definitive due to the experimental difficulties inherent in working with membrane-bound enzymes and substrates and inhibitors that are insoluble in water.

Recent studies have raised the possibility that these different cytochromes P-450 may have specific locations within the cell. Smooth microsome fractions from rat and mouse liver, which differ in density, show qualitative differences in their spectral characteristics.

In the insect *Musca domestica*, although purification attempts to date have yielded preparations of low yield and purity, the results do support the indirect evidence that more than one cytochrome P-450 occurs. The indirect evidence is as follows:

1. Genetic studies on insecticide-susceptible and -resistant strains have provided the strongest evidence (see Chapter 6).

2. Controlled tryptic digestion of microsomes shows changes in spectral characteristics apparently due to sequential destruction of different cytochromes.

3. Spectral differences are seen between microsomal fractions differing in density.

Considerations of multiplicity may be of considerable importance in several aspects to be discussed in subsequent chapters, including developmental changes, sex differences, inhibition, and induction. Any of these effects on cytochrome P-450 or mixed-function oxidase activity could involve either changes in the proportion of specific cytochromes or specificity differences between cytochromes.

Purification of cytochrome P-450 was, for many years, an elusive goal; however, during the past decade considerable progress has been made. The initial difficulty involved the instability of cytochrome P-450 on solubilization, which resulted in degradation to cytochrome P-420, an enzymatically inactive form.

This problem has been partially solved by the use of glycerol and dithiothreitol as protectants. Subsequent to solubilization, the hydrophobicity of the protein causes a tendency to aggregate, which is partially overcome by maintaining a low concentration of a suitable detergent, such as Emulgen 911, throughout the procedure. The presence of multiple forms also presents problems since ultimately they must be separated from each other and purified. The final problem involves the removal of bound detergent before reconstitution experiments can be carried out.

Using the above precautions and by judicious selection of traditional and recent methods for protein purification, it has been possible to purify cytochrome P-450 as well as the NADPH–cytochrome P-450 reductase described above from mammalian liver and lung. These methods include the following:

1. *Solubilization:* Various detergents have been used, but sodium cholate, with or without sonication, is by far the most common.
2. *Protein precipitation:* The two reagents most commonly used are ammonium sulfate and polyethylene glycol.
3. *Column chromatography:* The materials most commonly used are hydroxylapatite, DEAE-cellulose, CM-cellulose, and "affinity" columns based on *n*-octylamine and *n*-hexylamine. The latter, although originally designed as affinity columns, may be simply hydrophobic columns.

A typical protocol is shown in Figure 4.3. As a result of these methods, highly

Figure 4.3 Resolution of multiple forms of cytochrome P-450 from rabbit liver microsomes. Cytochrome P-450d is present after phenobarbital induction.
SOURCE: *Johnson and Muller-Eberhard, Drug Metabolism Concepts (D. M. Jerina, ed.), ACS Symposium Series No. 44. American Chemical Society: Washington, D.C., 1977, p. 77.*

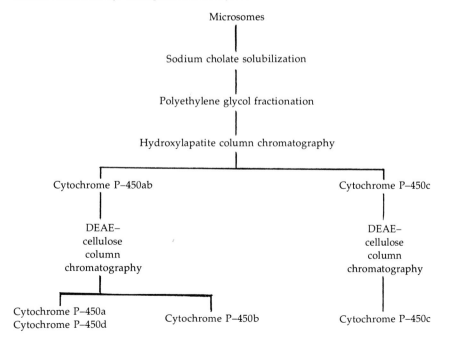

purified preparations of cytochrome P-450 with specific contents up to 22 nmoles/mg, and showing a single band on polyacrylamide gel electrophoresis following sodium dodecyl sulfate treatment, can now be prepared. These cytochromes have a molecular mass of about 50,000 daltons.

A number of investigators have demonstrated mixed-function oxidation of xenobiotics in systems reconstituted from purified cytochrome P-450, NADPH–cytochrome P-450 reductase, and phosphatidylcholine. Such systems will, in the presence of NADPH and oxygen, oxidize xenobiotics such as benzphetamine, often at rates comparable to microsomes. The fact that this minimum number of constituents is enzymatically active does not mean, however, that other microsomal constituents, such as cytochrome b_5, may not facilitate activity in vivo or that all substrates can be oxidized by this minimal system.

One important finding from such studies (the results of one study are shown in Table 4.1) is that the lack of specificity of the hepatic microsomal mixed-function oxidase system is not due to the presence of a mixture of several specific cytochromes P-450 since it appears that all of the cytochromes isolated are relatively nonspecific. The relative activity toward different substrates does, however, vary greatly from one to the other.

4.2.5. Microsomal Mixed-Function Oxidase Reactions

Although microsomal mixed-function oxidase reactions are basically similar in the role played by molecular oxygen and in the supply of electrons, the enzymes are markedly nonspecific, both substrates and products falling into many different chemical classes. It is convenient, therefore, to classify these activities on the basis of chemical reactions, bearing in mind that, not only do the classes often overlap, but the same substrate may undergo more than one oxidative reaction.

4.2.5a. Epoxidation and Aromatic Hydroxylation

Epoxidation is an extremely important microsomal reaction since not only can stable epoxides be formed, but arene oxides, the epoxides of aromatic rings, are

Table 4.1 Activities of Cytochrome P-450 Isolated (as Shown in Figure 4.3)

Substrate	Cytochrome			
	P-450a	P-450b	P-450c	P-450d
Benzphetamine	12	4	2	51
Benzo(a)pyrene	0.42	4.1	0.03	0.03
7-Ethoxyresorufin	0.04	0.4	0.4	0.003
Acetanilide	1.2	1.3	6.1	1.1

Source: Johnson and Muller-Eberhard, in Drug Metabolism Concepts (D. M. Jerina, Eds.), ACS Symposium Series 44, 1976. Washington, D.C.: American Chemical Society, 1977, p. 78.)

Note: NADPH–cytochrome P-450 reductase was present in excess. All enzyme activities are expressed in moles of product per mole of cytochrome P-450.

intermediates in aromatic hydroxylations. In the case of polycyclic hydrocarbons, these reactive intermediates are known to be involved in carcinogenesis.

The epoxidation of aldrin to dieldrin is the best known example of the metabolic formation of a stable epoxide:

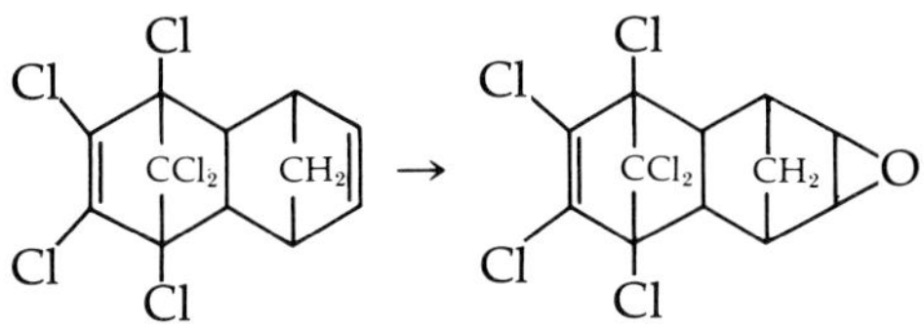

Aldrin   Dieldrin

The oxidation of naphthalene was one of the earliest understood examples of an epoxide as an intermediate in aromatic hydroxylation:

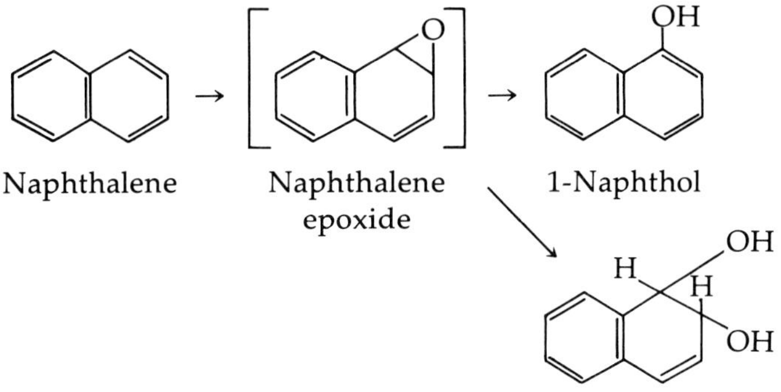

Naphthalene   Naphthalene   1-Naphthol
epoxide

Naphthalene-1,2-dihydrodiol

The epoxide can rearrange nonenzymatically to yield predominantly 1-naphthol, can interact with the enzyme epoxide hydrase to yield the dihydrodiol, or can interact with glutathione S-transferase to yield the glutathione conjugate, which ultimately is metabolized to a mercapturic acid. This reaction is also of importance in the metabolism of the insecticide carbaryl, which contains the naphthalene nucleus.

The proximate carcinogens arising from the metabolic activation of benzpyrene are now believed to be isomers of benzpyrene 7,8-diol-9,10-epoxide:

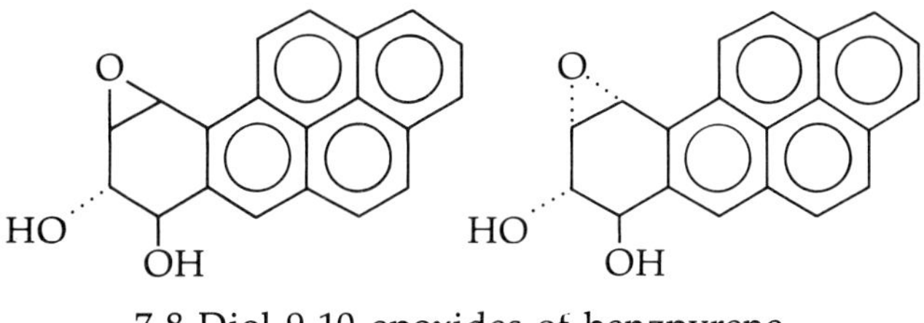

7,8-Diol-9,10-epoxides of benzpyrene

These metabolites appear to arise by the prior formation of the 7,8-epoxide, which gives rise to the 7,8-dihydrodiol through the action of epoxide hydrase.

This is further metabolized by the microsomal mixed-function oxidase system to the 7,8-diol-9,10-epoxides, which are both potent mutagens and unsuitable substrates for the further action of epoxide hydrase.

4.2.5b. Aliphatic Hydroxylations

Alkyl side chains of aromatic compounds are readily oxidized, often at more than one position, and provide good examples of this type of oxidation. The n-propyl side chain of n-propylbenzene can be oxidized, in the rabbit, at any of the three carbon atoms to yield 3-phenylpropan-1-o1 ($C_6H_5CH_2CH_2CH_2OH$) by ω-oxidation, benzylmethylcarbinol ($C_6H_5CH_2CHOHCH_3$) by $\omega-1$-oxidation, and ethylphenylcarbinol ($C_6H_5CHOHCH_2CH_3$) by α-oxidation. Further oxidation of these alcohols is also possible.

Alicyclic compounds, such as cyclohexane, are also susceptible to oxidation, in this case first to cyclohexanol and then *trans*-cyclohexane-1,2-diol.

In compounds with both saturated and aromatic rings, the former appears to be the most readily hydroxylated. For example, the major oxidation products of tetralin (5,6,7,8-tetrahydronaphthalene) in rabbit are 1- and 2-tetralol, whereas only a trace of the phenol, 5,6,7,8-tetrahydro-2-naphthol, is formed:

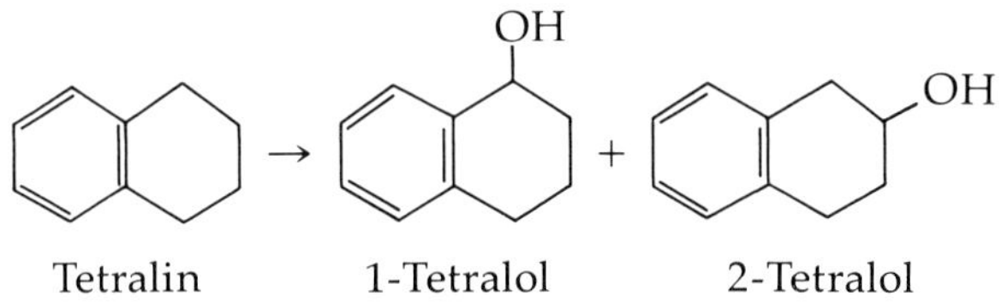

Tetralin   1-Tetralol   2-Tetralol

4.2.5c. Dealkylation: O-, N-, and S-Dealkylation

O-Dealkylation. Probably the best known example of O-dealkylation is the demethylation of p-nitroanisole. Due to the ease with which the product, p-nitrophenol, can be measured, it is a frequently used substrate for the demonstration of mixed-function oxidase activity. The reaction is believed to proceed via an unstable methylol derivative:

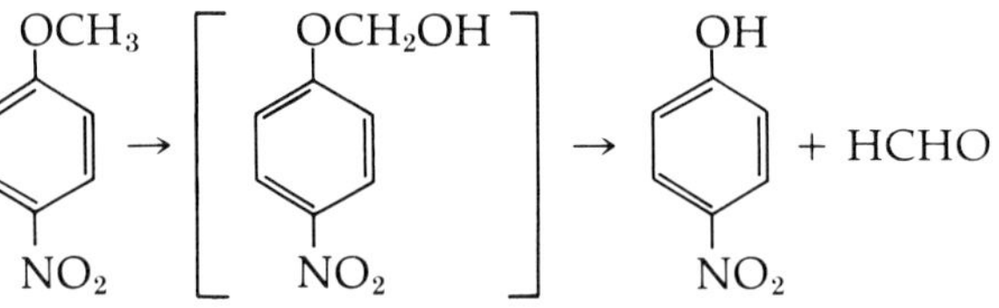

Other substrates of O-dealkylation include the drugs codeine and phenacetin and the insecticide methoxychlor.

The O-dealkylation of organophosphorus triesters differs from the above in that it involves the dealkylation of an ester rather than an ether. The reaction was first described for the insecticide chlorfenvinphos, but is now known to occur with a wide variety of vinyl, phenyl, phenylvinyl, and naphthyl phosphates and the thionophosphate triesters. At least one phosphonate, O-ethyl O-p-nitrophenyl phenylphosphonate (EPNO), is also metabolized by this mechanism. The proposed mechanism is shown below:

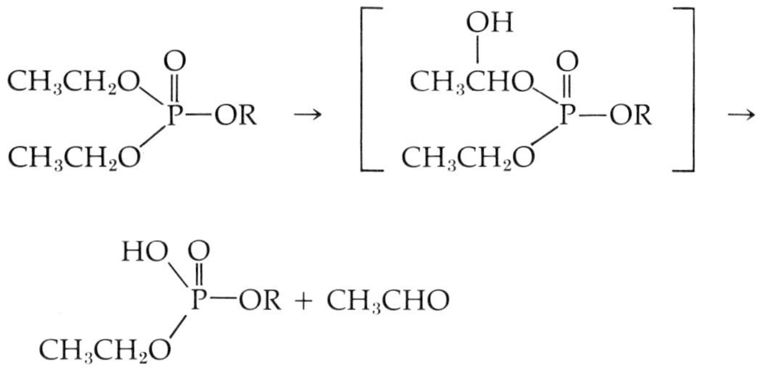

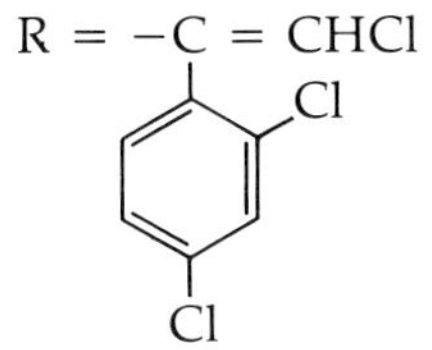

R = −C = CHCl

Chlorfenvinphos

N-Dealkylation. This is a common reaction in the metabolism of drugs, insecticides, and other xenobiotics. Both the N- and N, N-dialkyl carbamate insecticides are readily dealkylated and in some cases the methylol intermediates are stable enough to be isolated. N,N-dimethyl-p-nitrophenyl carbamate is a useful model compound for this reaction:

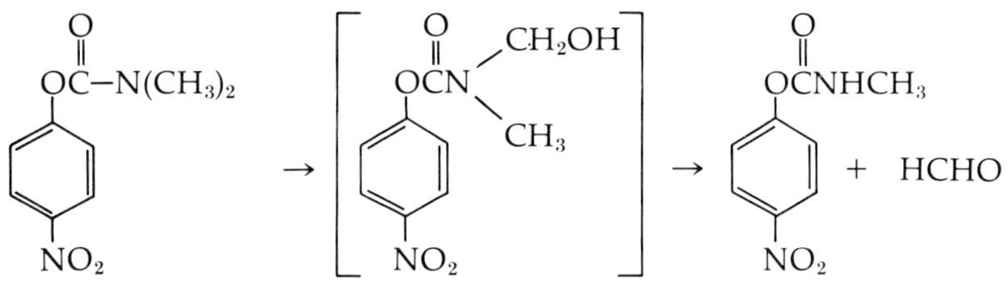

Another important example is the insecticide carbaryl, which undergoes several different microsomal oxidation reactions, including an attack on the N-methyl group. In this case the methylol compound is stable enough to be isolated or to be conjugated in vivo.

The drug aminopyrene undergoes two N-demethylations to form first monomethyl-4-aminoantipyrene and then antipyrene:

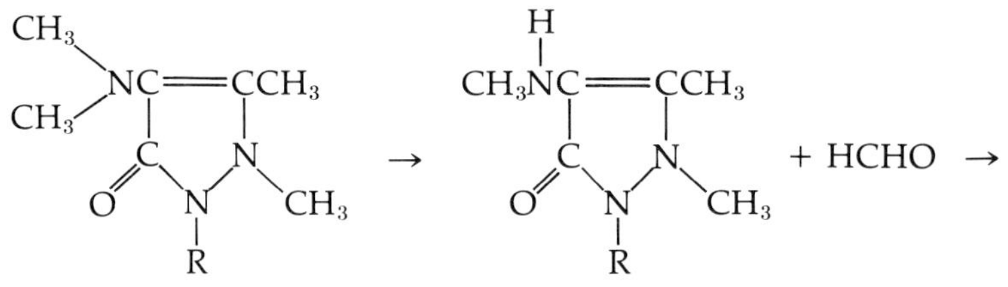

Aminopyrene   Monomethyl-4-aminoantipyrene

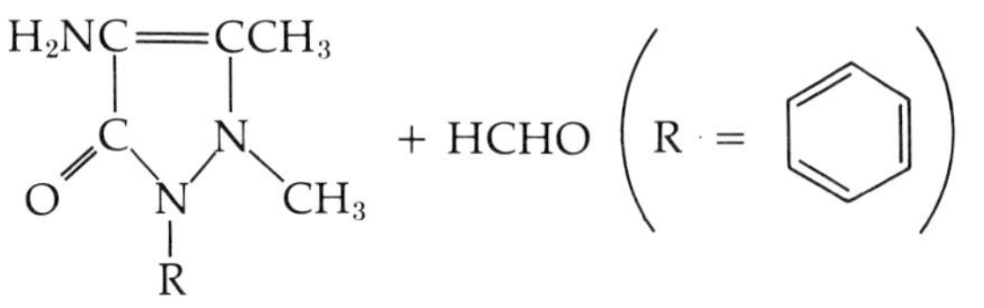

4-Aminoantipyrene

S-Dealkylation. This reaction is known to occur with a number of thioethers such as methylmercaptan, 6-methylthiopurine, etc.:

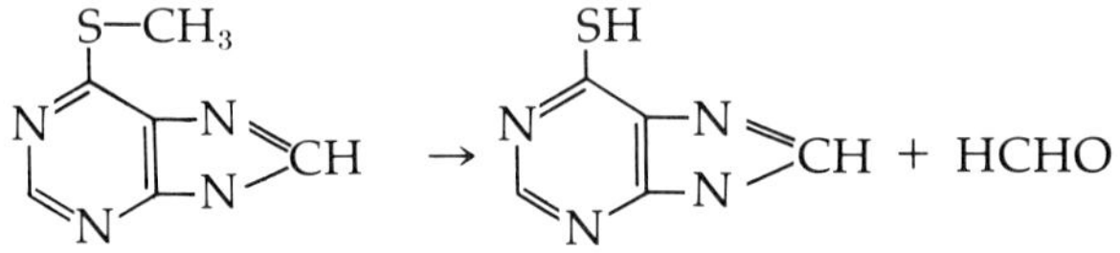

6-Methylthiopurine   6-Mercaptothiopurine

4.2.5d. N-Oxidation

N-oxidation can occur in a number of ways, including hydroxylamine formation, oxime formation, and N-oxide formation. The latter is primarily dependent on a flavoprotein enzyme found in the microsomes and will be discussed in Section 4.2.

Hydroxylamine formation. This reaction occurs with a number of amines, such as aniline and many of its substituted derivatives:

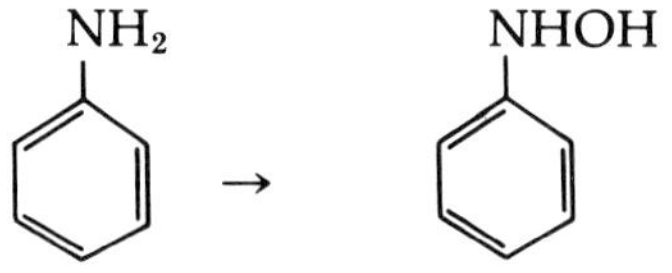

Aniline   Phenylhydroxylamine

In the case of 2-acetylaminofluorene, the product is a potent carcinogen and thus the reaction is an activation reaction:

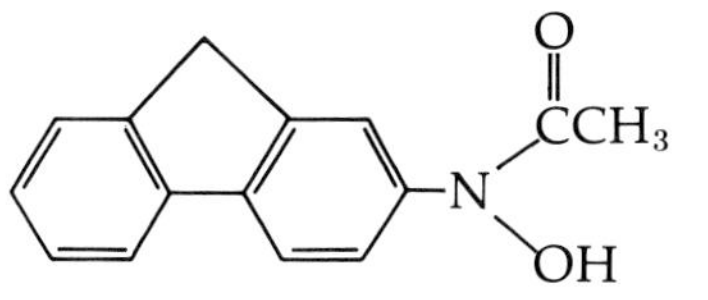

N-Hydroxy-2-acetylaminofluorene

Oxime formation. Oximes can be formed by the N-hydroxylation of imines and primary amines. Imines have, furthermore, been suggested as intermediates in the formation of oximes from primary amines:

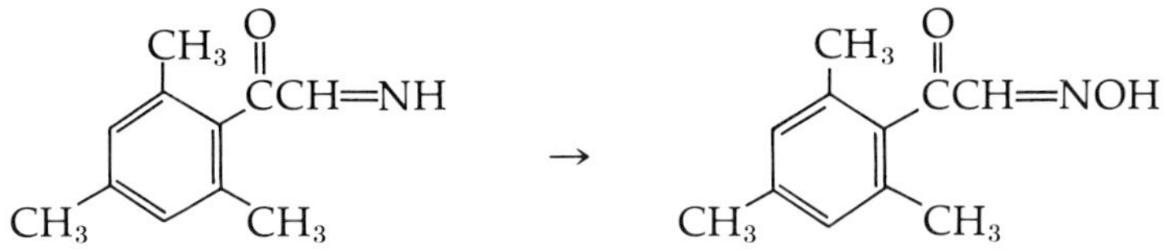

Trimethylacetophenone imine   Trimethylacetophenone oxime

4.2.5e. Oxidative Deamination

Oxidative deamination of amphetamine occurs in the rabbit liver but not to any extent in either the dog or rat, which tend to hydroxylate the aromatic ring:

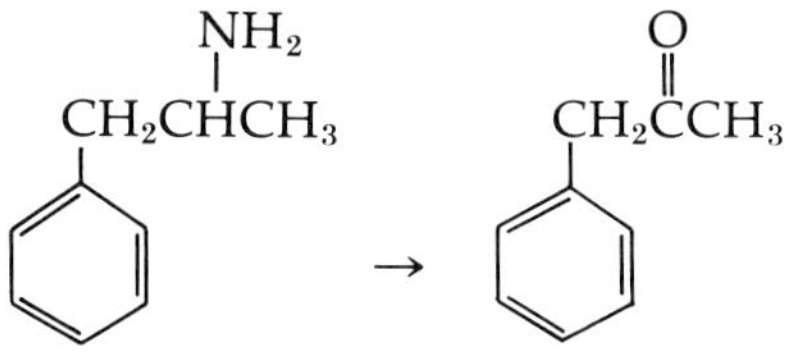

Amphetamine   Phenylacetone

A close examination of this reaction indicates that it is probably not an attack on the nitrogen but rather on the adjacent carbon atom, giving rise to a carbinol amine, which produces the ketone by elimination of ammonia:

$$R_2CHNH_2 \xrightarrow{O} R_2C(OH)NH_2$$

$$R_2C(OH)NH_2 \xrightarrow{-NH_3} R_2C = O.$$

The carbinol, by another reaction sequence, can also give rise to an oxime:

$$R_2C(OH)NH_2 \xrightarrow{-H_2O} R_2C = NH$$

$$R_2C = NH \xrightarrow{O} R_2CNOH.$$

The oxime can now be hydrolyzed to yield the ketone, which is thus formed by two different routes:

$$R_2CNOH \xrightarrow{H_2O} R_2C = O.$$

4.2.5f. S-Oxidation

Thioethers in general are oxidized by microsomal mixed-function oxidase enzymes to sulfoxides, some of which are further metabolized to sulfones. This reaction is very common among insecticides of several different chemical classes, including carbamates, organophosphates, and chlorinated hydrocarbons:

| Methiocarb | Methiocarb sulfoxide | Methiocarb sulfone |

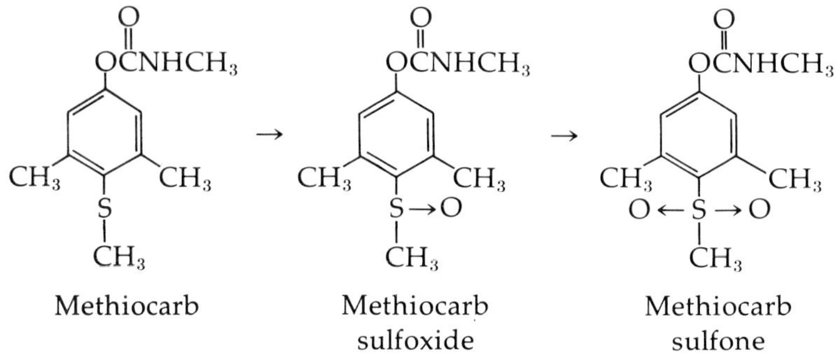

Organophosphates include phorate, demeton, and others, while among the chlorinated hydrocarbons, endosulfan is oxidized to endosulfan sulfate and methiochlor to a series of sulfoxides and sulfones to yield eventually the bis-sulfone.

S-Oxidation is also known among drugs, e.g., chloropromazine, while the solvent dimethylsulfoxide is further oxidized to the sulfone:

$$(CH_3)_2SO \rightarrow (CH_3)_2SO_2.$$

4.1.5g. P-Oxidation

This little-known reaction involves the conversion of trisubstituted phosphines to phosphine oxides. It is a typical cytochrome P-450–mediated mixed-function oxidation. Known substrates are diphenylmethylphosphine and 3-dimethyl-aminopropyl-diphenylphosphine:

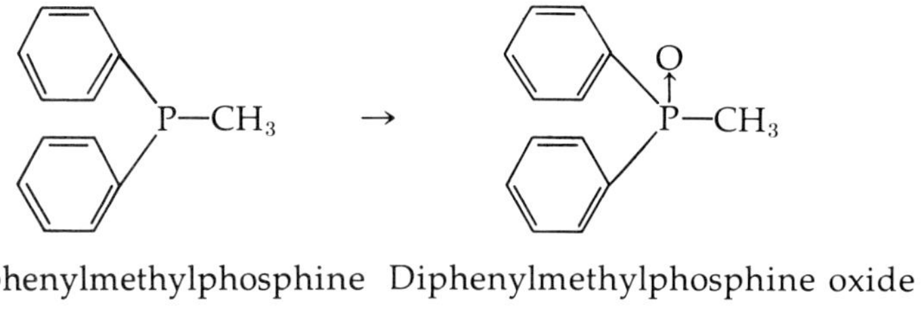

Diphenylmethylphosphine   Diphenylmethylphosphine oxide

4.2.5h. Desulfuration and Ester Cleavage

Phosphothionate and phosphorodithioate insecticides owe their insecticidal activity and their mammalian toxicity to an oxidative reaction in which the P$=$S group is converted to P$=$O, thereby converting compounds relatively inactive toward cholinesterases into potent cholinesterase inhibitors. This reaction is known for many organophosphorus compounds but has been studied most intensively in the case of parathion:

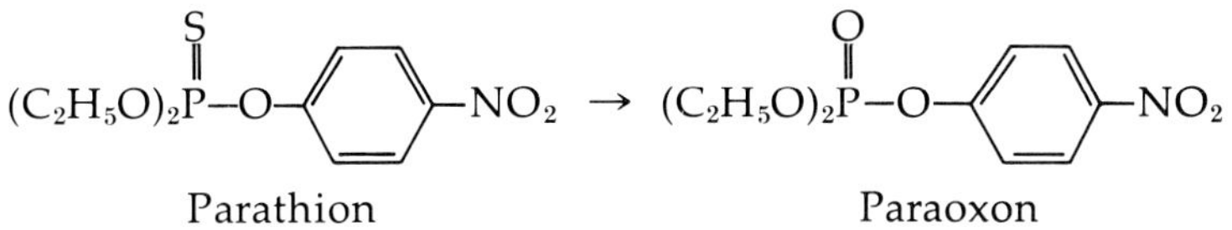

$$(C_2H_5O)_2\overset{\overset{\text{S}}{\|}}{P}-O-\!\!\left\langle\!\!\!\bigcirc\!\!\!\right\rangle\!\!-NO_2 \;\rightarrow\; (C_2H_5O)_2\overset{\overset{\text{O}}{\|}}{P}-O-\!\!\left\langle\!\!\!\bigcirc\!\!\!\right\rangle\!\!-NO_2$$

Parathion   Paraoxon

Much of the splitting of the phosphorus ester bonds in organophosphorus insecticides, which was formerly believed to be due to hydrolysis, is now known to be due to oxidative dearylation. This is a typical cytochrome P-450–dependent oxidation which requires NADPH and oxygen and is inhibited by CO:

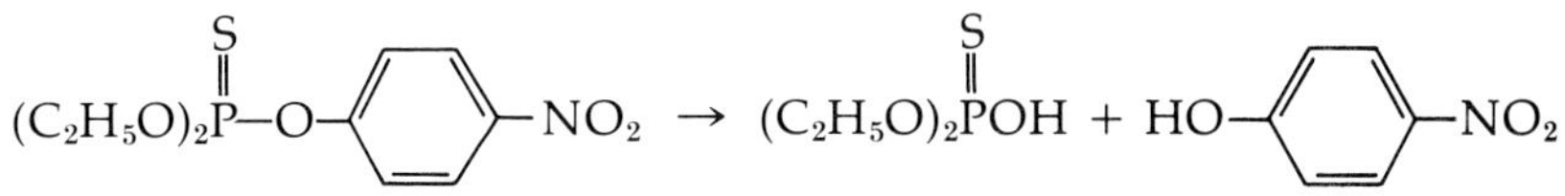

$$(C_2H_5O)_2\overset{\overset{\text{S}}{\|}}{P}-O-\!\!\left\langle\!\!\!\bigcirc\!\!\!\right\rangle\!\!-NO_2 \;\rightarrow\; (C_2H_5O)_2\overset{\overset{\text{S}}{\|}}{P}OH + HO-\!\!\left\langle\!\!\!\bigcirc\!\!\!\right\rangle\!\!-NO_2$$

The question of whether desulfuration and dearylation occur independently of each other, possibly catalyzed by two different cytochromes P-450, or whether they involve common intermediates is not yet resolved with certainty. However, persuasive evidence, including investigations with purified, reconstituted systems, has been brought forward to support the hypothesis that they involve a common intermediate of the "phosphooxythirane" $\left(\!\begin{smallmatrix}\text{S}\\ \diagup \ \diagdown \text{O}\\ \text{P}\end{smallmatrix}\!\right)$ type.

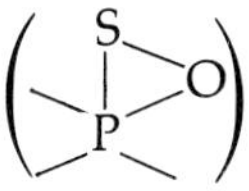

4.3. Other Microsomal Oxidations

Tertiary amines such as trimethylamine and dimethylaniline are metabolized to N-oxides by an amine oxidase that is not dependent on cytochrome P-450:

$$(CH_3)_3N \rightarrow (CH_3)_3NO.$$

This enzyme is a flavoprotein, located in the microsomes, which is dependent on NADPH and oxygen. The enzyme has been purified to homogeneity from pig liver microsomes. It has a molecular weight of 474,000 and contains 6 moles FAD/mole enzyme. This preparation is devoid of cytochrome P-450 and NADPH–cytochrome c reductase and is active toward a number of tertiary and some secondary amines.

From a toxicological point of view, it is of interest that this enzyme is responsible for the oxidation of nicotine to nicotine-1'-N-oxide, while the oxidation of nicotine to cotinine is catalyzed by two enzymes acting in sequence—cytochrome P-450 and a soluble aldehyde dehydrogenase:

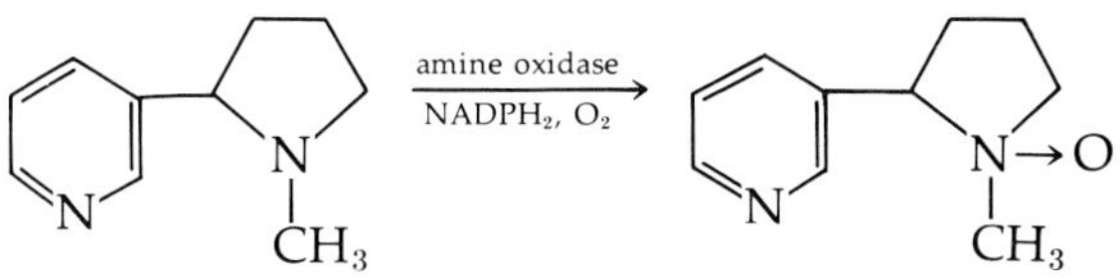

4.4. Nonmicrosomal Oxidations

In addition to the mixed-function oxidases, there are a number of other enzymes that are involved in the oxidation of foreign compounds. These oxidoreductases are located in either the mitochondrial fraction or the 100,000 g supernatant of tissue homogenates.

4.4.1. Alcohol Dehydrogenases

As a class of enzymes, the alcohol dehydrogenases catalyze the conversion of alcohols to aldehydes or ketones, e.g.,

$$RCH_2OH + NAD^+ \rightleftharpoons RCHO + NADH + H^+.$$

This should not be confused with the mixed-function oxidation of ethanol observed in liver microsomes. This reaction is reversible and carbonyl compounds can be reduced to alcohols. Alcohol dehydrogenase is probably the most important dehydrogenase involved in the metabolism of foreign alcohols and carbonyl compounds. The enzyme is found in the soluble fraction of the liver, kidney, and lung and requires NAD or NADP as a coenzyme. The reaction proceeds at a slower rate with NADP. In the intact organism the reaction proceeds to the right, since aldehydes are further oxidized to acids. The oxidation of aldehydes to acids by aldehyde oxidase is a vital detoxication reaction since aldehydes are usually toxic and, because of their lipid solubility, are not readily excreted.

Alcohol dehydrogenases will metabolize primary alcohols to aldehydes, n-butanol being the substrate oxidized at the highest rate. Secondary alcohols are oxidized to ketones but at a reduced rate. Butanol-2 is oxidized at one-third the rate of n-butanol. Tertiary alcohols are not readily oxidized.

A number of other dehydrogenases, described from various sources, play an important role in steroid, lipid, and carbohydrate metabolism. However, in general, their substrate specificity is narrow, and they are unlikely to be important in the metabolism of xenobiotics.

4.4.2. Aldehyde Dehydrogenase

The oxidation of aliphatic and aromatic aldehydes to their corresponding acids allows the acids to be excreted or conjugated in phase II reactions:

$$RCHO + NAD^+ \rightarrow RCOOH + NADH + H^+.$$

Aldehyde dehydrogenases have been isolated from a variety of sources, but probably the most important source is the liver, the enzyme from which can handle a wide variety of substrates. With a series of linear aliphatic aldehydes, the rate of oxidation increases as the carbonyl carbon becomes more positive.

In addition to liver aldehyde dehydrogenase, a number of other enzymes are present in the soluble fraction of liver homogenates that will oxidize aldehydes and certain N-heterocyclic compounds. Among these are aldehyde oxidase and xanthine oxidase, both flavoprotein enzymes containing molybdenum. These enzymes catalyze the oxidation of aldehydes formed by the deamination of endogenous amines by amine oxidases.

4.4.3. Amine Oxidases

The biological function of amine oxidases appears to involve the oxidation of biogenic amines formed during normal biological processes. In mammals, the monoamine oxidases are involved in the control of the serotonin: catecholamine ratios in the brain, which in turn influence sleep and EEG patterns, body temperature, and mental depression. Two groups of amine oxidases are involved in the oxidative deamination of naturally occurring amines as well as foreign compounds.

4.4.3a. Monoamine Oxidases

Monoamine oxidases (MAO) are flavoprotein enzymes located in the mitochondrial fraction of liver, kidney, and brain. The enzymes have also been found in blood platelets and intestinal mucosa. The MAO exist as a large group of similar enzymes with overlapping substrate specificities and inhibition patterns. The number is difficult to assess because of the great variety and variation within each tissue as well as in different animal species.

The general reaction catalyzed is

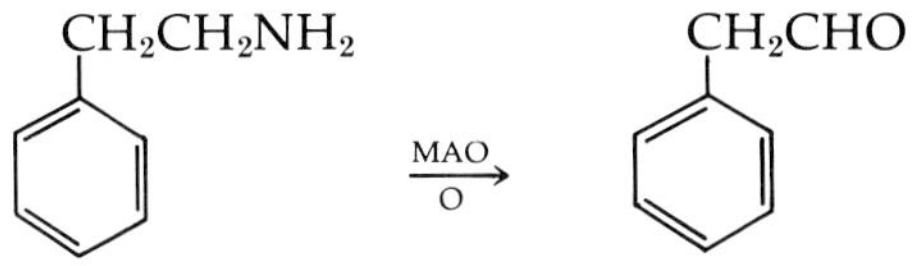

$$CH_2CH_2NH_2 \quad \xrightarrow[O]{MAO} \quad CH_2CHO$$

Phenylethylamine   Phenylacetaldehyde

MAO will deaminate primary, secondary, and tertiary aliphatic amines, the reaction rate being faster with the primary, and slower with the secondary and tertiary amines. Electron-withdrawing substituents on an aromatic ring increase the rate of deamination. Compounds that have a substituted methyl group on the α-carbon atoms are not metabolized by the MAO system (e.g., amphetamine and ephedrine).

4.4.3b. Diamine Oxidases

Diamine oxidases (DAO) also oxidize diamines to the corresponding aldehydes in the presence of oxygen. The DAO are pyridoxal phosphate proteins containing copper that are found in the soluble fraction of liver, intestine, kidney, and placenta. A typical DAO reaction is the oxidation of putrescine:

$$H_2N(CH_2)_4NH_2 \xrightarrow[O]{DAO} H_2N(CH_2)_3CHO + NH_3.$$

Putrescine

The rate of deamination is determined by the chain length, and with polymethylene diamines, $NH_2 - (CH_2)_n - NH_2$, the maximum rate occurs when $n = 4$ (putrescine) and $n = 5$ (cadaverine) and decreases to zero when $n = 9$ or more. At this stage, MAO become active and can oxidatively deaminate the diamines. It should be noted that although MAO can deaminate both substituted and primary amines, DAO can only deaminate primary amines.

4.5. Reduction Reactions

A number of functional groups, such as nitro, diazo, carbonyls, disulfides, sulfoxides, alkenes, etc., are susceptible to reduction. In many cases it is difficult to determine whether these reactions proceed nonenzymatically, by the action of biological reducing agents such as NADPH, NADH, FAD, etc., or through the mediation of functional enzyme systems.

4.5.1. Nitro Reduction

Aromatic amines are susceptible to reduction by both bacterial and mammalian nitroreductase systems:

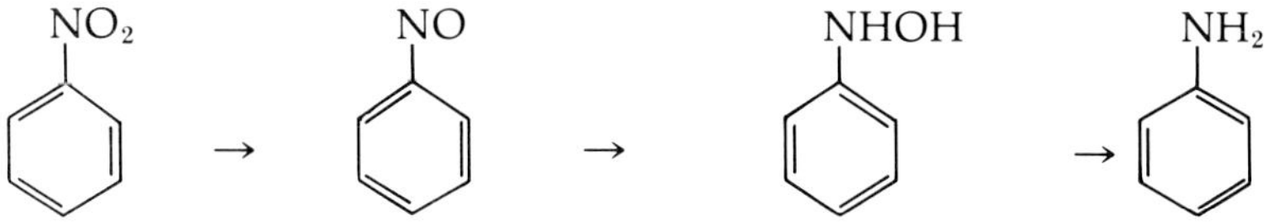

Nitrobenzene   Nitrosobenzene   Phenylhydroxylamine   Aniline

Nitroreductase activity has been demonstrated in liver homogenates as well as in the soluble fraction, while other studies have reported that nitroreductase activity has been found in all liver fractions evaluated. The reductase appears to be distributed in liver, kidney, lung, heart, and brain. The reaction utilizes both NADPH and NADH and requires anaerobic conditions. The reaction can be inhibited by the addition of oxygen. The reaction is stimulated by FMN and FAD, and at high flavin concentrations they can act simply as nonenzymatic electron donors. The reduction process probably proceeds via the nitroso and hydroxylamine intermediates as illustrated above.

4.5.2. Azo Reduction

Requirements for azoreductases are quite similar to those for nitroreductases; i.e., they require anaerobic conditions and NADPH and are stimulated by reduced flavins:

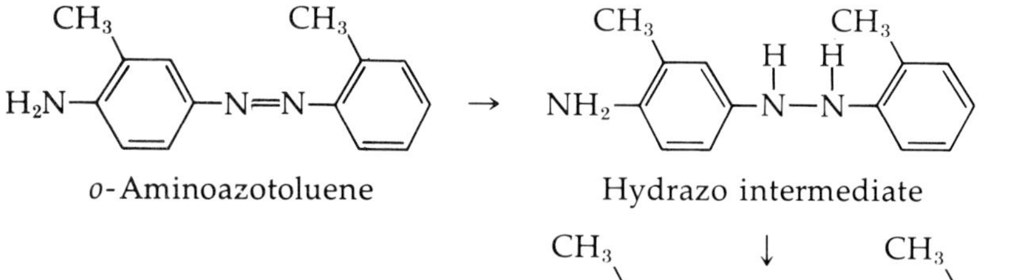

o-Aminoazotoluene   Hydrazo intermediate

The ability of mammalian tissue to reduce azo bonds is rather poor. With p-[2,4-(diaminophenyl)azo]benzenesulfonamide (Prontosil), in vivo reduction forms sulfanilamide. However, pretreatment with antibiotics destroys the intestinal bacteria, which results in a decrease in the formation of the amino compound. Generally, it would appear that both nitro and azo reduction as a function of specific tissues is of minor importance, and intracellular bacteria as well as intestinal bacteria are actually responsible for these reductions.

4.5.3. Reduction of Pentavalent Arsenic to Trivalent Arsenic

Pentavalent arsenic compounds such as tryparsamide appear to require reduction to the trivalent state for antiparasitic activity:

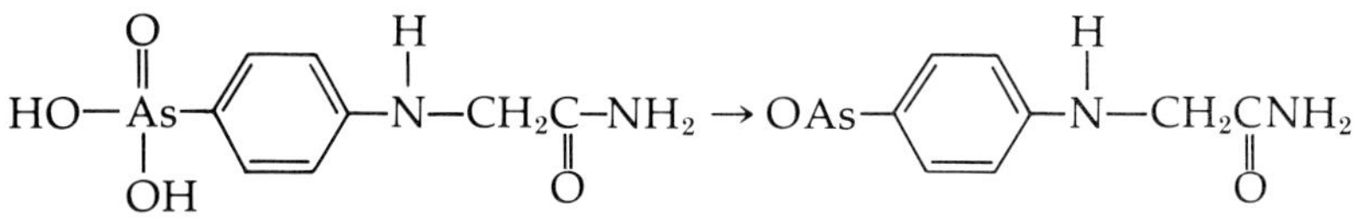

Tryparasamide

As^{+5} As^{+3}

Various arsenicals containing pentavalent arsenic have only slight in vitro antiprotozoal activity, whereas compounds containing trivalent arsenic are highly active.

4.5.4. Reduction of Disulfides

A number of disulfides are reduced in mammals to their sulfhydryl compounds. An example is disulfiram (Antabuse), a drug used for the treatment of alcoholism:

$$(C_2H_5)_2NCSS - SSCN(C_2H_5)_2 \xrightarrow{2H} \quad 2(C_2H_5)_2NCSSH$$

Disulfiram   Diethyldithiocarbamic acid

4.5.5. Ketone and Aldehyde Reduction

The reduction of ketones and aldehydes occurs via the reverse reaction of alcohol dehydrogenases (Section 4.4.1):

$$R_1R_2CO \rightarrow R_1R_2CHOH.$$

4.5.6. Sulfoxide and N-Oxide Reduction

The reduction of sulfoxides has been reported to occur in a number of mammalian systems. It appears that liver enzymes reduce sulfoxide or sulfonyl compounds to thioether or sulfides under anaerobic conditions:

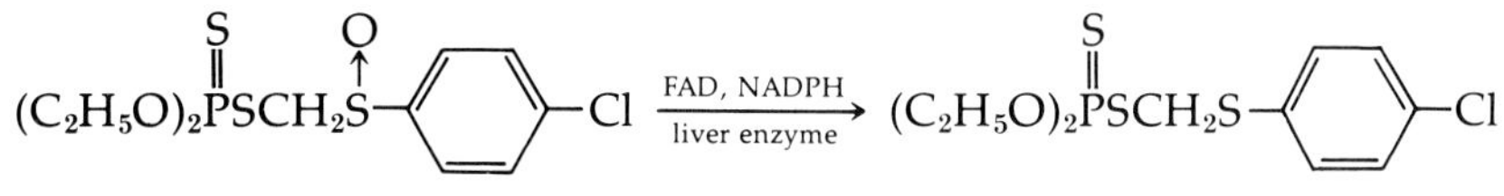

Carbophenothion sulfoxide   Carbophenothion

N-Oxides have been reported to be reduced by a bacterial reductase:

$(R)_3NO \rightarrow (R)_3N.$

4.5.7. Reduction of Double Bonds

Certain aromatic compounds have been reported to be reduced by intestinal flora as follows:

$$C_6H_5CH = CHCO_2H \xrightarrow{2H} C_6H_5CH_2CH_2CH_2OH.$$

Cinnamic acid

4.6. Hydrolysis

A large number of xenobiotics, such as esters, amides, or substituted phosphates that are composed of ester-type bonds, are susceptible to hydrolysis. Hydrolytic reactions are the only phase I reactions that do not utilize energy. Numerous hydrolases are found in blood plasma, liver, intestinal muscosa, kidney, muscle, and nervous tissue. Hydrolases are present in both soluble and microsomal fractions.

The general reactions are

$$\underset{\text{Ester}}{RC-O-R'} + H_2O \xrightarrow{\text{esterase}} \underset{\text{Acid}}{R-C-OH} + \underset{\text{Alcohol}}{HOR'}$$

$$RCONH_2 + H_2O \xrightarrow{\text{amidase}} RCOOH + NH_3$$

The acid and alcohol or amine formed on hydrolysis can be eliminated directly or conjugated by phase II reactions. In general, amide analogs are hydrolyzed at slower rates than the corresponding esters.

Tissue esterases have been divided into two classes, A-type esterases, which are insensitive, and the B-type esterases, which are sensitive to inhibition by organophosphorus esters. The A esterases include the arylesterases, whereas the B esterases include cholinesterases of plasma, acetylcholinesterases of erythrocytes and nervous tissue, carboxylesterases, lipases, etc. The nonspecific arylesterases that hydrolyze short-chain aromatic esters are activated by Ca^{2+} ions and are responsible for the hydrolysis of certain organophosphate triesters, e.g.,

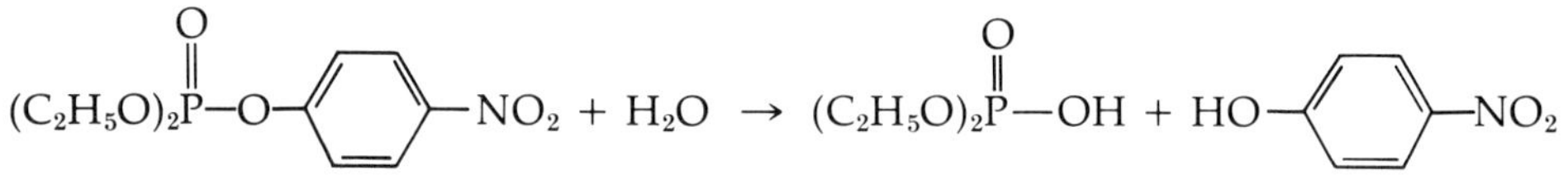

$$(C_2H_5O)_2P-O-\!\!\!\!\!\bigcirc\!\!\!\!\!-NO_2 + H_2O \rightarrow (C_2H_5O)_2P-OH + HO-\!\!\!\!\!\bigcirc\!\!\!\!\!-NO_2$$

Paraoxon

Certain hydrolases also are present in mammalian plasma and tissue that hydrolyze and subsequently detoxify chemical warfare agents such as the nerve gases tabun, sarin, and DFP:

$$O \qquad\qquad O$$
$$\parallel \qquad\qquad\quad \parallel$$
$$(i\text{-}C_3H_7O)_2PF \rightarrow (i\text{-}C_3H_7O)_2P\text{—}OH + HF.$$

DFP

A variety of foreign compounds, such as phthalic acid esters (plasticizers), phenoxyacetic and picolinic acid esters (herbicides), and pyrethroids and their derivatives (insecticides), as well as a variety of ester and amide derivatives of drugs, are detoxified by hydrolases found in plants, animals, and bacteria, i.e., the entire plant and animal kingdom.

In certain strains of insects that are resistant to malathion, the resistance mechanism is associated with a higher level of a carboxylesterase, which detoxifies malathion:

$$S \qquad\qquad\qquad\qquad\qquad\qquad S$$
$$\parallel \qquad\qquad\qquad\qquad\qquad\qquad \parallel$$
$$(CH_3O)_2PSCHCOOC_2H_5 + H_2O \rightarrow (CH_3O)_2PSCHCOOH + C_2H_5OH$$
$$\vert \qquad\qquad\qquad\qquad\qquad\qquad\qquad \vert$$
$$CH_2COOC_2H_5 \qquad\qquad\qquad\qquad CH_2COOC_2H_5$$

Malathion

4.7. Epoxide Hydration

Epoxide rings of certain alkene and arene compounds are hydrated enzymatically by epoxide hydrases to form the corresponding *trans*-dihydrodiols:

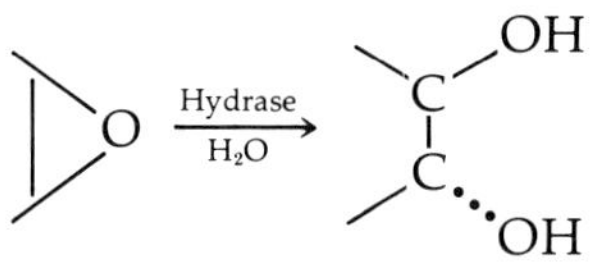

Certain labile epoxides that may be responsible for carcinogenesis are deactivated by the epoxide hydrases as well as the glutathione epoxide S-transferases (see Chapter 5). The enzyme(s) that mediate the hydration are located in the microsomal fraction of mammalian liver. The mechanism of hydration is optimal at alkaline pH and probably involves a nucleophilic attack of the −OH on the oxirane carbon. With styrene oxide as the substrate, the relative activity in the liver of several species is rhesus monkey > human = guinea pig > rabbit > rat > mouse. With the guinea pig and rat, low activity was also found in kidney, intestine, and lung, but no detectable activity was found in muscle, spleen, heart, and brain.

There is evidence that more than one epoxide hydrase exists in hepatic microsomes, based on different purification factors (different relative activities to various epoxide substrates).

4.8. DDT-Dehydrochlorinase

In the early 1950s it was demonstrated that DDT-resistant houseflies detoxified DDT mainly to its noninsecticidal metabolite DDE. The rate of dehydrohalogenation of DDT to DDE was found to vary between various insect strains as well as between individuals. This enzyme also occurs in mammals but has been studied more intensively in insects.

DDT-dehydrochlorinase, a reduced glutathione (GSH)-dependent enzyme, has been isolated from the high-speed supernatant of resistant houseflies. Although the enzyme-mediated reaction requires glutathione, the glutathione levels are not altered at the end of the reaction:

DDT   DDE

The lipoprotein enzyme has a molecular mass of 36,000 daltons as a monomer and 120,000 daltons as the tetramer. The K_m for DDT is 5×10^{-7} M with optimum activity at pH 7.4.

The enzyme system catalyzes the degradation of p,p-DDT to p,p-DDE or the degradation of p,p-DDD (2,2-bis(p-chlorophenyl)-1,1-dichloroethane to the corresponding ethylene TDEE (2,2-bis(p-chlorophenyl)-1-chloroethylene). o,p-DDT is not degraded by DDT-dehydrochlorinase, suggesting a p,p-orientation requirement for dehalogenation. In general, the DDT resistance of house fly strains is correlated with the activity of DDT-dehydrochlorinase, although other resistance mechanisms are known in certain strains.

At one time, it was believed that DDT-dehydrochlorinase, glutathione S-aryltransferase, and enzymes metabolizing the γ-isomer of hexachlorocyclothexane (γ-BHC) were one enzyme since experimental results suggested the existence of a nonspecific enzyme that catalyzed all these reactions. However, it has since been demonstrated that DDT-dehydrochlorinase is different from glutathione S-aryltransferase based on the following: a difference in electrophoretic mobility; a difference in stability and response to inhibitors; results of genetic studies; and purification of a house fly glutathione S-aryltransferase that lacks DDT-dehydrochlorinase activity. The glutathione S-aryltransferase enzyme preparation, however, still has the ability to metabolize γ-BHC.

Suggested Reading

Bend, J. R., Hook, G. E. R. Hepatic and extrahepatic mixed function oxidases. In Lee, D. H. K., Falk, H. L., Murphy, S. D. (Eds.). Handbook of Physiology, Section 9, Reactions to Environmental Agents. Bethesda, Md.: American Physiological Society. 1977

Brodie, B. B., Gillette, J. R., Ackerman, H. S. (Eds.). Handbook of Experimental Pharmacology, Vol. 28, Part 2, Concepts in Biochemical Pharmacology. Berlin: Springer, 1971. This volume contains the following articles of particular relevance to this chapter:

Estabrook, R. W. Cytochrome P-450—Its function in the oxidative metabolism of drugs. Chapter 38, p. 347.

Gillette, J. R. Reductive enzymes. Chapter 42, p. 349.

La Du, B. N., Snady, H. Esterases of human tissues. Chapter 50, p. 477.

Estabrook, R. W., Gillette, J. R., Leibman, K. C. (Eds.). Microsomes and Drug Oxidations (Proceedings of the Second International Symposium). Baltimore, Md.: Williams & Wilkins 1972.

Goldstein, A., A., Aronow, L., Kalman, S. M. Principles of Drug Action: The Basis of Pharmacology, Second Edition. New York: Wiley, 1974.

Jallow, D. R., Locsis, J. J., Snyder, R., Vainio, H. (Eds.). Biological Reactive Intermediates: Formation, Toxicity and Inactivation. New York: Plenum Press, 1977.

Jenner, P., Testa, B. Novel pathways in drug metabolism. Xenobiotica, 8 (1978), 1.

Jerina, D. M. (Ed.). Drug Metabolism Concepts. New York: American Chemical Society Symposium Series, 44, 1977. This symposium contains the following articles of particular relevance to this chapter:

Coon, M. J., Vermilion, J. L., Vatsii, K. P., et al. Biochemical studies on drug metabolism: Isolation of multiple forms of liver microsomal cytochrome P-450. p. 46.

Estabrook, R. W., Werringloer, J. Cytochrome P-450—Its role in oxygen activation for drug metabolism. p. 1.

Johnson, E. J., Muller-Eberhard, U. Resolution of multiple forms of rabbit liver cytochrome P-450. p. 72.

Moore, P. D., Koreeda, M., Wislocki, P. G. *In vitro* reactions of the diastereomeric 9,10-epoxides of (+) and (−)-trans-7,8-dihydroxy-7,8-dihydrobenzo(a)pyrene with polyguanylic acid and evidence for formation of an enantiomer of each diastereomeric 9,10-epoxide from benzo(a)pyrene in mouse skin. p. 127.

Kulkarni, A. P., Hodgson, E. Metabolism of insecticides by mixed function oxidase systems. Pharmacol. Ther. (in press).

Lee, A. Y. H., Levin, W. The resolution and reconstitution of the liver microsomal hydroxylation system. Biochem. Biophys. Acta 344(1974), 205.

Parke, D. V. The Biochemistry of Foreign Compounds. London: Pergamon Press, 1968.

Williams, R. T., Millburn, P. Detoxication mechanisms—The biochemistry of foreign compounds. In Blaschko, H. K. F. (Ed.). Physiological and Pharmacological Biochemistry, Biochemistry Series 1, Vol. 12. Baltimore, Md.: University Park Press, 1975.

Walter C. Dauterman

5

Metabolism of Toxicants
Phase II Reactions

5.1. Introduction

Foreign compounds containing functional groups such as hydroxyl, amino, carboxyl, epoxide, or halogen, or metabolites of phase I reactions, as well as many naturally occurring compounds, can undergo biosynthetic reactions referred to as conjugations or Phase II reactions. Biochemical conjugation is the union or coupling of a natural or foreign compound, or its Phase I metabolite, with a readily available endogenous conjugating agent derived from a carbohydrate, a protein source, or a sulfur component. In general, conjugation products are more polar, less lipid soluble, more readily eliminated from the organism, and less toxic.

Conjugations are generally energy dependent and are linked directly to high-energy intermediates. Williams[1] classified conjugation reactions into two classes based on whether an activated conjugating agent or an activated substrate was utilized in the biosynthesis:

Type I:

Activated conjugating agent (intermediate) + Substrate →
Conjugated product

Type II:

Activated substrate + Amino acid → Conjugated product

---

[1] Williams, R. T., The biogenesis of conjugation and detoxication products. In: Biogenesis of National Compounds (Bennfeld, P., Ed.). Oxford: Pergamon Press, 1967.

Type I reactions include the formation of glycosides and sulfates as well as methylated and acetylated conjugates, whereas type II reactions result in peptide conjugates.

5.2. Glycoside Conjugation

In order for glycoside conjugation to occur, two initial stages are required for both glucoside and glucuronide conjugation. The first is the formation of an activated intermediate, uridine diphosphate glucose (UDPG) and uridine diphosphate glucuronic acid (UDPGA):

$$\text{D-glucose-1-PO}_4 + \text{UTP} \xrightarrow[\text{pyrophosphorylase}]{\text{UDPG}} \text{UDP-}\alpha\text{-D-glucose} + \text{P}_2\text{O}_7{}^{4-} \quad (5.1)$$

$$\text{UDP-}\alpha\text{-D-glucose} + 2\text{ NAD} + \text{H}_2\text{O} \xrightarrow[\text{dehydrogenase}]{\text{UDPG}}$$

$$\text{(5.2)}$$

$$\text{UDP-}\alpha\text{-D-glucuronic acid} + 2\text{NADH}_2$$

Reactions (5.1) and (5.2) are associated with the soluble fraction of the liver and, to a lesser extent, the kidney, intestinal tract, and skin.

5.2.1. Glucuronides

The three steps of glucuronic acid conjugation involve the reaction of the active intermediate UDPGA with the aglycone.

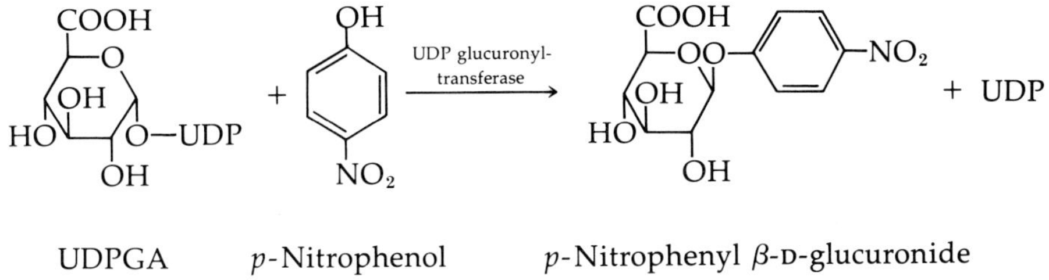

UDPGA   *p*-Nitrophenol   *p*-Nitrophenyl β-D-glucuronide

Reaction (5.3) is the result of nucleophilic displacement (SN_2 reaction) of the functional groups of the substrate with Walden inversion. UDPGA is in the α-configuration, and the glucuronide formed due to inversion is in the β-configuration. The enzyme UDP glucuronyltransferase is found in the microsomal fraction of the liver, kidney, intestinal tract, and skin.

A wide variety of reactions are mediated by glucuronyltransferases, depending on the structure of the aglycone. Structurally, *O*-glucuronides, *N*-glucuronides, and *S*-glucuronides have been isolated and characterized.

5.2.1a. O-Glucuronides

Ether type. This type of glucuronide occurs with primary, secondary, and tertiary alcohols and phenols, e.g.,

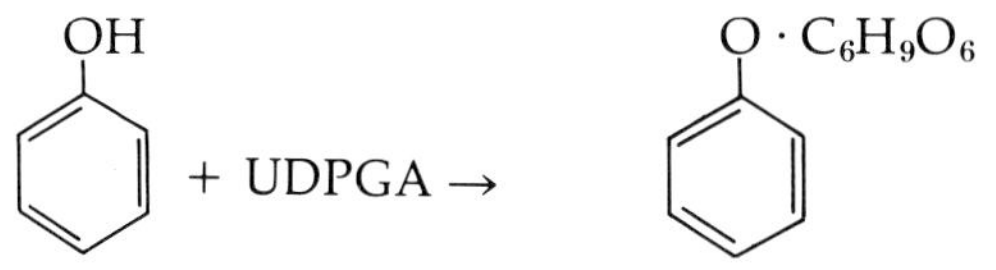

Phenol → Phenyl β-D-glucuronide

Ester. The conjugates are formed from carboxylic acids:

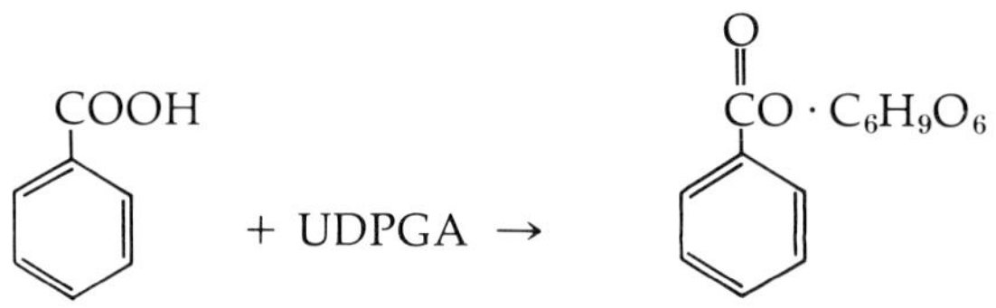

Benzoic acid + UDPGA → Benzoyl β-D-glucuronide

Hydroxylamino. When 2-acetylaminofluorene is metabolized by the mixed-function oxidase system, the amino group becomes hydroxylated at the nitrogen group and then conjugated with UDPGA:

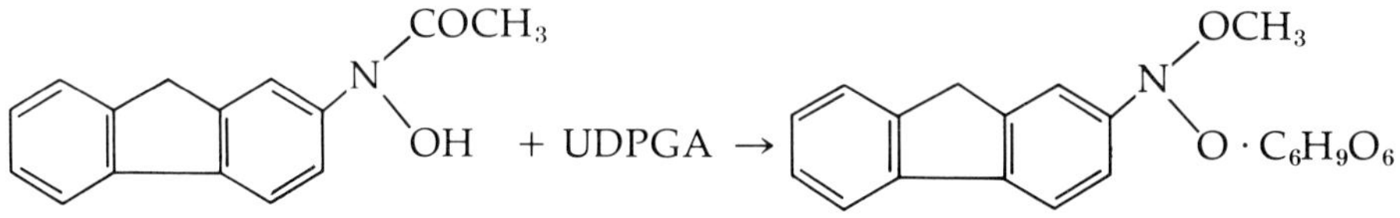

N-Hydroxy-2-acetylaminofluorene + UDPGA → N-Hydroxy-2-acetylaminofluorenyl β-D-glucuronide

5.2.1b. N-Glucuronides

Several types of N-glucuronides have been identified, in which the glucuronyl moiety is attached to the nitrogen. They include the following functional groups: aromatic amino group, sulfonamide group, carbamyl group, and heterocyclic nitrogen group:

Aromatic amino type:

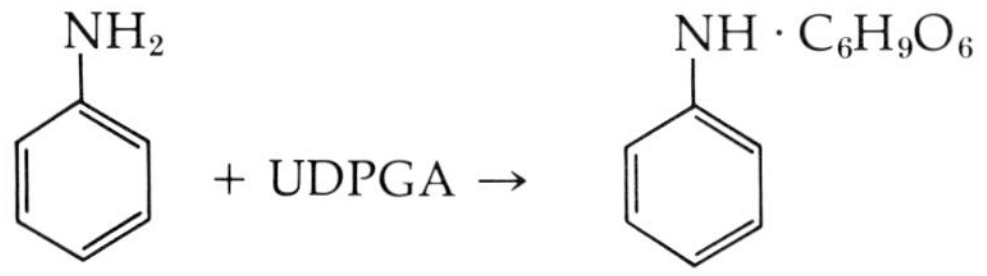

Aniline + UDPGA → Aniline glucuronide

Carbamyl type:

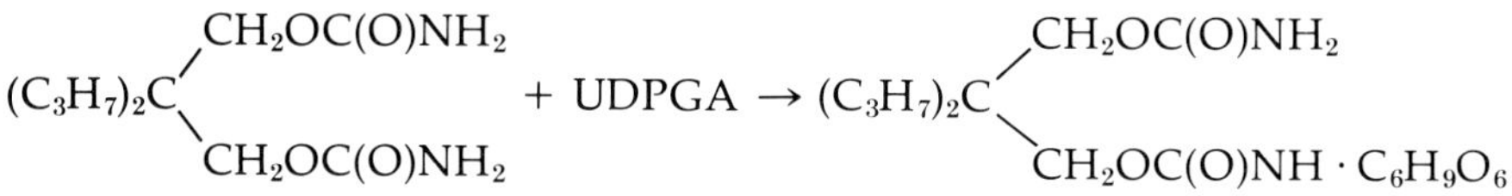

Meprobamate + UDPGA → Meprobamate glucuronide

Sulfonamide type:

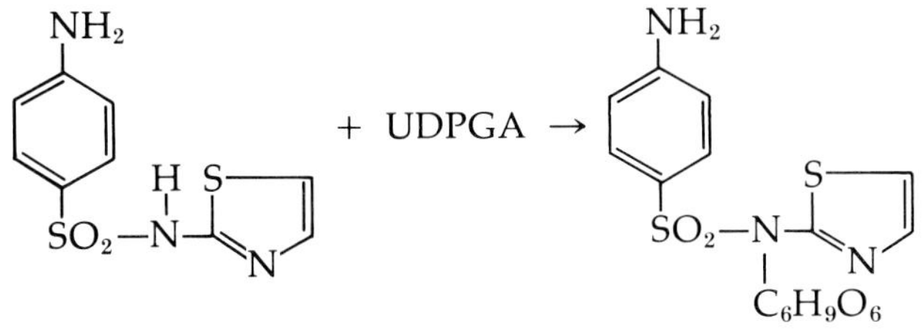

Sulfathiazole   Sulfathiazole — *N*-glucuronide

Heterocyclic type

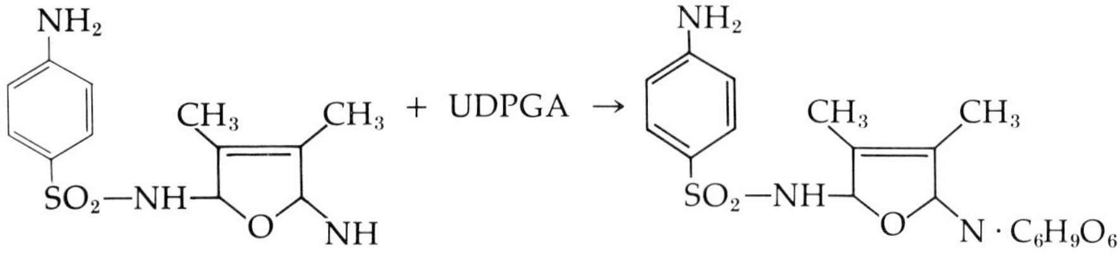

Sulfisoxazole   Sulfisoxazole-N-glucuronide

5.2.1c. S-Glucuronides

There are also a number of thiol compounds that are conjugated with glucuronic acid:

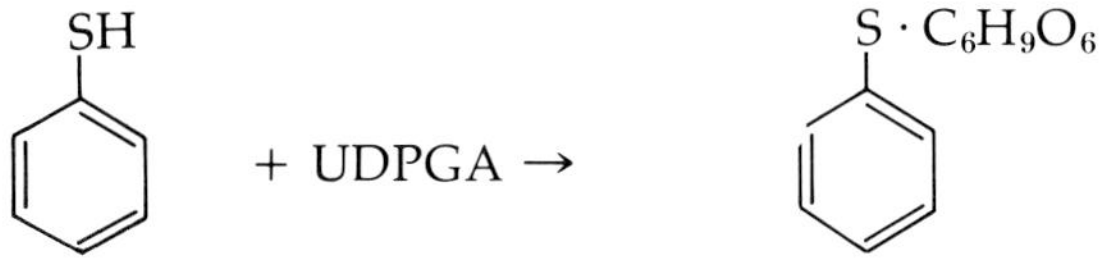

Thiophenol   Thiophenyl β-D-glucuronide

S-glucuronides are not found too often, but are similar to the *N*-glucuronides in that they are acid labile.

UDP glucuronyltransferases are a group of closely related enzymes with similar properties. The cat is able to form glucuronide conjugates of thyroxine and bilirubin but is unable to form other glucuronides. Cats are able to excrete injected glucuronides and also have a sufficient amount of UDPG. Therefore, it appears that glucuronyltransferases for certain xenobiotics are lacking in the cat. As a group of enzymes, the UDP glucuronyltransferases are difficult to solubilize and in general are quite unstable after partial purification. Therefore, much of the data on substrate specificity has been obtained using crude homogenates.

5.3. Sulfate Conjugation

Sulfate ester formation is known to occur with primary, secondary, and tertiary alcohols, phenols, and arylamines. Sulfate esters, in terms of biological conjugations, are in reality half-esters, i.e., $ROSO_3$, which are completely ionized, very water soluble, and quickly eliminated from the organism.

Conjugation via the sulfate route requires a great deal of energy. The activation of the sulfate ion by ATP kinase has an absolute requirement for Mg^{2+}:

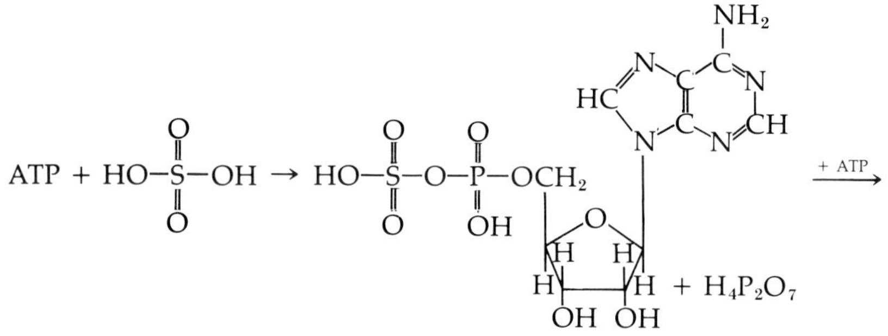

Adenosine 5'-phosphosulfate

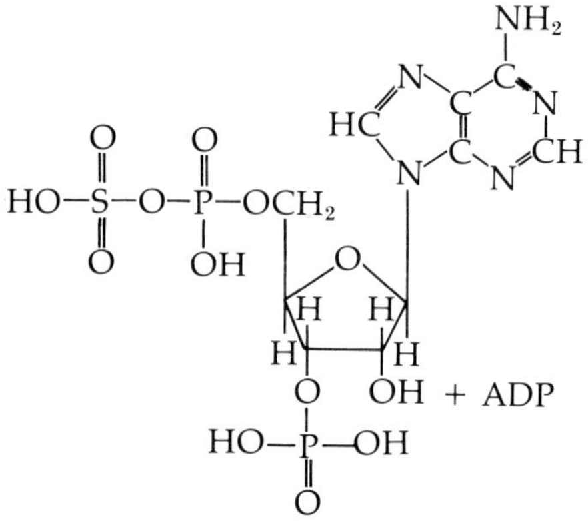

Adenosine 3'-phosphate-5'-phosphosulfate (PAPS)

The enzymes responsible for PAPS formation have been found in the soluble fraction of the adrenal, brain, intestinal mucosa, kidney, liver, muscle, ovaries, and testis.

The sulfating agent (PAPS) with a group of sulfotransferases and the following xenobiotics will form sulfate conjugates:

Aryl Sulfates:

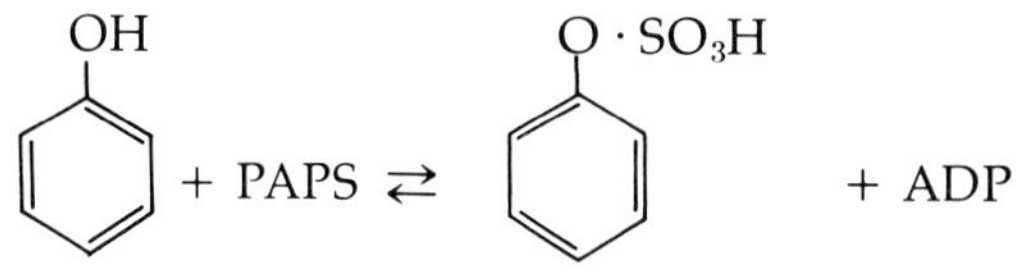

Phenol   Phenyl sulfate

Alkyl sulfates:

$$C_2H_5OH + PAPS \rightleftarrows C_2H_5OSO_3H + ADP$$

Ethanol   Ethyl sulfate

Sulfamates:

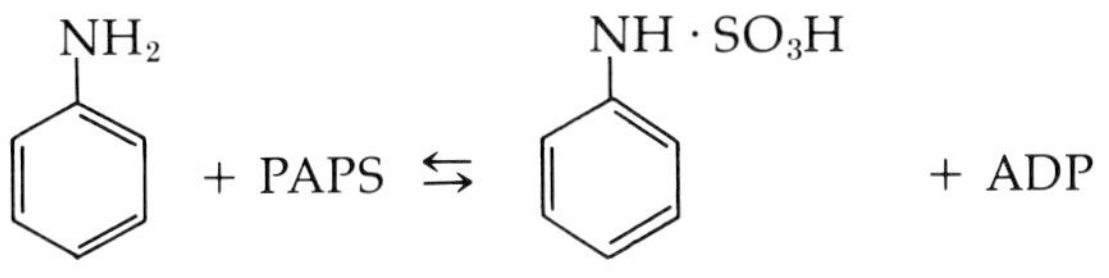

Aniline   Phenyl sulfamate

It appears that a number of sulfotransferases exist. No sulfotransferase has been obtained in a pure state, and the enzymes have usually been studied as crude tissue preparations. Therefore, it is not certain how many separate enzymes actually exist. With xenobiotics, phenol sulfotransferases, alcohol sulfotransferases, and arylamine sulfotransferases appear to be the most important. Phenol sulfotransferase is found in the soluble fraction of mammalian liver, kidney, and intestinal mucosa, whereas some alcohol sulfotransferases have only been found in mammalian livers. A number of other sulfotransferases are known, such as steroid sulfotransferase, choline sulfotransferase, mucopolysaccharide sulfotransferase, and cerebroside sulfotransferase. However, of these, probably only the steroid sulfotransferase may play a role in detoxication of foreign compounds.

5.4. Methyltransferases

Methylation is a common biochemical reaction involving the transfer of methyl groups from three major coenzymes to amines, phenols, and thiol compounds to form N-, O-, and S-methyl conjugates. The coenzymes that provide methyl groups for transfer are S-adenosylmethionine, N^5-methyltetrahydrofolate derivatives, and vitamin B_{12} (methylcorrinoid) derivatives. Of these coenzymes, S-adenosylmethionine is probably the most important for xenobiotic methylation. S-Adenosylmethionine is synthesized from L-methionine and ATP. In all cases involving methylation, products are less water soluble than the parent compound, except for the tertiary amines. Even with the decrease in water solubility, methylation generally is considered a detoxication reaction.

Transmethylation reactions can be classified according to substrates.

5.4.1. N-Methylation

There are several enzyme systems that catalyze the N-methylation of natural and foreign amines. A highly specific enzyme, imidazole-N-methyltransferase, methylates histamine:

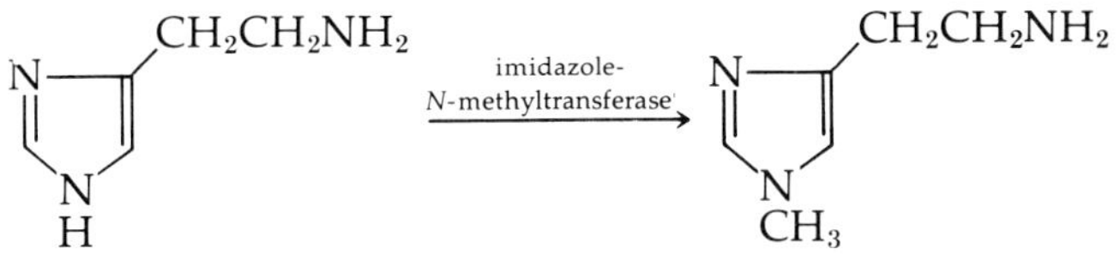

Histamine N-Methylhistamine

Phenylethanolamine-N-methyltransferase, located in the soluble fraction of the adrenal, medulla, heart, and brain, catalyzes the methylation of noradrenaline and other phenylethanolamine derivatives but cannot methylate phenyl ethylamine:

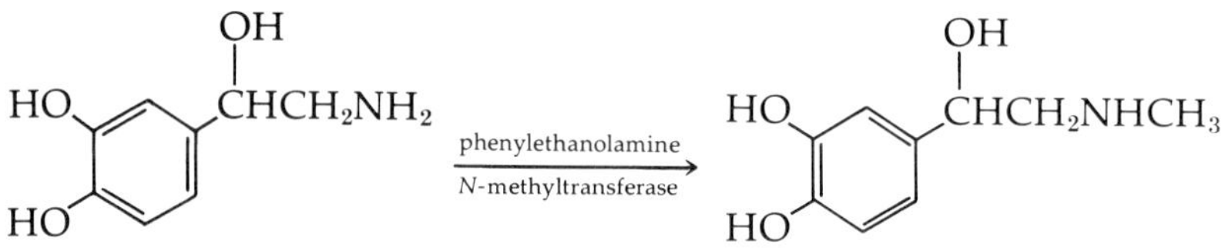

Noradrenaline   Adrenaline

Nonspecific N-methyltransferases have been isolated in the soluble fraction from rabbit lung. Other tissues that have activity include the adrenals, kidney, and, to a lesser degree, the liver and the spleen. The nonspecific N-methyltransferase methylates serotonin, tryptamine, and foreign amines such as normorphine, nornicotine, and norcodeine. Certain heterocyclic tertiary amines such as pyridine are also methylated to form quaternary salts:

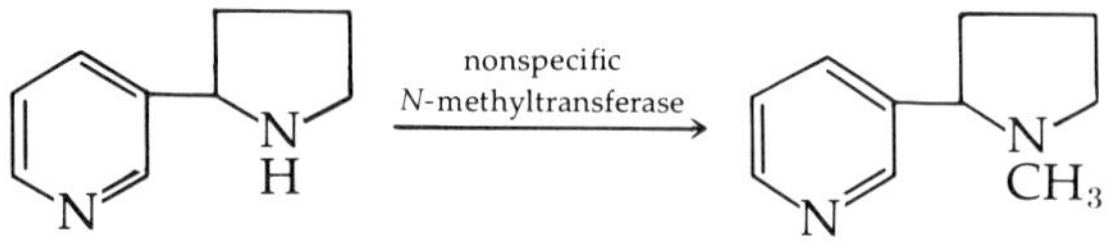

Nornicotine   Nicotine

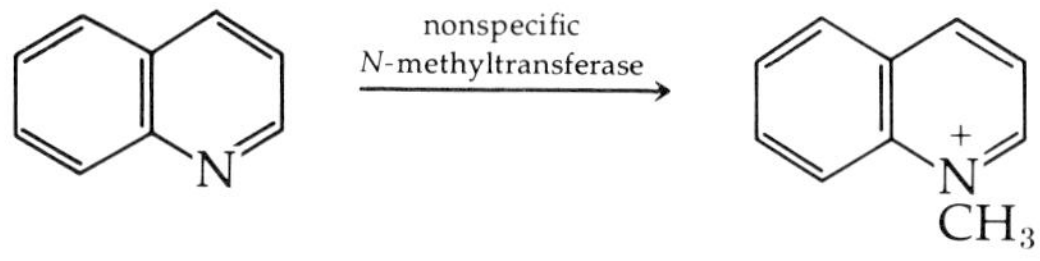

Quinoline   N-Methylquinoline

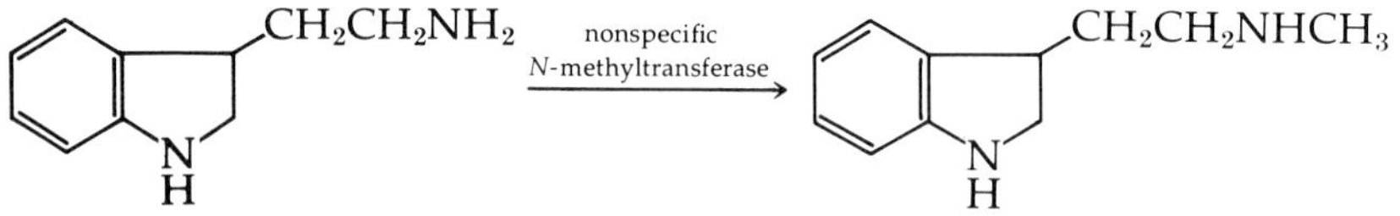

Tryptamine   N-Methyltryptamine

5.4.2. O-Methylation

Catechol-O-methyltransferase is localized in the soluble fraction of rat liver, skin, blood, kidney, glandular tissue and nervous tissue. The reaction requires S-adenosylmethionine and Mg^{2+} or other divalent ions:

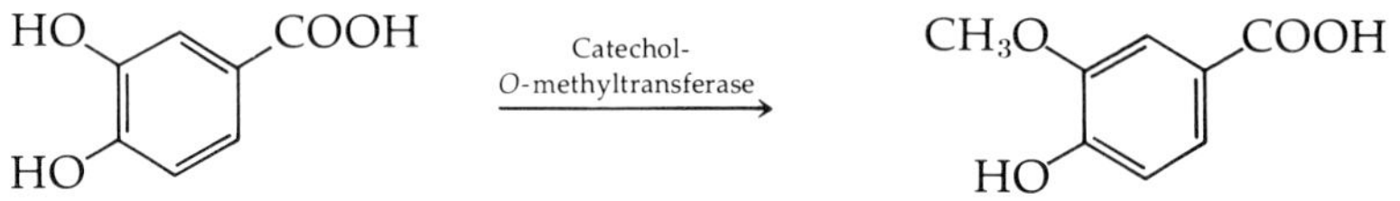

3,4-Dihydroxybenzoic acid   3-Methoxy-4-hydroxybenzoic acid

This enzyme catalyzes the methylation of epinephrine, norepinephrine, and other catechol derivatives. With this enzyme, methylation generally occurs at the *meta* position, but in some cases it will occur at the *para* position.

Recently, a phenol-*O*-methyltransferase that methylates a wide variety of simple alkyl-, methoxy-, and halophenols has been described. The enzyme is present in microsomes from mammalian liver and lung. The methylation is inhibited by SKF-525, *p*-chloromercuribenzoate, and *N*-ethylmaleimide:

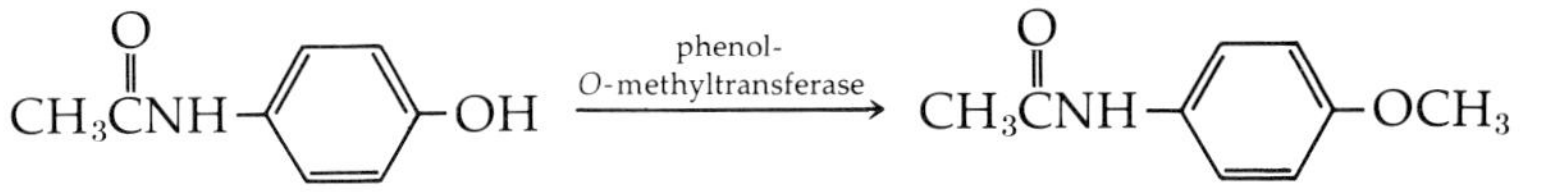

$$CH_3\overset{\overset{\text{O}}{\|}}{C}NH\text{—}\langle\bigcirc\rangle\text{—OH} \xrightarrow[\text{\textit{O}-methyltransferase}]{\text{phenol-}} CH_3\overset{\overset{\text{O}}{\|}}{C}NH\text{—}\langle\bigcirc\rangle\text{—OCH}_3$$

| Hydroxyacetanilide | *p*-Methoxyacetanilide |

A hydroxyindole-*O*-methyltransferase enzyme has been localized in the soluble fraction of the pineal gland of mammals, birds, reptiles, amphibians, and fish. The enzyme has also been found in the brain of amphibians and the eyes of fish, amphibians, reptiles, and some birds. The enzyme is responsible for the methylation of *N*-acetylserotonin and requires *S*-adenosylmethionine:

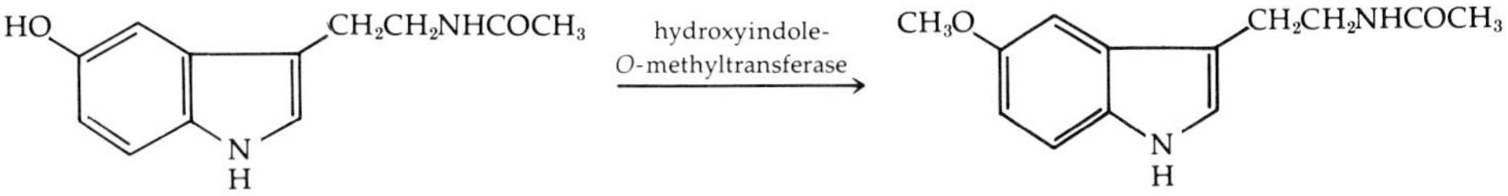

| *N*-acetylseratonin | Melatonin |

A number of other 5-hydroxyindoles, such as *N*-methylserotonin, bufotenine, and some 5,6-dihydroxyindoles, are all methylated at the 5 position but to a lesser extent.

5.4.3. *S*-Methylation

Methyl groups are also transferred to thiol groups of certain xenobiotics, but the reaction appears to be of minor importance. *S*-Methylation has been demonstrated with methyl and ethyl mercaptan, mercaptoethanol, thiouracil, mercaptoacetic acid and dimercaprol (BAL).

$$\text{HSCH}_2\text{CH}_2\text{OH} \xrightarrow{\text{\textit{S}-methyltransferase}} \text{CH}_3\text{SCH}_2\text{CH}_2\text{OH}$$

| Mercaptoethanol | S-Methylthioethanol |

5.4.4. Biomethylation of Elements

Biomethylation of toxic elements in the environment is an important biotransformation mechanism. A variety of metals, i.e., mercury, lead, tin, pallidium, platinum, thallium, and gold, as well as the metalloids, i.e., arsenic, selenium, tellurium, and sulfur, are methylated. The coenzymes reported to be the methyl donors for biomethylation are S-adenosylmethione and vitamin B_{12} (methylcorrinoid derivatives):

$$Hg^{2+} \quad \rightarrow \quad CH_3Hg^+ \quad \rightarrow (CH_3)_2Hg$$

Inorganic   Monomethyl   Dimethyl
mercury   mercury   mercury

5.5 Glutathione S-Transferases

A large number of foreign compounds are metabolized into mercapturic acids, conjugates of L-acetylcysteine, and eliminated via biliary excretion. Mercapturic acids were first reported in 1875, but it was not until the 1950s that it was demonstrated that the cysteine portion of the conjugate came from reduced glutathione (GSH). The general scheme of mercapturic acid biosynthesis is given in Figure 5.1.

The overall reaction involves the conjugation of foreign compounds possessing electrophilic centers with GSH followed by transfer of the glutamate group,

Figure 5.1 Mercapturic acid biosynthesis

RX + HSCH₂CHC(O)NHCH₂COOH
|
NHC(O)CH₂CH₂C(NH₂)COOH
|
      Glutathione S-transferase
|
RSCH₂CHC(O)NHCH₂COOH
|
NHC(O)CH₂CH₂(NH₂)COOH
|
      γ-glutamyltranspeptidase
|
RSCH₂CHC(O)NHCH₂COOH
|
NH₂
|
      cysteinyl glycinase
|
RSCH₂CH(NH₂)COOH
|
      acetylase
|
RSCH₂CHCOOH
|
HNC(O)CH₃

mercapturic acid

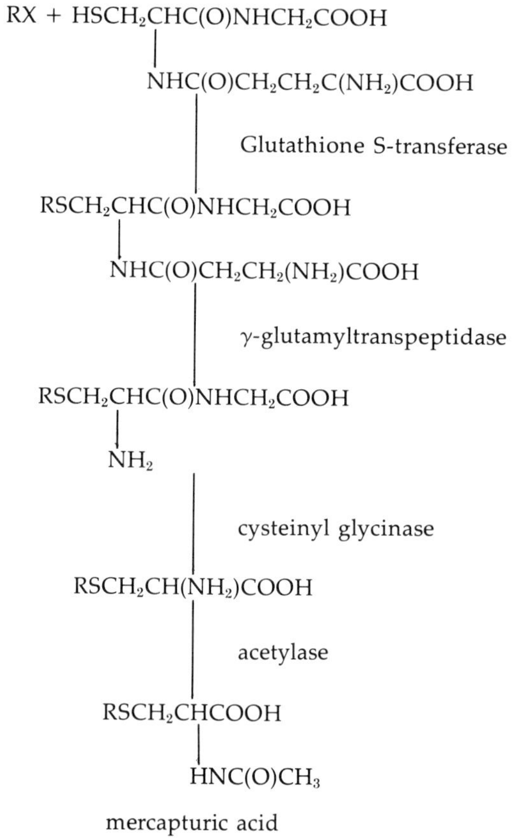

loss of glycine, and finally acetylation. As can be seen, a number of enzymes are involved in the mercapturic acid pathway. The GSH conjugation, the initial reaction, does not require the use of a high-energy intermediate. However, the synthesis of GSH from the various amino acid components and the N-acetylation of the cysteine conjugate does require ATP.

The initial step is mediated by a group of enzymes referred to as glutathione S-transferases, which are involved in the conjugation of GSH with certain foreign compounds.

The role of the glutathione S-transferases is to conjugate toxic electrophiles with endogenous GSH and therefore protect critical nucleophiles such as proteins and nucleic acids. GSH conjugates are anionic and have the necessary properties for biliary excretion, especially with molecular weights greater than 300 (Chapter 9).

The glutathione S-transferases seem to be distributed quite widely, e.g., in mammals, insects, fish, aquatic invertebrates, plants, and possibly bacteria. In mammals, the highest concentration of the enzymes is found in the soluble fraction of the liver. No sulfur-containing compounds other than GSH, will mediate this reaction.

A sufficient amount of GSH appears to be present in various mammalian tissues, plants, and insects to act as a component of a functional glutathione S-transferase system. However, depletion of hepatic GSH, which results when compounds that are reactive with GSH are administered, can have an important toxicological effect, such as a dramatic increase in toxicity when the organism is exposed to additional foreign compounds.

Glutathione S-transferases were initially classified according to their substrate specificity and pH optima. Some substrates used for the classification were as follows:

Glutathione S-alkyltransferase:

$$CH_3I \quad + GSH \rightarrow CH_3\text{-}SG$$

Methyl iodide

Glutathione S-aryltransferase:

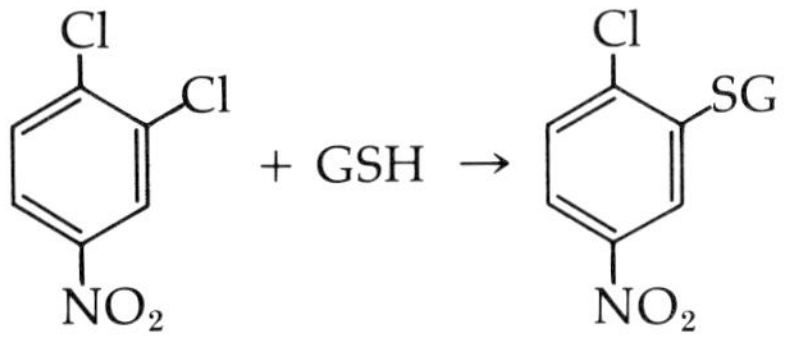

3,4-Dichloronitrobenzene (DCNB)

Glutathione S-aralkyltransferase:

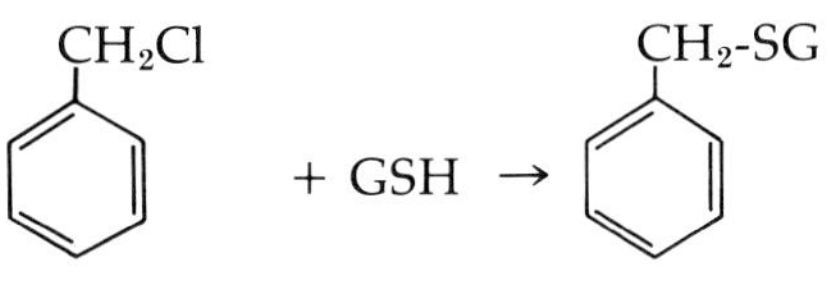

Benzyl chloride

Glutathione S-alkenetransferase:

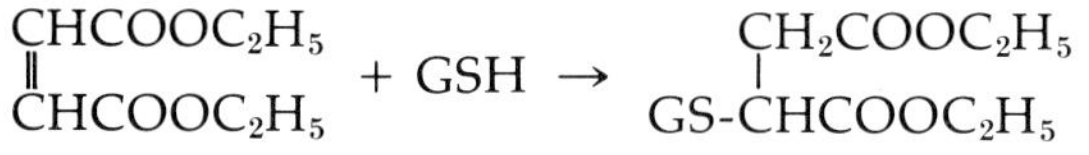

$$\begin{array}{c} CHCOOC_2H_5 \\ \| \\ CHCOOC_2H_5 \end{array} + GSH \rightarrow \begin{array}{c} CH_2COOC_2H_5 \\ | \\ GS\text{-}CHCOOC_2H_5 \end{array}$$

Diethyl maleate

Glutathione S-epoxidetransferase:

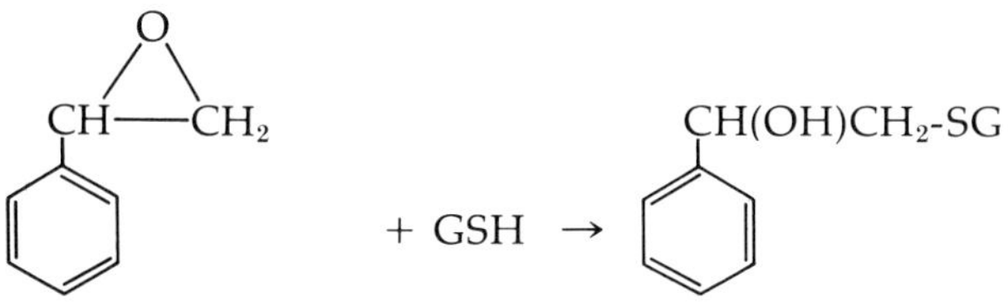

1,2-Epoxyethylbenzene

Recently, the presence of multiple forms of glutathione S-transferases have been reported from livers of the rat, mouse, and man and in insects. Five forms of glutathione S-transferases have been purified to apparent homogeneity from the soluble fraction of both the rat liver and human liver. The molecular masses of the transferases were 45,000–50,000 daltons, and they were composed of two subunits with a molecular mass of 23,000–25,000 daltons.

.The isolated enzymes showed a pattern of overlapping substrate specificity. For example, 1-chloro-2,4-dinitrobenzene and several other substrates were found to be substrates for the entire family of purified enzymes. Therefore, the previous nomenclature is not applicable, and a system based on elution position from a CM-cellulose column or an increase in isoelectric point is being utilized. Glutathione S-transferase B has been reported to be identical to a protein that binds bilirubin, cortisol, and other toxic substances and is known as a ligandin, a major binding protein of liver.

5.6. Acylation

Foreign carboxylic acids and amides undergo biological acylation in mammalian species to form amide conjugates before excretion. This reaction renders the compound less water soluble than the parent compound but generally decreases toxicity.

Acylation reactions are of two general types. The first involves an activated conjugating intermediate (type I reaction) and the foreign compound.

5.6.1 Acetylation

Foreign amines are acetylated by acetyl-coenzyme A (CoA) to form acetylated derivatives.

$$CH_3COSCoA + RNH_2 \rightarrow RNHCOCH_3 + CoASH$$

Acetyl-CoA   Amine   Conjugated   CoA
                          amine

The acetylation involves the enzyme N-acetyltransferase, which has been found in the soluble fraction of liver and associated with the reticuloendothelial cells of liver, spleen, and lung as well as with the intestinal mucosa. Evidence exists for more than one N-acetyltransferase based on the acetylating capacity of mammalian tissue.

Acetylation of amino, hydroxy, and sulfur compounds occurs quite readily in vivo. Acetylation of $-OH$ groups has been demonstrated with choline, while the acetylation of $-SH$ groups is known to occur in the formation of acetyl-CoA. At the present time, the acetylation of hydroxy or thiol groups present in foreign compounds is not known. Aromatic amines, sulfonamides, and certain amino acids are N-acetylated, while aliphatic and phenyl-substituted aliphatic amines are not acetylated.

The ability to acetylate foreign compounds is influenced by developmental and genetic factors in addition to species differences. There are rapid and slow acetylators in both human and rabbit populations that are genetically determined. New borns have low levels of acetyltransferase activity that increase during development.

It has also been demonstrated that slow acetylators are likely to be more susceptible than fast acetylators to adverse effects from xenobiotics that are inactivated by acetylation.

5.6.2. Amino Acid Conjugation

The second type of acylation reaction is a type II reaction involving the activation of foreign carboxylic acids in the presence of ATP and CoA to form acyl S-CoA derivatives that then acylate the α-amino group of certain amino acids to form peptide conjugates:

$$CoASH + RCOOH \xrightarrow{ATP} RCOSCoA$$

| CoA | Acid | Acyl-CoA |

$$RCOSCoA + H_2NCH_2COOH \longrightarrow RCONHCH_2COOH$$

| Acyl-CoA | Glycine | Glycine conjugate |

Peptide conjugation has been reported to occur with glycine and glutamine in mammals and certain primates. In other organisms, different amino acids are utilized in peptide conjugation. Ornithine is utilized by reptiles and some birds, while ticks utilize arginine and glutamine, insects use alanine, glycine, serine, and glutamine, and fish use taurine.

The activating enzyme system is present in human and rat liver mitochondria and is presumably identical to the fatty acid–activating enzyme system. The acyltransferase has been found in both mitochondria and the soluble fraction. An acyltransferase has been purified from beef liver mitochondria that is able to mediate the transfer of various aliphatic (C_2–C_{10}) and aromatic acyl-CoA derivatives. The molecular mass of the 53-fold purified enzyme was estimated to be 190,000 daltons. Tests for various acyl acceptors showed that it was specific for glycine. Another purified rat liver glycine acyltransferase preparation had a different pH optimum than the beef liver enzyme. Evidence would indicate that more than one acyltransferase may be present in various tissues.

5.6.3. Deacetylation

Enzymes that deacetylate N-acetylated xenobiotics have been found in the liver and kidney of many species. The aromatic deacetylase is known as arylacylamidase, which cleaves the conjugate and forms the starting compound:

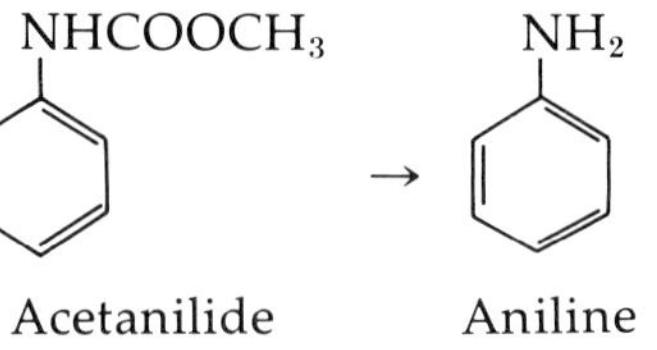

NHCOOCH$_3$ NH$_2$

$\rightarrow$

Acetanilide   Aniline

Deacetylation occurs in various species, and there is a large difference in the amount of deacetylase activity among species, within different strains of the same species, and among individuals of the sample population.

Acetylation and deacetylation reactions are independent of one another and act in opposite directions. Therefore, it is difficult to evaluate the importance of acetylation in vivo in certain animal species because of the two competing systems. This is not difficult with the dog because the dog has an active deacetylase system but is deficient in N-acetyltransferase activity. The rabbit has high N-acetyltransferase activity but has negligible deacetylase activity. Therefore, the rabbit excretes large amounts of acetylated amines. In other animals with both systems operating it is difficult to determine which reaction predominates in vivo.

5.7. Phosphate Conjugation

The biosynthesis of phosphate esters is a general phenomenon found in all intermediary metabolism. However, phosphate conjugates of xenobiotics are rarely encountered. At present it appears that insects are the only major group of animals that utilize this mechanism as a phase II reaction.

An active phosphotransferase preparation has been obtained from gut tissue of the Madagascar cockroach. The enzyme requires ATP and Mg^{2+} for phosphorylation of 1-naphthol and p-nitrophenol:

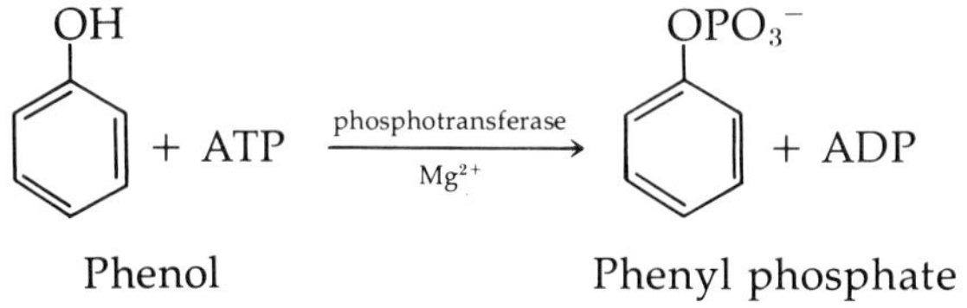

OH   OPO$_3^-$

$+$ ATP $\xrightarrow[\text{Mg}^{2+}]{\text{phosphotransferase}}$ $+$ ADP

Phenol   Phenyl phosphate

Suggested Reading

Arias, I. M., Jakoby, W. B. (Eds.). Glutathione: Metabolism and Function. New York: Raven Press, 1976. This volume contains the following articles of particular relevance to this chapter:

Chasseud, L. F. Conjugation with glutathione and mercapturic acid excretion. Chapter 7, p. 77.

Jakoby, W. B., Habig, W. H., Keen, J. H., Ketley, J. N., Pabst, M. J. Glutathione S-transferases: Catalytic aspects. Chapter 12, p. 189.

Brodie, B. B., Gillette, J. R., Ackerman, H. S. (Eds.). Handbook of Experimental Pharmacology, Vol. 28, Part 2, Concepts in Biochemical Pharmacology. Berlin: Springer, 1971. This volume contains the following articles of particular relevance to this chapter:

Axelrod, J. Methyltransferase enzymes in the metabolism of physiologically active compounds and drugs. Chapter 56, p. 609.

Dutton, G. J. Glucuronide-forming enzymes. Chapter 45, p. 378.

Roy, A. B. Sulphate conjugation enzymes. Chapter 53, p. 536.

Weber, W. W. Acetylating, deacetylating and amino acid conjugation enzymes. Chapter 54, p. 564.

Goldstein, A., Aronow L., Kalman, S. M. Principles of Drug Action: The Basis of Pharmacology, Second Edition. New York: Wiley, 1974.

Arun P. Kulkarni and
Ernest Hodgson

6

Comparative Toxicology

6.1. Introduction

Comparative toxicology is the study of the variation in toxicity of exogenous chemicals toward different organisms, either of different genetic strains or of different taxonomic groups. Thus, the comparative approach can be used in the study of any aspect of toxicology, such as absorption, metabolism, mode of action, and acute or chronic effects. However, most comparative data exist in two areas—acute toxicity and the metabolism of toxic compounds.

Although most toxicologists are interested in a specific toxic event or mechanism and use only the most convenient experimental animal, the comparative approach is extremely valuable. Its value can be summarized in four areas:

Selective toxicity. If toxic compounds are to be used for controlling diseases, pests, and parasites, it is important to develop selective biocides toxic to the target organism and less toxic to other organisms, particularly man. The most obvious examples are those herbicides that interfere with photosynthesis: such compounds frequently having little effect on animals. Among biocides used to control animals, such as insecticides, nematocides, rodenticides, etc., the toxicity to nontarget organisms is frequently high. An exception is the insecticide malathion, which is less toxic to mammals because a carboxylesterase cleaves one of the carboxyl ester linkages. This enzyme is usually lacking in insects.

Experimental models. Comparative studies of toxic phenomena are necessary to select the most appropriate model for extrapolation to man. Taxonomic proximity does not necessarily indicate which will be the best experimental animal, since, in some cases, primates are less valuable than other mammals. In any event, the expense and handling problems associated with primates are such that alternative animals are absolutely necessary.

Environmental xenobiotic cycles. Much of the current concern over toxic compounds springs from their occurrence in the environment as a result of industrial, agricultural, or domestic processes. Different organisms in the complex ecological foodwebs metabolize compounds at different rates and to different products; the metabolic end products are released back to the environment, either to be further metabolized by other organisms or to exert toxic effects of their own. Clearly, it is desirable to know the range of metabolic processes possible.

There have been several attempts to simplify the ecological complexities by constructing laboratory microecosystems that could be used to simulate many of the characteristics of complex natural ecosystems. Usually ^{14}C-labeled compounds and their metabolites are followed through the plants and terrestrial and aquatic animals involved in the microecosystem. R. L. Metcalf pioneered this approach and has been one of its most successful practitioners.

Comparative biochemistry. Comparative toxicology can play a role in the science of comparative biochemistry. It has been said that the proper role of comparative biochemistry is to put evolution on a molecular basis, and detoxication enzymes, like other enzymes, are suitable subjects for study. Detoxication enzymes were probably essential in the early stages of animal evolution since secondary plant products, even those of low toxicity, are frequently lipophilic and as a consequence would, in the absence of detoxication enzymes, accumulate in lipid membranes and lipid depots. Consideration of the distribution and functions of cytochrome P-450 throughout the plant and animal kingdoms would indicate that it is an ancient enzyme that most often serves to metabolize xenobiotics.

Although the development of drugs is properly the province of pharmacology, their development involves comparative toxicology since many preliminary studies are carried out on a variety of experimental animals. Of the many variables that affect the toxicological action of a chemical agent, only species and genetic constitution are considered here; information on other factors may be found in other chapters.

6.2. Variations among Taxonomic Groups

Although the ultimate explanation of comparative differences must be at the level of biochemical genetics, they are manifested at many other levels, which are summarized below.

6.2.1. In Vivo Toxicity

Toxicity is a term used to describe the adverse effects of chemicals on living organisms. Depending upon the degree of toxicity, an animal may die or suffer injury to certain organs or have a specific functional derangement in a subcellular organelle. Sublethal effects of toxicants are often reversible and in many cases can be measured by biochemical tests.

Numerous biocides are introduced into the environment to combat parasites and pests. Available data on the toxicity of selected pesticides to rats suggest that herbicides, in general, provide the greatest human safety by selectively killing weeds. Similarly, destruction of lower organisms such as pathogenic plant fungi has been quite successful without jeopardizing human safety. However, as the evolutionary position of the target species approaches that of man the human safety factor is narrowed considerably. Thus, as far as man and other mammals are concerned, biocide toxicity seems to be in the following progression: herbicides = fungicides < molluscicides < acaricides < nematocides < insecticides < rodenticides. This relationship is obviously oversimplified since astonishing differences in lethality are observed when members of each group of biocides are tested against laboratory test animals and target species. For example, the insecticide DDT shows remarkable differences in its toxicity to animal species that are phylogenically close as well as those that are distantly related. As compared to mammals, with LD_{50} values in the range of 40–500 mg/kg, birds, with LD_{50} values of 800–4000 mg/kg, seem to tolerate relatively higher doses, while insects and marine organisms are extremely susceptible.

Interspecific differences are also known for some naturally occurring poisons. Nicotine, for instance, effectively kills many insect pests, yet tobacco leaves constitute a normal diet for several species. Most strains of rabbit eat *Belladona* leaves with impunity, while other mammals are easily poisoned. Scorpion venom paralyzes prey, but its ingestion by scorpions has no effect. Natural immunity to HCN poisoning in millipedes and the high resistance to the powerful axonal blocking agent tetrodotoxin in puffer fish are further interesting examples of the tolerance of animals to the toxins they produce.

The specific organ toxicity of chemicals also exhibits wide species differences. Although carbon tetrachloride, a highly potent hepatotoxicant, induces liver damage in many species, chickens are practically immune to it. Some strains of mice, although showing typical liver necrosis with carbon tetrachloride, show no signs of increased lipid peroxidation in the endoplasmic reticulum. Dinitrophenol causes cataracts in humans, ducks, and chickens but not in other experimental animals. Birth defects occur in dogs and guinea pigs fed diets containing carbaryl, but the same is not true in hamsters and rabbits, even at higher doses. The eggshell thinning associated with DDT poisoning in birds is observed in falcons and mallard ducks, whereas this reproductive toxicity is not observed in gallinaceous species. Delayed neurotoxicity caused by organophosphates such as leptophos and tri-*o*-cresyl phosphate can be easily demonstrated in chickens but can be produced only with difficulty in common laboratory mammals.

Species variation in toxicity may be reflected in metabolism if a major metabolite is either more or less toxic than the parent compound. For example, 1-isonicotinoyl-2-acetylhydrazine, the major metabolite of isoniazid in man, is considerably less toxic than the parent compound. This explains the higher toxicity of isoniazid to dogs, which cannot acetylate isoniazid.

6.2.2. In Vivo Metabolism

Many ecological and physiological factors affect the rates of penetration, distribution, biotransformation, and excretion of chemicals and thus govern their biological fate in the body. In general, xenobiotic absorption, tissue distribution, and penetration across the blood–brain barrier and other barriers are dictated by their physicochemical nature and, therefore, tend to be similar in various animal species. The biological effect of a chemical depends upon the concentration of its active form and its duration inside the body. This is governed, in turn, by the rates of its biotransformation and excretion and the magnitude and nature of its binding to tissue macromolecules. Logic dictates that substantial differences in these variables should confer species specificity in the biological response to any metabolically reactive xenobiotic. By the same token, highly polar compounds, such as strong acids or bases, those compounds that undergo spontaneous transformations, especially at physiological pH values (e.g., thalidomide), as well as those that are extremely resistant to metabolism (e.g., mirex) might be expected to display a lack of species specificity.

6.2.2a. Binding to Macromolecules

Xenobiotics may bind to many macromolecules either at the target site or elsewhere. Modes of toxic action usually involve the combination of the administered chemical or its metabolites with a specific macromolecule. Enough difference may exist in the sensitivity of such target sites to permit, in some cases, the division of animals into target and nontarget species on this basis. Thus, compared to the mouse, the 22-fold lower toxicity of paraoxon to the frog is paralleled by a 79-fold lower sensitivity of its acetylcholinesterase to inhibition. This unusual insensitivity in the frog is also noted toward the carbamate eserine. Other examples, including insensitivity of the millipede to the respiratory inhibitor cyanide and resistance in spider mites to ATPase inhibition by organotin compounds, also support the view that selectively may be due to target site variation.

Binding to nontarget sites is also important since it renders the xenobiotic biologically inactive. Reversibly bound molecules may be released under suitable biochemical conditions, thus affecting the duration of actin of a toxicant.

A number of xenobiotics bind avidly to various proteins in the blood, particularly to serum albumin, as well as to numerous tissue proteins. Species differences in the binding of chemicals are not only related to the absolute quantities and relative proportions of different classes of proteins, but are also dependent on differences in composition and conformation within classes, such as the albumins. In general, xenobiotics tend to bind more tightly to serum proteins in man than in other mammals. Interestingly, however, the species trend in metabolic inactivation is in the opposite direction.

6.2.2b. Biological Half-Life

The biological half-life is governed by the rates of metabolism and excretion and thus reflects the most important variables explaining interspecies differences in toxic response. Striking differences between species can be seen in the biological half-lives of various drugs. Humans, in general, metabolize xenobiotics more slowly than various experimental animals. For example, phenylbutazone is metabolized slowly in man, with a half-life averaging 3 days. However, in the monkey, rat, guinea pig, rabbit, dog, and horse, the drug is metabolized readily, with half-lives ranging between 3 and 6 hr.

Large differences in the effective therapeutic dose between human and other animals may not be due to differences in the relative sensitivity of the target sites to the drug but instead to interspecific variation in the rate and pattern of metabolism. If this is the case, a given response should appear at a plasma concentration that is similar in all species, even though the dose required to produce this concentration may vary greatly. The data given in Table 6.1 for the muscle relaxant carisoprodol indicate that, although an equivalent dose produces marked differences in the duration of the loss of reflex, all species display essentially the same plasma concentration on recovery from the drug's effect.

The interdependence of metabolic rate, half-life, and pharmacological action can also be seen from the data in Table 6.1 for hexobarbital. The duration of sleeping time is directly related to the biological half-life and is inversely proportional to the in vitro degradation capacity of liver enzymes from the respective species. Thus, mice inactivate hexobarbital readily, as reflected in the smallest biological half-life in vivo and the shortest sleeping time, while the reverse is true in dogs.

6.2.2c. In Vivo Metabolite Production

Xenobiotics, once inside the body, undergo a series of biotransformations. Those reactions that introduce a new functional group into the molecule, either by oxidation, reduction, or hydrolysis, are designated phase I reactions, while the conjugation reactions by which phase I metabolites are combined with endogenous substrates in the body are referred to as phase II reactions. Chemicals may undergo any one of these reactions or any combination of them, either simultaneously or consecutively. Since biotransformations are catalyzed by a large number of enzymes, it is to be expected that they would vary between

Table 6.1 Variation Among Species in the Mode of Action of Carisoprodol and Hexobarbital Metabolism

Drug	Species	Pharmacological action		Enzyme activity (μg/g liver/hr)	Plasma level on recovery (μg/ml)
		Loss of righting reflex (hr)			
Carisoprodol	Mouse	0.2		—	130
	Rat	1.5		—	125
	Rabbit	5.0		—	100
	Cat	10.0		—	125
		Half-life (min.)	*Sleeping time (min.)*		
Hexobarbital	Mouse	19	12	598	—
	Rabbit	60	49	196	—
	Rat	140	90	134	—
	Dog	260	315	36	—

species. Qualitative differences imply the occurrence of different enzymes, whereas quantitative differences, on the other hand, imply variations in the rate of biotransformation along a common metabolic pathway resulting from differences in enzyme levels, in the extent of competing reactions, in the amount of natural enzyme inhibitor(s), or in the efficiency of enzymes capable of reversing the reaction.

Phase I reactions. The case of oxidation, the most studied class of phase I reactions, will be considered first. Even in the case of a xenobiotic undergoing oxidation primarily by a single reaction, there may be remarkable species differences in relative rates. Thus, in humans, rats, and guinea pigs, the major route of papaverine metabolism is *O*-demethylation to yield phenolic products, but very little of these products are formed in dogs.

Aromatic hydroxylation of aniline is another example. In this case, both *ortho* and *para* positions are susceptible to oxidative attack yielding the respective aminophenols. The biological fate of aniline has been studied in many animal species and striking selectivity in hydroxylation position has been noted (Table 6.2). These data show a trend in that carnivores, in general, display a high aniline *ortho*-hydroxylase ability with a *para/ortho* ratio of ≤ 1, while rodents exhibit a striking preference for the *para* position, with a *para/ortho* ratio of from 2.5 to 15. Along with extensive *p*-aminophenol, substantial quantities of *o*-aminophenol are also produced from aniline administered to rabbits and hens.

Coumarin is susceptible to aromatic hydroxylation at four different positions, and the formation of 7-hydroxycoumarin or umbelliferone is the primary reaction in rabbits. The rat produces the same four metabolites, but to a much smaller extent; humans, in contrast, convert up to 90% of the administered dose into 7-hydroxycoumarin.

The major metabolic pathway is not always the same in any two animal

Table 6.2 In Vivo Aromatic Hydroxylation of Aniline in Females of Various Animal Species

Class	Order	Species	Percent dose excreted as aminophenol		Para/ortho ratio
			Ortho	*Para*	
Mammalia	Carnivora	Dog	18.0	9.0	0.5
		Cat	32.0	14.0	0.4
		Ferret	26.0	28.0	1.0
	Rodentia	Rat	19.0	48.0	2.5
		Mouse	4.0	12.0	3.0
		Hamster	5.5	53.0	10.0
		Guinea pig	4.2	46.0	11.0
		Gerbil	3.2	48.0	15.0
	Lagomorpha	Rabbit	8.8	50.0	6.0
Aves	Galliformes	Hen	10.5	44.0	4.0

Source: Parke, Biochem. J. 77 (1960), 493.

species. For example, the mouse hydrolyzes 6-propylthiopurine to mercaptopurine, and thus the drug is a potent carcinogen in the mouse. Humans, on the other hand, oxidize the drug in two positions, without hydrolysis, and the end products are not carcinogenic. Similarly, 2-acetylaminofluorene may be metabolized in mammals by two alternative routes, N-hydroxylation, yielding the carcinogenic N-hydroxy derivative, and aromatic hydroxylation, yielding the noncarcinogenic 7-hydroxy metabolite. The former is the metabolic route in the rat, rabbit, hamster, dog, and human species, in which the parent compound is known to be carcinogenic. In contrast, the monkey carries out aromatic hydroxylation and the guinea pig appears to deacetylate the N-hydroxy derivative, and thus both escape the carcinogenic effects.

Rats exhibit a remarkable ability to hydroxylate amphetamines, whereas biotransformation proceeds primarily via oxidative deamination in other species, including man. The primary metabolite resulting from the deamination of amphetamine is susceptible to further degradation by oxidation, reduction, and enol formation, and wide species differences are encountered (Figure 6.1). Rats metabolize amphetamine exclusively by aromatic hydroxylation and very little, if any, of either the parent compound or its metabolites are excreted in the urine. Although the amount of unchanged amphetamine excreted in rabbits and guinea pigs does not differ significantly, in guinea pigs all the deaminated drug is rapidly oxidized to metabolite IV, while in rabbits this process occurs relatively slowly. Reduction, leading to the formation of an alcoholic product, also occurs in the rabbit.

Several animal species, including man, carry out reactions involving reduction of azo linkages, aldehydes, ketones, and nitro groups, as well as replacement of halogens by hydrogen and reduction of double bonds. Many enzymes catalyze these reactions, and, like oxidative enzymes, variations in them contribute to the selective action of xenobiotics.

The drug chloramphenicol, which contains an aromatic nitro group, undergoes reduction to an arylamine. This reaction occurs extensively in the rat but is of very low magnitude in man. The biotransformation of carbomal (2-bromo-2-ethylbutylurea) into 2-ethylbutylurea involves the replacement by hydrogen of the bromine attached to the carbon atom. The compound simultaneously undergoes an oxidative reaction. Compared to the rat or dog, the mouse metabolizes this compound very rapidly, producing nearly equal quantities of two metabolites. The rat and the dog display a preference for reduction and produce 2-ethylbutylurea in quantities that exceed those of the oxidation product, hydroxycarbomal, by a large margin.

The hydrolysis of esters by esterases and of amides by amidases constitutes one of the most common enzymatic reactions of xenobiotics in man and other animal species. Both the number of enzymes involved in hydrolytic attack and the number of chemicals acting as substrates for them are large. It is therefore not surprising to observe interspecific differences in the disposition of xenobiotics due to variations in these enzymes.

Deesterification of reserpine in vivo liberates methyl reserpate. Rats carry out this reaction extensively, but only if the drug is administered orally. In dogs and monkeys this reaction is of minor importance. The rat's intestinal mucosa possesses an esterase capable of splitting reserpine that is absent in dogs and

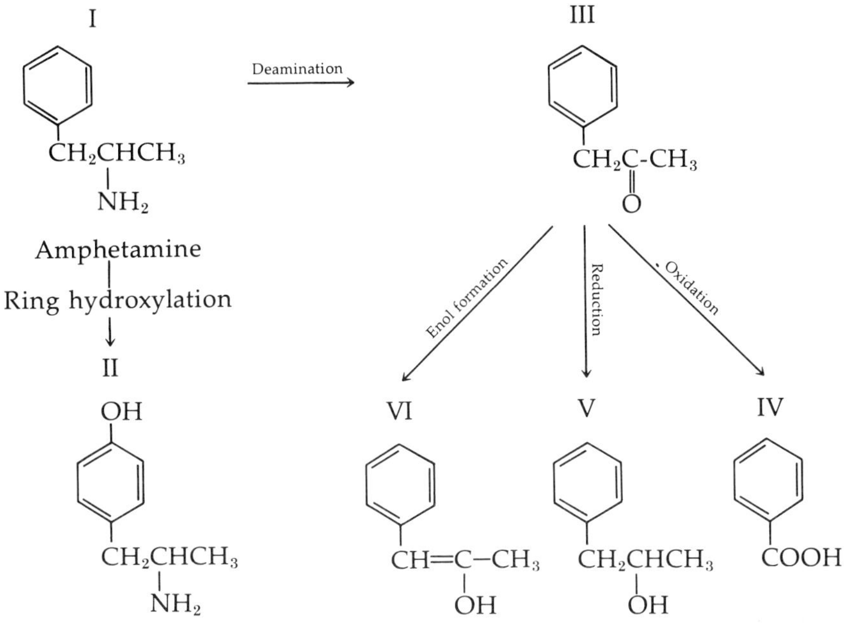

Figure 6.1 Amphetamine metabolism in several animal species.

| Species | Metabolites excreted in the urine | | | | |
	I	II	III	IV	V
Man	30	3	3	20	0
Rhesus monkey	25	6	0	29	0
Dog	30	6	1	28	1
Rabbit	13	6	22	23	8
Guinea pig	18	1	0	65	0
Mouse	30	15	0	31	0
Rat	3	60	0	3	0

monkeys. Similarly, atropinesterase is absent in the mouse and human, while it is present in the liver, but not the plasma, of guinea pigs. Rabbits are the only species investigated that possess this enzyme in the plasma.

As with esters, there are wide differences between species in the rates of hydrolysis of various amides in vivo. Fluoroacetamide is less toxic than the parent acid to mice but not to the American cockroach. This is explained by the faster release of fluoroacetate in insects as compared to mice. The systemic acaricide 2-fluoro-N-methyl-N-(1-naphthyl) acetamide (Nissol) is another example in which a close relationship between toxicity and the rate of hydrolysis to release fluoroacetate can be found. The guinea pig is 60–130-fold more sensitive to Nissol than the rat or mouse, and the activation rate is 30–45-fold higher in the guinea pig than in the rat or mouse. The insecticide dimethoate is susceptible to the attack of both esterases and amidases, yielding nontoxic products. In the rat and mouse both reactions occur, whereas sheep liver contains only the amidase and that of guinea pig only the esterase. The relative rates of these degradative enzymes in insects are very low as compared to mammals, and this correlates well with the high toxicity of dimethoate to insects.

Phase II reactions. The various phase II reactions are concerned with the conjugation of primary metabolites of xenobiotics produced by phase I reactions. A number of factors alter or govern the rates of phase II reactions, and these will be considered in light of their role in interspecific differences in xenobiotic metabolism.

Although the final disposition of xenobiotics, frequently in the form of conjugates, occurs via urine, feces, lungs, sweat, saliva, milk, hair, nails, placenta, etc., comparative data are available only with regard to the first two routes. Interspecific variation in the pattern of biliary excretion may determine species differences to the extent to which compounds are eliminated in the urine or feces. It is a common observation that fecal excretion of a chemical or its metabolites tends to be higher in species that are generally good biliary excretors, such as the rat and dog, than in species that are poor, such as the rabbit, guinea pig, and monkey. For example, the fecal excretion of stilbestrol in the rat accounts for 75% of the dose, while in the rabbit about 70% can be found in the urine. Dogs, like humans, metabolize indomethacin to a glucuronide, but, unlike humans, which excrete it in the urine, dogs primarily excrete it in the feces—apparently due to inefficient renal and hepatic blood clearance of the glucuronide. It can be presumed that these differences may involve species variation in enterohepatic circulation, plasma levels, and biological half-life.

Interspecific differences in the magnitude of biliary excretion of a xenobiotic largely depend upon molecular weight, the presence of polar groups in the molecule, and the extent of conjugation. Compounds, involving conjugates, with molecular weights of less than 300 are poorly excreted in bile by most laboratory animals (Table 6.3). Based on fragmentary evidence, humans also appear to be ineffective biliary excretors of simple aromatic compounds. A marked species difference is noted for biliary excretion of chemicals with molecular weights around 300. Thus, the biliary excretion of succinylsulfathiazole is 20–30-fold greater in the rat and the dog than in the rabbit and the guinea pig, and over 100-fold higher than in the pig and the rhesus monkey. The cat and sheep are intermediate and excrete about 7% of the dose in the bile. Similar but less dramatic species differences in biliary excretion are obvious with molecules with molecular weights between 445 and 495. This trend in species variation disappears in the biliary excretion of relatively high molecular weight (above 500) substances, although the magnitude of excretion in the bile is generally high in all animal species tested (Table 6.3).

The evidence reported in a few studies suggests some relationship between the evolutionary position of a species and its conjugation mechanisms (Table 6.4). In humans and most mammals the principal mechanisms involve

Table 6.3 Biliary Excretion of Xenobiotics in Various Animal Species

Compound	Molecular weight	Percent dose in bile[a]					
		Rat	Guinea pig	Rabbit	Dog	Cat	Hen
Aniline	93	5.7	5.6	2.6	0.3	1.6	2.7
Benzoic acid	122	1.2	1.7	0.7	0.8	1.2	0.5
4-Aminohippuric acid	194	1.4	6.7	3.0	3.4	0.7	0.5
4-Acetamidohippuric acid	236	1.3	0.4	1.5	3.5	0.9	0.4
Methylenedisalicylic acid	288	54.0	4.0	5.0	65.0	—	—
Succinylsulfathiazole	355	29.0	1.0	1.0	20.0	7.0	25.0
Stilboestrol glucuronide	445	95.0	20.0	32.0	65.0	77.0	93.0
Sulfadimethoxine N^1-glucuronide	487	43.0	12.0	10.0	43.0	—	—
Phenophthalein glucuronide	495	54.0	6.0	13.0	81.0	34.0	71.0
Dichloromethotrexate	523	80.0	—	38.0	80.0	—	—
Indocyanine green	775	60–82	—	94.0	97.0	—	—

[a] Three or six hours after ip or iv administration of a comparable dose.

Table 6.4 Occurrence of Common and Unusual Conjugation Reactions

Conjugating group	Common	Unusual
Carbohydrate	Glucuronic acid (animals)	N-Acetylglucosamine (rabbit)
	Glucose (insects and plants)	Ribose (rats and mice)
Amino acids	Glycine	Glutamine (insects and man)
	Glutathione	
	Methionine	Ornithine (birds)
		Arginine (ticks and spiders)
		Glycyltaurine and glycylglycine (cat)
		Serine (rabbit)
Acetyl	Acetyl group from acetyl-CoA	
Formyl		Formylation (dog and rat)
Sulfate	Sulfate group from PAPS	
Phosphate		Phosphate monoester formation (dog and insects)

glucuronic acid, glycine, glutamine, and sulfate conjugations, mercapturic acid synthesis, acetylation, methylation, and thiocyanate synthesis. In some species of birds and reptiles ornithine conjugation replaces that with glycine, and in plants, bacteria, and insects conjugation with glucose instead of glucuronic acid results in the formation of glucosides. In addition to these predominant reactions, certain other conjugative processes are found involving specific compounds in only a few species. These reactions include conjugation with phosphate, taurine, N-acetylglucosamine, ribose, glycyltaurine, serine, arginine, formic acid, and succinate. Certain species of spiders use glutamic acid and arginine for the conjugation of aromatic acids.

From the evolutionary standpoint, similarity might be expected between humans and other primate species, as opposed to the nonprimates. This phylogenic relationship is obvious from the data given in Table 6.5 involving the relative importance of glycine and glutamine conjugation of arylacetic acids. The conjugating agent in man is exclusively glutamine, and the same is essentially true with Old World monkeys. New World monkeys, however, employ both the glycine and glutamine pathways. Most nonprimates and lower primates selectively carry out glycine conjugation. A similar evolutionary trend is also observed in the N^1-glucuronidation of sulfadimethoxine and in the aromatization of quinic acid; both reactions occur extensively in man and their importance decreases as one goes down the evolutionary scale. When the relative importance of metabolic pathways is considered, one of the simplest cases of an enzyme-related species difference in the disposition of a substrate, under-

Table 6.5   Conjugation of Arylacetic Acids in Various Species

Compound	Class	No. of species tested	Percent dose excreted in 24 hr as conjugated	
			Glutamine	Glycine
Phenylacetic acid	Man	—	92–94	0
	Old World monkeys	8	30–90	0.1–1.0
	New World monkeys	3	64–80	1–10
	Lemurs	2	0	80–87
	Nonprimates	10	0	80–100
Indolylacetic acid	Man	—	10–21	0
	Old World monkeys	3	32–53	0
	New World monkeys	3	19–41	7–26
	Lemurs	2	0	14–49
	Nonprimates	8	0	25–70
p-Chlorophenylacetic acid	Man		92	0
	Rhesus monkey		45	0.4
	Capuchin monkey		36	1.4
	Rat		0	97
p-Nitrophenylacetic acid	Man		0	0
	Rhesus monkey		0	0
	Rat		0	68

Source: Williams, Biochem. Soc. Trans. 2 (1974), 359.

going only one conjugative reaction, is the acetylation of 4-aminohippuric acid. In the rat, guinea pig, and rabbit the major biliary metabolite is 4-acetamidohippuric acid; the cat excretes nearly equal amounts of free acid and its acetyl derivative; and the hen excretes mainly the unchanged compound. In the dog 4-aminohippuric acid is also passed into the bile unchanged since this species is unable to acetylate aromatic amino groups.

A xenobiotic undergoing the same conjugation reaction but at different sites offers the opportunity for regioselectivity. The involvement of two similar but different enzymes is strongly suggested and must be considered when evaluating interspecies differences. This case can be illustrated by sulfanilamide disposition. Two sites on the molecule are available for acetylation, yielding the N^1- and N^4-monoacetyl and the N^1,N^4-diacetyl derivatives:

Sulfanilamide

Sulfanilamidopyrimidine

The extent to which these products are formed varies from species to species. Thus, all three acetylated products are produced by most animal species tested but in different proportions. Acetylation in the dog proceeds exclusively at the N^1 position, while the rhesus monkey displays a greater preference for the N^4 position. Excretion of this drug in humans resembles that observed in the rat, mouse, or pigeon. Biliary excretion of aniline presents another good example of this type. The main metabolites in the bile of the rat, guinea pig, rabbit, and hen are 4-aminophenol and its glucuronide, and small amounts of the 2-isomer and its glucuronide, while cat bile contains only 2-aminophenol. The last mentioned species difference is not surprising since *ortho*-hydroxylation of aniline is higher in the cat than *para*-hydroxylation, and glucuronide conjugation appears to be at a low level.

The relative importance of various conjugation mechanisms in different animal species can also be seen from the urinary excretion of methoxy derivatives of 6-sulfanilamidopyrimidine. Biotransformation of these compounds yields N^4-acetyl, N^1-glucuronide, and N^4-sulfate conjugates in different proportions in various species. N^4-Acetylation is the predominant metabolic pathway in the rabbit except for the 2,5-dimethoxy analog, which is excreted essentially unchanged. The same is true in the rat, except that the amount of excreted free drug is greater than in the rabbit. In the monkey, acetylation is extensive with the 4- and/or 5-methoxy analogs, while glucuronidation predominates with the 2,4-dimethoxy derivative. The metabolic pattern in man is comparable to that in the monkey, although less N^4-acetylation and greater excretion of unchanged 4,5-demethoxy derivative occurs.

Defective operation of phase II reactions usually causes a striking species difference in the disposition pattern of a xenobiotic. The origin of such species variations is usually either the absence or a low level of the enzyme(s) in question and/or its obligatory cofactors.

Glucuronide synthesis is one of the most common detoxication mechanisms is most mammalian species. However, the cat and closely related species have a defective glucuronide-forming system. Although cats form little or no glucuronide from o-aminophenol, phenol, p-nitrophenol, 2-amino-4-nitrophenol, 1- or 2-naphthol, and morphine, they readily form glucuronides from phenolphthalein, bilirubin, thyroxine and certain steroids. Recently, based on substrate specificity, polymorphism of UDP glucuronyl-transferase has been demonstrated in rat and guinea pig liver preparations. Defective glucuronidation of certain substrates in the cat is therefore probably related to the absence of the appropriate transferase rather than that of the active intermediate, UDP glucuronic acid, which is known to occur in cat liver in normal concentrations, or to the presence of an endogenous inhibitor. Insects are incapable of synthesizing glucuronide conjugates. This may be due to the lack of UDP glucuronyltransferase, UDPGA, or UDP glucose dehydrogenase, which converts UDP glucose into UDPGA.

Similarly, the failure to observe acetylation of aromatic amines and hydrazines in dogs can be explained on the basis of enzyme multiplicity. Dog liver apparently does not possess all of the N-acetyltransferases. This is evidenced by the dog's ability to acetylate aliphatic amino groups and the α-amino group of amino acids as well as the sulfonamide group of sulfanilamide. The fox, on the other hand, cannot acetylate sulfanilamide. In addition to the lack of a specific transferase, the presence of endogenous inhibitors may also contribute to the defective operation of this mechanism in the dog and the fox.

Studies on the metabolic fate of phenol in several species have indicated that four urinary products are excreted (Figure 6.2). Although extensive phenol metabolism takes place in most species, the relative proportion of each metabolite produced varies from species to species. In contrast to the cat, which selectively forms sulfate conjugates, the pig excretes phenol exclusively as the glucuronide. However, this defect in sulfate conjugation in the pig is restricted to only a few substrates and may be due to the lack of a specific phenyl sulfotransferase since the formation of substantial amounts of the sulfate conjugate of 1-naphthol clearly indicates the occurrence of other forms of sulfotransferase.

Certain peculiar mechanisms, involving conjugation with sugar derivatives and amino acids, have been uncovered during comparative investigations that are not only restricted to certain species but also to a limited number of chemicals. This may, however, be a reflection of inadequate data, and the possibility exists that future investigations may demonstrate a wider distribution.

A few species of birds and reptiles employ ornithine for the conjugation of aromatic acids rather than glycine, as in mammals. For example, the turkey, goose, duck, and hen excrete ornithuric acid as the major metabolite of benzoic acid, whereas pigeons and doves excrete it exclusively as hippuric acid. Similarly, the hen produces primarily diphenylacetylornithine from phenylacetic acid with only a little phenylaceturic acid, whereas in the pigeon the latter is the major metabolite. In addition, the pigeon also produces small amounts of

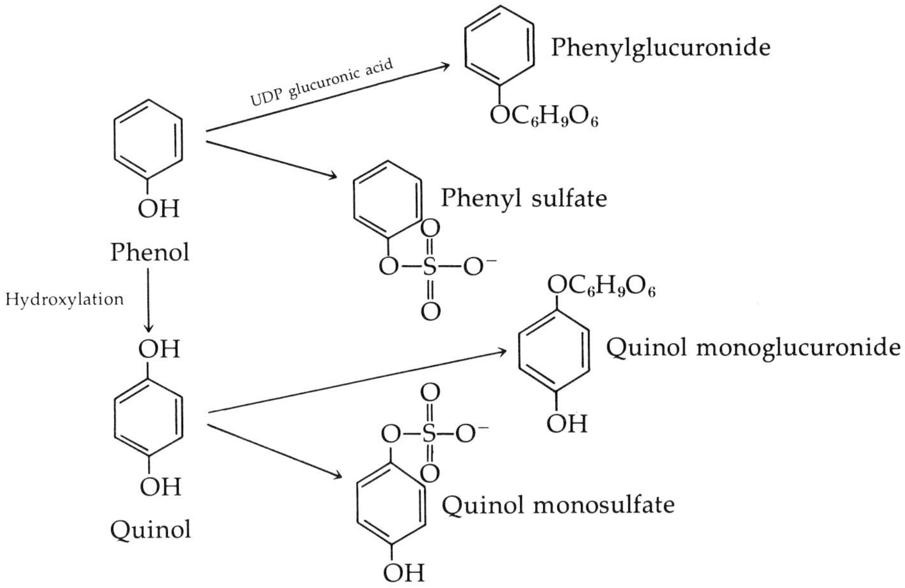

Figure 6.2 represented by the chemical scheme showing Phenol being converted via UDP glucuronic acid to Phenylglucuronide ($OC_6H_9O_6$), to Phenyl sulfate, and via Hydroxylation to Quinol, which forms Quinol monoglucuronide ($OC_6H_9O_6$) and Quinol monosulfate.

| Species | Percent of 24-hr excretion as | | | |
| | Glucuronide | | Sulfate | |
	Phenol	Quinol	Phenol	Quinol
Pig	100	0	0	0
Indian fruit bat	90	0	10	0
Rhesus monkey	35	0	65	0
Cat	0	0	87	13
Human	23	7	71	0
Squirrel monkey	70	19	10	0
Rat tail monkey	65	21	14	0
Guinea pig	78	5	17	0
Hamster	50	25	25	0
Rat	25	7	68	0
Ferret	41	0	32	28
Rabbit	46	0	45	9
Gerbil	15	0	69	15

Figure 6.2 Species variation in the metabolic conversion of phenol in vivo.

phenylacetyltaurine. Taurine conjugation with bile acids, phenylacetic acid, and indolylacetic acid seems to be a minor process in most species, but in the pigeon and ferret it occurs extensively. Other infrequently reported conjugations include serine conjugation of xanthurenic acid in rats, excretion of quinaldic acid as quinaldylglycyltaurine and quinaldylglycylglycine in the urine of the cat but not of the rat or rabbit, phosphate conjugation of 2-naphthylamine in the dog but not in the rat or rabbit, and conversion of furfural to furylacrylic acid in the dog and rabbit but not in the rat, hen, or human.

The dog and human but not the guinea pig, hamster, rabbit, or rat excrete the carcinogen 2-naphthyl hydroxylamine as a metabolite of 2-naphthylamine, which, as a result, has carcinogenic activity in the bladder of humans and dogs. Similarly, man is unique in forming an unusual metabolite, the azoxybenzene, from 2-(methoxyethoxy)-5-acetaminoacetophenone. This metabolite is not found in the dog or rat. The formation of O-benzyl benzaldozine from benzyl carbethoxyhydroxamate occurs in the human and rat but not in the monkey, cat, or guinea pig.

Reversibility of reactions. The absolute level of a conjugate formed in vivo depends not only upon the components of the synthetic reaction but also on the efficiency of the conjugate-splitting enzymes. Enzyme pairs such as β-glucuronidase–glucuronyl transferase or arylsulfatase-sulfotransferase, acting in a concerted fashion, may affect the biotransformation of xenobiotics in vivo. In a few cases, differences in the capacity to reverse a particular reaction contribute to variations between species. In the metabolism of imipramine, for example, the methylation of desmethylimipramine back to the parent drug is catalyzed by an enzyme present in the lungs of rabbits, but not in those of rats. Acetylation of isoniazid and sulfamethazine offers another good example. The rates of these reactions in the squirrel monkey were found to be only one-half to one-third of those observed in the rhesus monkey; this observation explained by the fact that the squirrel monkey possesses a competing deacetylation mechanism apparently absent in the rhesus monkey.

Endogenous inhibitors. The presence of endogenous inhibitors has been invoked to explain the absence of, or extremely low, xenobiotic-metabolizing activity in preparations of placenta of the tissues of fetal and new born animals, as well as those from mature animals of some species. Thus, the inability of lobster hepatopancreas microsomes to metabolize parathion and the failure of chicken liver microsomes to activate carbon tetrachloride may be related to endogenous inhibitors; unfortunately, however no attempts have been made to isolate and characterize them.

Several studies have established a close inverse relationship between lipid peroxidation and the xenobiotic-metabolizing ability of liver microsomes of laboratory animals. There is a marked species difference in lipid peroxidation, the relative rates being rat < guinea pig < mouse < rabbit. Recently, an inhibitor of this reaction was isolated from rat liver cytosol and characterized, but no quantitative data are available on its occurrence in other species.

Physiological levels of catecholamines and related compounds have been demonstrated to be potent inhibitors of house fly glutathione S-transferase. Another example of endogenous inhibitors involves the O-demethylation of isomeric methoxyoxindoles. This reaction is catalyzed by liver microsomes of the rabbit but not those of the rat or guinea pig; these observations are explained by the presence of heat-labile inhibitor(s) in liver extracts of the rat and guinea pig that are not found in liver extracts of the rabbit.

Gut flora. The gastrointestinal tract of animals harbors numerous species of microorganism. Over 100 species and subspecies of microbes are typically found in humans, while other mammals contain similarly diverse flora. Although variations in the gut flora in different animal species are well known, their importance in xenobiotic disposition is not fully established. Biliary excretion of conjugated xenobiotics is the major mechanism of disposition in human and other animals. The gut possesses several conjugate-hydrolyzing enzymes such as β-glucuronidase, arylsulfatase, glutathionase, etc., and their origin appears to be, at least in part, microbial. In addition, many reductive, hydrolytic, and other reactions are performed by these microorganisms, and some of the enzymes are reported to be inducible. Following an oral dose of quinic acid to man or Old World monkeys, extensive conversion to benzoic acid and its subsequent excretion as hippuric acid occurs. In contrast, intraperitoneally injected quinic acid is excreted unchanged by the rhesus monkey. Furthermore, suppression of the gut flora by neomycin pretreatment depresses the excretion of hippuric acid from orally administered quinic acid. Aromatization of quinic acid to benzoic acid, a process dependent upon gut flora, displays remarkable interspecies differences. This reaction occurs extensively in man and the Old World monkeys but does not occur to an appreciable extent in primates lower on the evolutionary scale than the Old World monkeys or in nonprimate species.

The insecticide mirex is extremely refractory to metabolism by animals and recent evidence indicates that the only known metabolite may, in fact, be produced by the gut flora.

6.2.3. In Vitro Metabolism and Biochemical Considerations

Numerous variables simultaneously modulate the in vivo metabolism of xenobiotics, and therefore their relative importance cannot easily be studied. This problem is alleviated to some extent by in vitro studies of the underlying enzymatic mechanisms responsible for qualitative and quantitative species differences. Quantitative differences may be directly related to the absolute amount of active enzyme present and the affinity and specificity of the enzyme toward the substrate in question. Since many other factors alter enzymatic rates in vitro great caution must be excercised in interpreting data in terms of species variation.

6.2.3a. Phase I Reactions

Microsomes represent a mixture of fragments originating from smooth (SER) and rough (RER) endoplasmic reticulum. Species differences exist in the distribution of these microsomal subfractions as well as in the capacity of the enzymes associated with them. In monkey, rat, and guinea pig liver microsomes the SER/RER ratio for specific enzyme activities varies between 1.5 and 3.0, while in the rabbit, ratios as high as 5 can be observed. The mouse exhibits a fairly even distribution. In addition to these differences, variations in the chemical composition of the membranes have also been reported.

Species variation in the oxidation of xenobiotics, in general, is quantitative (Table 6.6), while qualitative differences, such as the total lack of parathion

Table 6.6 Species Variation in Microsomal Oxidation of Xenobiotics In Vitro

Substrate oxidation	Rabbit	Rat	Mouse	Guinea pig	Hamster	Chicken	Trout	Frog
Coumarine 7-hydroxylase (nmole/mg/hr)	0.86	0.00	0.00	0.45	—	—	—	—
Biphenyl 4-hydroxylase (nmoles/mg/min)	3.00	1.50	5.70	1.40	3.80	1.70	0.22	1.15
Biphenyl 2-hydroxylase (nmoles/mg/min)	0.00	0.00	2.20	0.00	1.80	0.00	0.00	0.15
2-Methoxybiphenyl demethylase (nmoles/mg liver/hr)	5.20	1.80	3.40	2.20	2.30	2.00	0.60	0.40
4-Methoxybiphenyl demethylase (nmoles/mg liver/hr)	8.00	3.00	3.20	2.30	2.30	1.70	0.40	0.90
p-Nitroanisole O-demethylase (nmoles/mg/15 min)	32.00	4.93	20.33	—	—	11.33	—	—
2-Ethoxybiphenyl deethylase (nmoles/mg liver/hr)	5.30	1.60	1.40	2.10	2.50	1.70	0.60	0.40
4-Ethoxybiphenyl deethylase (nmoles/mg liver/hr)	7.80	2.80	1.80	2.30	1.80	1.50	0.40	0.90
Ethylmorphine N-demethylase (nmoles/mg/min)	4.00	11.60	13.20	5.40	—	—	—	—
Aldrin epoxidase (nmoles/mg/min)	0.34	0.45	3.35	—	—	0.46	0.006	—
Parathion desulfurase (nmoles/mg/min)	2.11	4.19	5.23	8.92	7.75	—	—	—

oxidation by lobster hepatopancreas microsomes, are seldom observed. Although the amount of cytochrome P-450 or the activity of NADPH–cytochrome c/P-450 reductase (Table 6.7) seem to be related to the oxidation of certain substrates, this explanation is not always satisfactory. Several steps in the mixed-function oxidation of xenobiotics have been believed to be rate limiting but later dismissed in light of new evidence. It now appears that the cleavage of the C-H bond, one of the final steps, may indeed be the rate-limiting step in substrate oxidation. If this is true, qualitative differences in the nature of the forms of cytochrome P-450 with which the oxidizable substrate interacts appear to provide the most logical explanation for species variation.

Several lines of evidence indicate that there are multiple forms of microsomal cytochrome P-450 in each species, and that these forms differ from one species to another. An indirect reflection of this difference is the observation that the optimal temperature for in vitro oxidation of foreign compounds by hepatic microsomes from warm-blooded species (e.g., mammals) is around 37°C, whereas the enzymes from cold-blooded species (e.g., fishes) perform best at much lower temperatures, and the enzymes from birds are most active at 40–43°C.

Inhibitors provide further indirect evidence of cytochrome P-450 multiplicity in that they are more effective in some animal species than in others and they may exert their effects by different mechanisms in the same species depending upon the substrate. Thus, SKF-525A exhibits competitive inhibition of aminopyrine N-demethylation and hexobarbital hydroxylation but inhibits

Table 6.7 Species Variation in the Components of Microsomal Electron Transport Pathways

Species	Cytochrome P-450 (ΔA/mg protein)	NADPH-cytochrome c reductase (ΔA/5 min/mg protein)	NADPH oxidase (ΔA/5 min/mg protein)
Mouse	0.09	1.44	0.16
Rat	0.10	1.56	0.14
Rabbit	0.12	1.85	0.14
Guinea pig	0.10	—	—
Pig	0.06	3.32	0.20
Sheep	0.08	0.66	0.03
Chicken	0.02	2.03	0.11
Bobwhite quail	0.03	4.03	0.38
Japanese quail	0.04	3.32	0.23
Turkey	0.03	1.64	0.10
Large mouth bass	0.02	—	—
Drosophila	0.01	0.99	0.16
Tobacco hornworm	0.01	3.69	0.09
Mosquito	—	0.28	0.14
Housefly, CSMA	0.03	2.75	0.22
Housefly, Fc	0.03	3.43	0.35

Source: Kulkarni et al., Comp. Biochem. Physiol. 54B (1976), 509.

aniline hydroxylation by rat hepatic microsomes noncompetitively. In contrast to this, it displays noncompetitive inhibition of all these reactions with rabbit liver enzymes and quasi-competitive inhibition of the first two reactions with mouse liver preparations.

More direct evidence in support of the above contention includes both qualitative and quantitative species-related differences in the substrate difference spectrum of microsomal cytochrome P-450. Difference spectra are presumed to be a direct reflection of enzyme–ligand complex formation. If the cytochromes P-450 of all animals were alike, similarity in spectral size and the ratio of type II/type I binding would be expected. However, a wide species variation is evident (Table 6.8). Thus, in a closely related group of chlorinated hydrocarbons, DDT, dicofol, and DDD, DDT gives the smallest type I spectrum in all species tested, dicofol exhibits the largest type I difference spectrum with microsomes from sheep, rats, and Fc houseflies, and DDD displays the largest spectral response with microsomes from mice and rabbits. It should be noted, however, that several studies have failed to establish any relationship between spectral magnitude and substrate oxidation rate. Species-dependent qualitative differences in the spectral response of a xenobiotic can be illustrated with menazon. This organophosphorus insecticide causes no detectable difference spectrum formation in microsomes from CSMA houseflies but exhibits a type I difference spectrum in those from Fc houseflies, a type II in mouse liver microsomes, and a mixture of types I and II in rat, rabbit, and sheep liver microsomes. Other compounds, such as allethrin, bioallethrin, and carbaryl, display similar species-dependent variations.

Table 6.8 Spectral Interactions of Insecticides with Cytochrome P-450 of Mammalian and Insect Microsomes

	Sheep		Rabbit		Rat		Mouse		Housefly, Fc		Housefly, CSMA	
Insecticide	Type	Size	Type	Size	Type	Size	Type	Size	Type	Size	Type	Size
Nicotine	II	0.434	II	0.540	II	0.505	II	0.522	II	0.412	II	0.255
Rotenone	a	0.094	a	0.130	ND	—	ND	—	ND	—	ND	—
Allethrin	I	0.270	I	0.160	I	0.362	I	0.278	b	0.300	b	0.286
p,p'-DDT	I	0.166	I	0.076	I	0.103	I	0.112	I	0.120	ND	—
TDE	I	0.283	I	0.219	I	0.310	I	0.330	I	0.100	ND	—
Kelthane	I	0.314	I	0.057	I	0.345	I	0.295	I	0.154	ND	—
Carbaryl	I	0.174	c	0.088	I	0.270	I	0.200	I	0.133	ND	—
Baygon	I	0.362	I	0.104	I	0.105	I	0.215	I	0.136	ND	—
Zectran	I	0.261	I	0.171	I	0.200	I	0.103	I	0.115	ND	—
Menazon	d	—	d	—	d	—	II	0.101	I	0.148	ND	—
Zinophos	II	0.377	II	0.321	II	0.242	II	0.312	II	0.321	II	0.166
Malathion	I	0.269	I	0.093	I	0.263	I	0.150	I	0.228	ND	—

Source: Kulkarni et al., J. Agric. Food Chem. 23 (1975), 177. Reprinted with permission from the Journal of Agricultural and Food Chemistry. © 1975 by the American Chemical Society.

Symbols: a, absorption minimum at 395 nm and maximum at 415 nm in sheep or at 417 in rabbit; b, absorption minimum at 445–447 nm and maximum 415–418 nm; c, ΔA calculated as difference in A at 407 and 427 nm; d, see text for details; ND, no detectable spectrum formation.

Immunochemical studies, sodium dodecyl sulfate–polyacrylamide gel electrophoresis of microsomes, subfractionation of microsomes on sucrose density gradients, susceptibility to trypsinolysis and purification following solubilization, etc., all support the multiplicity of microsomal cytochrome P-450. However, due to differences in methodology and different enzyme sources, numerical comparisons are precluded, and the relationship to species-dependent differences is not yet clearly established.

Reductive reactions, like oxidations, are carried out by enzyme preparations of different species at different rates. Microsomes from mammalian liver are as much as 18 times higher in azoreductase activity and more than 20 times higher in nitroreductase activity than those from fish liver. Although relatively inactive in nitroreductase, fish can reduce the nitro group of parathion, suggesting multiple forms of reductase enzymes.

Enzymatic hydration of epoxides is catalyzed by epoxide hydrase, an enzyme that is chiefly associated with microsomes and is involved in both detoxication and intoxication reactions. With styrene oxide as a substrate, the relative activity in several animal species is rhesus monkey > human = guinea pig > rabbit > rat > mouse. Studies on insecticidal cyclodiene enantiomers indicate that rat liver and house fly microsomes possess low hydrase activity toward these substrates, whereas pig and rabbit liver microsomes are more active.

Blood and various organs of man and other animals contain esterases capable of acetylsalicylic acid hydrolysis. A comparative study has shown that the liver possesses the highest activity in all animal species studied except the guinea pig in which activity in the kidney is more than twice that in the liver. Human liver is least active, while the enzyme in guinea pig liver is the most active. Mammalian serum contains an arylester hydrolase, called "A esterase," that catalyzes paraoxon hydrolysis to yield diethylphosphoric acid and p-nitrophenol. The enzyme activities in sera from nine mammalian species reveal remarkable differences. Rabbit serum possesses the highest A esterase activity and mouse serum has the lowest. Rabbit serum is approximately 35 times more active than human serum. The relatively low toxicity of some of the new synthetic pyrethroid insecticides appears to be related to the ability of mammals to hydrolyze their carboxyester linkages. Thus, mouse liver microsomes catalyzing (+)-transresmethrin hydrolysis are more than 30-fold more active than insect microsomal preparations. The relative rates of hydrolysis of this substrate in enzyme preparations from various species are mouse ≫ milkweed bug ≫ cockroach ≫ cabbage looper > housefly.

The metabolic detoxication of the organophosphorus insecticide dimethoate offers another interesting example. Its toxicity depends upon the rate at which it is hydrolyzed in vivo. This toxicant undergoes two main metabolic changes, one carried out by an esterase and the other by an amidase, both of which detoxify the compound as follows:

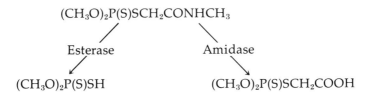

$$(CH_3O)_2P(S)SCH_2CONHCH_3$$

Esterase   Amidase

$$(CH_3O)_2P(S)SH \qquad (CH_3O)_2P(S)SCH_2COOH$$

Rat and mouse liver carry out both reactions, but only the amidase reaction occurs in sheep liver, while the guinea pig liver enzyme selectively deesterifies dimethoate. The detoxication ability of the livers of different animal species is as follows: rabbit > sheep > dog > rat > cattle > hen > guinea pig > mouse > pig; these rates are roughly inversely related to the toxicity of dimethoate to the various species. Insects degrade this compound much more slowly than mammals and hence are highly susceptible to dimethoate.

6.2.3b. Phase II Reactions

Hepatic microsomes of several animal species possess UDP glucuronyltransferase activity and, with p-nitrophenol as a substrate, a 12-fold difference in activity due to species variation is evident. The relative activity of untreated microsomes is guinea pig > rabbit > man > rat > beef > mouse. Phospholipase-A activates the enzyme 12–16-fold in the rat, rabbit, guinea pig, and mouse but only 3–4-fold in bovine and human liver microsomes, while activation parallels the treatment of microsomes with p-chloromercuribenzoate, with the exception of the rat. These results indicate that the amount of constraint on the activity of this enzyme is variable in different animal species.

Comparative study of the relative distribution of glutathione S-transferase in dialyzed liver cytosol from different animal species shows a wide variation in activity (Table 6.9). The activity of this family of enzymes is very low in the human adult and fetus. In general, both the mouse and guinea pig appear to be more efficient in this respect than other species. The remarkable ability of the guinea pig to form the initial conjugate contrasts with its inability to form mercapturic acids.

Table 6.9   Relative Distribution of Glutathione S-Transferases in Dialyzed liver Supernatant Fractions from Different Animals

Species	Glutathione S-transferase activity[a]				
	Alkyl	Aryl	Aralkyl	Epoxide	Alkene
Rat ($♀$)	1.00	1.00	1.00	1.00	1.00
Dog ($♀,♂$)	0.16	2.80	0.69	0.42	0.39
Guinea pig ($♂$)	0.50	2.46	3.14	1.06	0.93
Mouse ($♂$)	1.16	2.40	0.82	1.42	1.62
Rabbit ($♂$)	0.36	1.40	0.47	0.14	0.22
Ferret ($♂$)	0.11	1.00	0.13	0.38	0.52
Pigeon ($♂$)	3.56	0.80	1.43	0.47	0.36
Hamster ($♂$)	0.56	0.40	0.82	0.80	0.90
Human adult ($♀$)	0.26	0.08	0.21	0.19	0.13
Human fetus ($♂$)	0.23	0.00	0.30	0.23	0.12

Source: Reprinted from Chasseaud, Drug Metab. Rev. 2 (1973), 185 by courtesy of Marcel Dekker, Inc., N.Y.

[a] The substrate and the absolute enzyme activities (μmoles thiol lost per minute per gram liver) for the rat liver were as follows: alkyl, methyl iodide, 3.0; aryl, dichloronitrobenzene, 0.5; aralkyl, benzyl chloride, 2.3; epoxide, 2,3-epoxypropyl phenyl ether, 2.1; alkene, diethyl maleate, 7.5.

6.3. Selectivity

Selective toxic agents have been successfully developed to protect crops, animals of economic importance, and man from the vagaries of pests, parasites, and pathogens. Such selectivity is conferred primarily through distribution and comparative biochemistry.

Selectivity through differences in uptake permits the use of an agent toxic to both target and nontarget cells, provided that lethal concentrations accumulate only in target cells leaving nontarget cells unharmed. An example is the accumulation of tetracycline by bacteria, but not by mammalian cells, the result being drastic inhibition of protein synthesis in the bacteria, leading to death.

In most cases, however, selectivity is closely associated with differences in the metabolism of the target and nontarget organism. The highly selective antibacterial action of sulfonamide drugs is based on the fact that pathogenic bacteria cannot absorb folic acid or its derivatives from the surrounding medium but depend upon its biosynthesis from p-aminobenzoic acid, a process blocked by the drug. Humans, on the other hand, cannot synthesize folic acid but absorb it directly from food.

Schistosome worms are parasitic in man and their selective destruction by antimony is accounted for by the differential sensitivity of phosphofructokinase in the two species. The enzyme from schistosomes is more susceptible to inhibition by antimony than the mammalian enzyme. Similarly, selective inhibition of dihydrofolate reductase from the malarial parasite *Plasmodium berghei* is the basis for the action of antimalarial drugs. Acetylcholinesterase in the worm *Haemonchus contortus*, which parasitizes the gut of the sheep, is irreversibly inhibited by the organophosphorus compound haloxon. The sheep enzyme is only temporarily affected and rapidly recovers.

Sometimes both target and nontarget species metabolize a xenobiotic by the same pathways but differences in rates determine selectivity. Malathion, an extensively used selective insecticide, is activated metabolically to the cholinesterase inhibitor malaoxon. In addition to this activation reaction, several detoxicating reactions occur simultaneously. Thus, carboxylesterase hydrolyzes malathion to form the monoacid, phosphatases hydrolyze the P—O—C linkages to yield nontoxic products, and glutathione S-alkyltransferase converts malathion to desmethylmalation. All of these reactions occur both in insects and mammals. However, although activation by oxidative desulfuration is rapid in both insects and mammals, hydrolysis is rapid in mammals but slow in insects. Thus, the accumulation of malaoxon in insects but not in mammals results in selective toxicity. Similarly, in the case of dimethoate, the mammalian carboxyamidases readily hydrolyze the amide linkage, but insects are almost unable to do this. High vertebrate efficiency in detoxication has helped greatly in the development of selective organophosphorus compounds. Thus, haloxon, trichlorfon, and dichlorvos may be given orally to cattle, sheep, pigs, horses, and poultry for the control of various parasitic worms and obnoxious insects.

A few examples are also available in which the lack of a specific enzyme in some cells in the human body has enabled the development of a therapeutic agent. For example, guanase is absent from the cells of certain cancers but abundant in healthy tissue; as a result, 8-azaguanine can be used therapeutically.

The use of unnatural analogs has also proved quite successful in the development of selective agents. In this case the target enzyme utilizes the analog in place of its normal substrate or coenzyme, thus preventing the normal function of the enzyme. The action of these compounds is usually reversed by the normal metabolite. Examples include the use of drugs such as azaserine, cytarabine, allopurinol, ephedrin, methyldopa, and salbutamol for the treatment of certain human diseases.

Distinct differences in cells with regard to the presence or absence of target structures or metabolic processes offer suitable opportunities for exploitation. Herbicides such as phenylureas, simazine, etc. block the Hill reaction in chloroplasts and thereby kill plants without harm to animals. The unique characteristics of bacterial cell walls make them vulnerable to antibiotics that prevent synthesis of new cell wall, causing lysis. Cuticular tanning is vital for insect survival, and therefore interference in this process selectively kills insects. The successful development of juvenile hormone mimics as insecticides is also based on the principle of exploiting unique metabolic pathways for selectivity.

6.4. Genetic Differences

Not all humans react alike to a given dose of a chemical agent, nor do experimental animals. This variation in individual response has long been a stumbling block to the assessment of the potency of drugs or toxicants. Just as the xenobiotic-metabolizing ability in different animal species seems to be related to evolutionary development and therefore to different genetic constitutions, different strains within a species may differ from one another in their ability to metabolize xenobiotics.

6.4.1. In Vivo Toxicity

The toxicity of several organic solvents has been found to vary in different strains of laboratory animals. For example, stocks of mice exposed to chloroform vapor during a laboratory accident showed different death rates in the males of different strains as follows: 75% in DBA_2, 51% in DBA_1, 32% in C_3H, and 10% in BALC. The males of six other strains survived the exposure.

Mouse strain C_3H is resistant to histamine. Thus, the LD_{50} is 1523 mg/kg in C_3H/Jax mice as compared to 230 in Swiss/ICR mice; i.e., the animals of the former strain are 6.6 times less susceptible to the effects of histamine. Striking strain differences in the toxicity of thiourea, a compound used in the treatment of hyperthyroidism, are seen in different strains of the Norway rat. Harvard and wild Norway rats were 11 and 335 times more resistant, respectively, than rats of the Hopkins strain.

Although iproniazid is nontoxic to mice of the Swiss, C57BL, and DBA/2 strains, AKR mice exhibit severe hepatic injury and high mortality. The rate of inactivation of isoniazid shows polymorphism. "Slow inactivators" are homozygous for a recessive gene; this is believed to lead to the lack of the hepatic enzyme acetyltransferase, which in normal homozygotes or heterozygotes (rapid inactivators) acetylates isoniazid as one step in the metabolism of this drug. This effect is also seen in man, the gene for slow inactivation showing marked differences in distribution between different human populations. It is very low in Eskimos and Japanese, but up to 80% of blacks and some European populations are either heterozygous or homozygous for the slow inactivation gene. Slow inactivators develop symptoms of hepatotoxicity and polyneuritis at the dosage necessary to maintain adequate blood levels in fast inactivators. Although a similar situation occurs in rabbits, it is interesting to note that in slow acetylating rabbits the level of blood p-aminobenzoic acid N-acetyltransferase associated with erythrocytes and lymphocytes averages approximately 2.5 times that in rapid acetylating rabbits. Thus, it is evident that in the rabbit isoniazid acetylation by the liver enzyme and acetylation of p-aminobenzoic acid by the blood enzyme are inversely related.

A study of 15 mouse strains for the development of fibrosarcosoma following injection of 1 mg methylcholanthrene revealed that in males tumor incidence varied from 91% in CHI and C_3H mice to 14% in the I strain. In females, the incidence was lower and the trend was apparently reversed in a few strains.

The development of strains resistant to insecticides is an extremely widespread phenomenon that is known to occur in over 200 species of insects and mites and resistance of up to several hundred-fold has been noted. The different biochemical and genetic factors involved have been extensively studied and well characterized (Chapter 19). Relatively few vertebrate species are known to have developed pesticide resistance. Susceptible and resistant strains of pine voles exhibit a 7.4-fold difference in endrin toxicity. Similarly, pine mice of a strain resistant to endrin were reported to be 12-fold more tolerant than a susceptible strain. Studies with the organophosphates Gophacide and chlorophacinone, on the other hand, showed that the toxicity was greater to animals resistant to endrin than to endrin–susceptible animals. Other examples include the occurrence of organochlorine insecticide–resistant and –susceptible strains of mosquito fish, and resistance to *Belladona* in certain rabbit strains.

6.4.2. Metabolite production

Strain variation in response to hexobarbital also depends upon its degradation rate. For example, male mice of the AL/N strain are long sleepers, and this trait is correlated with slow inactivation of the drug by these animals. The reverse is true in CFW/N mice, which have a short sleeping time due to rapid hexobarbital oxidation. This close relationship is further evidenced by the fact that the level of brain hexobarbital at awakening is essentially the same in all strains. Similar strain differences have been reported for zoxazolamine paralysis in mice.

Data on benzo(a)pyrene hydroxylation show up to fivefold strain differences. Studies on the induction of aryl hydrocarbon hydroxylase by 3-methylcholanthrene have revealed several responsive and nonresponsive mouse strains, and it is now well established that the induction of this enzyme is controlled by a single gene. In the accepted nomenclature, Ah^b represents the allele for responsiveness, whereas Ah^d denotes the allele for nonresponsiveness. Although numerous monooxygenase reactions appear to be associated with the Ah locus, tumorigenesis initiated by 7,12-dimethylbenz(a)anthracene or benzo(a)pyrene, as well as the activity of a closely related microsomal enzyme, epoxide hydrase, were not.

Similar genetic studies on phase II reactions in mice are apparently lacking, although toxicity studies in vivo suggest that the differences do exist.

In rats, both age and sex seem to influence strain variation in xenobiotic metabolism. Male rats exhibit about twofold variation between strains in hexobarbital metabolism, whereas female rats may display up to sixfold variation, depending on their age. Whether the ability to metabolize hexobarbital is related to the metabolism of other substrates was tested in short and long sleepers of the same strain, and the data (Table 6.10) indicate a positive correlation, while the interstrain differences were maintained.

A well-known interstrain difference in phase II reactions is that of glucuronidation in Gunn rats. This is a mutant strain of Wistar rats that is characterized by a severe, genetically determined defect of bilirubin glucuronidation. Their ability to glucuronidate o-aminophenol or o-aminobenzoic acid is partially defective. This deficiency does not seem to be related to an inability to form UDPGA or to the presence of inhibitors, but to the lack of a specific UDP glucuronyltransferase. It has been demonstrated that Gunn rats can conjugate aniline by N-glucuronidation and can form the O-glucuronide of p-nitrophenol. This supports the growing evidence in favor of the multiplicity of UDP glucuronyltransferases.

In contrast to the 2–3-fold variation in xenobiotic biotransformation rates in rats and mice, rabbit strains may exhibit up to 20-fold variation (Table 6.11). This is particularly true of hexobarbital, amphetamine, and aminopyrine metabolism. Relatively smaller differences between strains occur with chlorpromazine metabolism. Wild rabbits and California rabbits display the greatest differences from other rabbit strains in hepatic drug metabolism.

Extensive studies have been carried out on the biochemical genetics of house fly strains with respect to insecticide toxicity and metabolism. Marked strain-specific differences in microsomal cytochrome P-450 and its relationship to the higher oxidase activity observed in resistant strains of the house fly have been reported (Chapter 19).

6.4.3. Enzyme Differences

The nature and amount of microsomal cytochrome P-450 have not been extensively studied in different strains of vertebrates. The only thorough investigations, those of the Ah locus, which controls aryl hydrocarbon hydroxylase induction, have shown that, in addition to quantitative differences in the amount

Table 6.10 Strain Variation in In Vitro Drug Metabolism in the Rat

Rat strain	Hexobarbital sleeping time (min)	Substrate metabolized (nmoles/mg protein)			
		Hexobarbital	o-Nitroanisole	Aminopyrine	Acetanilide
Long-Evans	50	31.6	9.1	2.2	8.5
	26	41.5	11.1	3.6	10.0
Sprague	55	30.0	6.6	1.1	8.8
Dawley	29	42.9	8.4	2.1	12.4
Buffalo	65	24.9	7.5	1.1	5.8
	32	36.4	8.9	2.0	7.4
Fischer	43	41.4	10.4	2.0	12.8
	19	47.9	12.2	2.9	16.6
Wistar	56	35.2	8.2	1.8	11.4
	30	44.6	10.2	3.0	15.4

Source: Mitoma et al., Proc. Soc. Exp. Biol. Med. 125 (1967), 284.

Table 6.11   Drug Metabolism by Hepatic Enzymes of Various Rabbit Strains

Substrate	Activity (nmoles substrate metabolized/mg protein/hr) in indicated rabbit strain					
	Dutch	English	Jack	Cali- fornia	New Zealand	Cotton- tail
Hexobarbital	141	173	220	248	254	19
Aniline	35	129	121	64	95	72
l-Amphetamine	154	87	102	55	82	8
p-Nitrobenzoic acid	89	67	92	22	122	50
Zoxazolamine	155	153	71	200	162	139
Chlorpromazine	152	139	100	159	143	147
Codeine	148	85	79	232	84	161
3,4-Benzpyrene	24	35	9	48	30	51
Aminopyrine	73	221	—	122	78	15

Source: Crom et al., Proc. Soc. Exp Biol. Med. 118 (1965), 872.

of cytochrome P-450 in the hepatic microsomes from different strains of mice, inducibility is associated with newly formed cytochrome P-450 (P-448).

The major differences in microsomal cytochrome P-450 between insecticide-resistant and -susceptible strains of the housefly are given in Table 6.12. A comparison of strains based on the size and peak location of the carbon monoxide, type I, type II, type III, n-octylamine, and ethyl isocyanide difference spectra reveal several points that, taken together, provide strong evidence for both qualitative and quantitative differences between strains. Ligand interaction of more than 100 other xenobiotics with cytochrome P-450 from resistant and susceptible house fly strains have been reported and lend strong support to the results given in Table 6.12.

Based on the data from crosses of house flies of susceptible strains (with visible mutant markers) with those of resistant strains, it is apparent that at least four genes, three on chromosome II and one on chrosome V, are required to explain the spectral variants alone. Moreover, the gene on chromosome V required for type I binding appears to be similar to the gene for the same trait on chromosome II in another strain, suggesting that translocation from chromosomes II to V may have occurred. Chromosomes II and V have long been associated with resistance to insecticides in the house fly (Chapter 19).

Table 6.12   Spectral Characteristics of Microsomal Cytochrome P-450 in Insecticide-Resistant and -Susceptible Strains of the Housefly, *Musca domestica*

Difference spectrum	Susceptible	Resistant
CO spectrum (λ_{max}, nm)	451–452	448–449
Relative P-450 level (CO spectrum)	100	150–200
Formation of type I difference spectrum	Absent	Present
Type II n-octylamine difference spectrum	Double trough	Single trough
Relative magnitude of type III ethyl iso-cyanide 455-nm peak	100	60–70

6.5. General Conclusions

Although differences in the ability to metabolize xenobiotics are well known at all taxonomic levels, a consistent rationalization of the overall findings, either in terms of known evolutionary relationships or in terms of the genetics of individual species, is not yet possible. It is clear, however, that the importance of comparative toxicology to the development of selective biocides and to a proper understanding of the environmental role of xenobiotics makes further studies imperative.

Although it is true that a man is neither a mouse nor any other experimental animal, the skilled use of comparative toxicology may reduce human risks and keep to an absolute minimum the necessity to carry out experiments on man.

Suggested Reading

Albert, W. Selective Toxicity: The Physico-chemical Basis of Therapy. London: Chapman and Hall, 1973.

Baker, S. B., Tripod, J., Jacob, J. (Eds.). The problem of species difference and statistics in toxicology. In Proceedings of the European Society for the Study of Drug Toxicity, XI. Amsterdam: Excerpta Medica 1970.

Elliott, R. W. Genetics of drug resistance. In Mihich, E. (Ed.). Drug Resistance and Selectivity: Biochemical and Cellular Basis. New York: Academic Press, 1973, p. 41.

Hodgson, E. Comparative toxicology: Cytochrome P-450 and mixed function oxidase activity in target and non-target organisms. Essays Toxicol. 7 (1976), 73.

Hucker, H. B. Species differences in drug metabolism. Ann. Rev. Pharmacol. 10 (1970), 99.

Nebert D. W., Felton, J. S. Importance of genetic factors influencing the metabolism of foreign compounds. Fed. Proc. 35 (1976), 1133.

Schwartz, H. S., Mihich, E. Species and tissue differences in drug selectivity. In Mihich, E. (Ed.). Drug Resistance and Selectivity: Biochemical and Cellular Basis. New York: Academic Press, 1973, pp. 413–452.

Smith, R. V. Metabolism of drugs and other foreign compounds by intestinal microorganisms. World Rev. Nutr. Diet. 29 (1978), 60.

Williams, R. T. Interspecies variations in the metabolism of xenobiotics. Biochem. Soc. Trans. 2(1974), 359.

Walter C. Dauterman

7

Physiological Factors Affecting Metabolism of Xenobiotics

7.1. Introduction

A foreign compound is usually metabolized by several different pathways involving phase I and II reactions, giving rise to a variety of different metabolites. The rate at which each reaction proceeds and its relative importance may be affected by a variety of factors resulting in changes in the pattern of metabolism as well as differences in toxicity. Genetic and environmental factors and the physiological state of the organism may affect the metabolism of xenobiotics. In this chapter the physiological factors will be discussed.

7.2. Age and Development

At birth there is a marked increase in the activity of many enzymes located in mammalian liver. Previously, the mother's metabolic enzymes have handled the detoxication and metabolism of foreign compounds for both mother and fetus. The increase in enzyme activity is usually initiated by birth of the animal. Premature delivery or prolongation of the gestation period has no effect on the time of development of certain enzyme levels.

The developmental aspects of the hepatic monooxygenase system have been studied extensively. The capacity of hepatic tissues to catalyze the xenobiotic monooxygenase reaction appears to be extremely low or absent in the late second trimester or third trimester and to increase after birth. No striking differences in hepatic drug metabolism are obvious between immature males and females. This general trend has been observed in such species as the mouse, rat, rabbit, hamster, guinea pig, opossum, swine, and ferret and is shown schematically in Figure 7.1. The general similarities rather than the differences are shown in this figure. The specific developmental patterns for each animal may vary according to the substrate, strain, and sex, as well as the technique used in the preparation of the subcellular fractions.

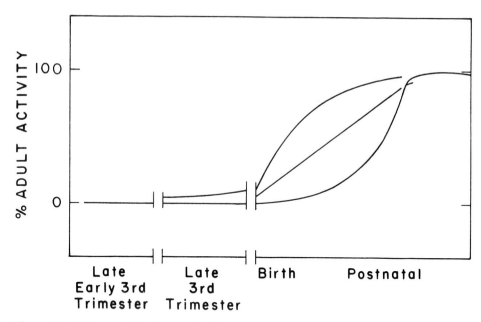

Figure 7.1   Pattern of development of monoxygenase system in nonprimate mammalian liver.

The various components of the hepatic monooxygenase system (cytochrome P-450, NADPH–cytochrome P-450 reductase, NADPH–cytochrome c reductase, NADPH, etc.) have varying developmental sequences. β-Glucuronidase activity (deglucuronidation) is higher than glucuronidation during prenatal development and the converse is found in the adult.

Two days after birth, NADPH reaches adult levels in the rat, whereas cytochrome P-450 approaches maximum activity in about 30 days. In the rabbit and swine the postnatal sequence of development of cytochrome P-450 and the activity of NADPH–cytochrome P-450 reductase parallel each other. However, in the rat and ferret the maturation of cytochrome P-450 reductase lags behind the increased development of cytochrome P-450. Biphenyl 4-hydroxylation parallels NADPH–cytochrome c reductase in the ferret and reaches a maximum 7–14 days after birth. Ethylmorphorine N-demethylase, aniline hydroxylase, and biphenyl 2-hydroxylase reach maximum activities 56 days after birth and parallel the cytochrome P-450. Epoxide hydrase activity is barely detectable in hepatic tissue from fetuses and 1-day-old neonate rats. However, enzyme activity increases rapidly to adult levels within 25 days.

A number of phase II reactions are also age dependent. Glucuronidation of many substrates is low or undetectable in fetal mammalian tissue preparations but increase with age, reaching "adult" activity just before birth. The rate of development is dependent upon the species, tissue, and substrate. The inability of newborns of most mammals, except the rat, to form glucuronides is associated with deficiencies in glucuronyltransferase activity and the coenzyme, UDPGA. Slow excretion of the glucuronide conjugate may also hinder its formation. The blood serum of newborn babies may contain pregnanediol, which is an inhibitor of glucuronide formation. This inhibition as well as low levels of the conjugating system are responsible for neonatal jaundice.

Other conjugation reactions that are impaired, or are low in the newborn, generally involve the utilization of amino acids or a polypeptide. Glycine conjugation is low because there is a lack of available glycine. Glycine reaches normal levels 30 days after birth in the rat and after 8 weeks in humans. Conjugation with reduced glutathione is also impaired in fetal and neonatal guinea pigs and is associated with the limited amount of available glutathione. With perinatal rats, glutathione S-transferase activity in serum is barely detectable but increases rapidly until approximately 35 days of age, after which the increase is slower until adult levels are obtained (Figure 7.2). The developmental pattern reported for serum is identical to that found in rat liver. Both the amount of reduced glutathione and the amount of glutathione S-transferase activity also increase with time during the development of the housefly from egg to adult.

Nonspecific liver carboxylesterase has been found to be low in prenatal guinea pigs but to increase to adult levels 21 days after birth. Sulfate conjugation and acetylation appear to be fully functional in the fetus and at the same level of activity as in the adult. Therefore, it would appear that compounds that are normally conjugated in adults as glucuronides are probably conjugated in young animals as sulfates or acetyl derivatives.

The direct effect of old age on the metabolism of xenobiotics has not been extensively studied. In rats the monooxygenase system reaches a maximum 30 days after birth, and approximately 250 days later the activity starts to decline slowly. This decrease in activity may be associated with a decrease in sex hormones. Glucuronidation also decreases in old animals, whereas monoamine oxidase activity in rats increases during aging.

Figure 7.2 Developmental pattern of serum glutathione S-transferase activity in female rats.

SOURCE: *Mukhtar and Bend, Life Sciences 21 (1977), 1277.*

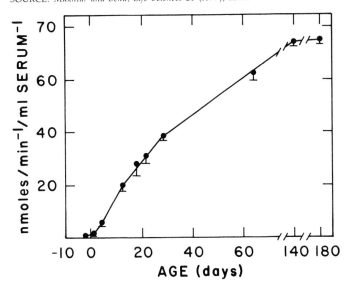

7.3. Sex Differences

The rate of metabolism of foreign compounds varies according to the sex of the organism. Sex differences in xenobiotic metabolism by mammalian liver appear with the onset of puberty and are usually maintained throughout the adult life of most mammals. Adult male rats metabolize many foreign compounds at higher rates than female rats, e.g., hydroxylation of hexobarbital, N-demethylation of aminopyrine, glucuronide formation of o-aminophenol, and formation of glutathione conjugates of aryl substrates. With other substrates such as aniline and zoxazolamine, no sex difference in aromatic hydroxylation is observed. When compared to rats, the sex difference in drug metabolism in vitro is less pronounced or absent in other species, including man. The differences between males and females with regard to metabolism by microsomal enzymes has been shown to be under the control of sex hormones. Enzyme activity is decreased by castration in the male, and administration of androgens to castrated animals increases the activity of the sex-dependent enzymes without increasing the sex-independent ones. Hexobarbital hydroxylation, aminopyrine N-demethylation, and pentobarbital oxidation are sex-dependent reactions, whereas aniline and zoxazolamine hydroxylations are considered to be sex independent. Castration or administration of androgens does not alter the metabolism of xenobiotics in rabbits or mice.

Sex differences in enzyme activity are also dependent upon which tissues are assayed. Hepatic microsomes from adult male guinea pigs are less active in p-nitrophenol conjugation than those from females (Table 7.1), whereas those from male rats were more active in o-nitrophenol conjugation. An equal amount of conjugating activity was found in microsomes isolated from the lungs, kidneys and small intestines of male and female guinea pigs.

Sex differences in toxicity between males and females of various species are well documented. Examples of xenobiotics that are more toxic to females than to males include O-ethyl O-p-nitrophenyl phenylphosphonothionate (EPN) (rat), dinitrophenol (cat), warfarin (rat), benzene (rabbit), folic acid (mouse), and strychnine (rat). There are also cases in which the male is more susceptible than the female; examples are nicotine (mouse), lead (rat), epinephrine (rat), digoxin (dog), and ergot (rat). In many of these examples, the sex effect occurs in a single species and in some instances in a particular strain of that species.

The sex-related differences in toxicity of a foreign compound depend on

Table 7.1   Glucuronidation of p-Nitrophenol in Adult Guinea Pigs

Tissue	p-Nitrophenol conjugated (nmoles/min/mg microsomal protein $\pm$ SD)	
	Male	Female
Liver	47.1 ± 1.5	78.0 ± 12.6
Lung	1.1 ± 0.2	1.8 ± 0.9
Kidney	18.5 ± 3.7	17.6 ± 1.3
Small intestine	0.6 ± 0.3	0.6 ± 0.1

Source: Lucier et al., Drug Metab. Dispos. 5 (1977), 279. © 1977 American Society for Pharmacology and Experimental Therapeutics.

whether enzymatic transformation is influenced by sex hormones. Hexobarbital is metabolized faster by male rats than female rats, and thus females have longer sleeping times. Aldrin is much more toxic to male rats than to female rats because aldrin is metabolized faster to the epoxide, dieldrin, by the male, and dieldrin is more toxic than the parent compound. Parathion is metabolized faster by the female rat than the male to paraoxon, which is more toxic than the parent compound, and therefore the female is more susceptible to parathion than the male.

7.4. Hormones

7.4.1. Thyroid Hormone

The deficiency or administration of hormones can also alter metabolism. Pretreatment of rats with thyroxine alters the hepatic microsomal drug metabolizing enzymes. The activity of microsomal NADPH–oxidase and NADPH–cytochrome c reductase in both male and female rats increases, but the magnitude of increase is greater in female than in male rats. The content of cytochrome P-450 decreases in male rats but is not significantly altered in female rats. Hyperthyroidism decreases the sex-dependent reactions and appears to interfere with the action of androgen to increase the activity of the sex-dependent, drug-metabolizing enzymes.

No sex difference has been found in the effect of thyroxine in mice and rabbits. With thyroxine-treated mice, aminopyrine N-demethylase, aniline hydroxylase, and hexobarbital hydroxylase activities decrease, while p-nitrobenzoic acid reductase is not altered. In thyroxine-treated rabbits, the activity of hexobarbital hydroxylase is not altered, whereas the activities of aniline hydroxylase and p-nitrobenzoic acid reductase increase. The different effects of hyperthyroidism would indicate that thyroxine treatment is related to different responses of the NADPH-dependent electron transport system in these species. The amount of cytochrome P-450 is slightly lower in both mice and rabbits, whereas NADPH oxidase and NADPH–cytochrome c reductase increase in thyroxine-treated rabbits, but are not significantly altered in thyroxine-treated mice.

Thyroidectomized male rats have an increased response to hexobarbital and zoxazolamine. The content of cytochrome P-450 is not decreased in thyroidectomized male rats, but the binding capacity of cytochrome P-450 with hexobarbital is slightly decreased. Thyroid hormone also affects the activity of other enzymes. Liver monoamine oxidase activity is reduced upon administration of L-thyroxine, while kidney monoamine oxidase increases. Thyroxine has no effect on the concentration of glutathione S-transferase B in normal rats, but its administration to either thyroidectomized or hypophysectomized rats results in a return to normal levels. Hyperthyroidism decreases the capacity for p-aminobenzoic acid acetylation. Glucuronidation of o-aminophenol increases in hypothyroid animals.

7.4.2. Adrenal Hormones

Removal of adrenal glands from male rats results in a decrease in activity of hepatic microsomal enzymes. Adrenalectomy of male rats impairs the metabolism of aminopyrine and hexobarbital, whereas adrenalectomy of female rats does not decrease the metabolism of any of the substrates. The administration of cortisone or prednisolone restores activity to normal levels. The content of cytochrome P-450 decreases slightly in liver microsomes of adrenalectomized male rats, whereas the amount of NADPH–cytochrome c reductase and NADPH–cytochrome P-450 reductase fall significantly.

7.4.3. Insulin

The metabolism of a variety of foreign compounds by liver microsomes from male rats with alloxan diabetes is reduced. The in vitro metabolism of hexobarbital and aminopyrine is decreased in alloxan-diabetic male rats, while it is increased in diabetic female rats. Aniline hydroxylase is increased in both male and female rats with alloxan diabetes. The metabolism of hexobarbital and aminopyrine is not depressed in castrated male and female rats with alloxan diabetes, but administration of methyltestosterone decreases metabolism in the castrated male and female rat. Diabetes interferes with the action of androgens to increase the sex-dependent activity of xenobiotic-metabolizing enzymes in rats. The binding capacity of cytochrome P-450 is decreased in liver microsomes from diabetic male rats. Studies on the drug-metabolizing enzyme systems in diabetic male and female mice have shown no sex difference. The activities of aminopyrine N-demethylase, hexobarbital hydroxylase, and aniline hydroxylase increase in both male and female diabetic mice.

A decrease in glucuronidation is associated with diabetic animals. The content of UDPGA is found to be lower in livers of diabetic rats as a result of a decrease in the activity of UDPGA dehydrogenase. However, the amount of glucuronyltransferase was not altered. Administration of insulin increases glucuronidation.

7.4.4. Other Hormones

Pituitary hormones regulate the function of thyroid, adrenal, and sex glands. Hypophysectomy in male rats results in a decrease in the activity of drug-metabolizing enzymes. Administration of adrenocorticotropic hormone (ACTH) to male rats also results in a decrease in activity of the sex-dependent metabolizing enzymes. In contrast, in female rats aminopyrine N-demethylase is slightly increased while other enzyme activities are not altered by ACTH treatment.

Daily rhythmic variations in xenobiotic metabolism by rats, mice, rabbits, and hamsters have been demonstrated both in vivo and in vitro. Activity profiles show a peak during early morning hours and a decrease during noon hours. This rhythmic variation in xenobiotic-metabolizing enzymes is related to serum corticosterone levels. An adrenalectomy or a constant supply of serum corticosterone abolishes the daily rhythmic variation.

7.5. Pregnancy

A large number of enzymes have decreased activity during pregnancy. Catechol-O-methyltransferase and monoamine oxidase activities in rat liver decrease during pregnancy. Glucuronide conjugation of xenobiotics is reduced during late pregnancy because of the increase of progesterone and pregnanediol, which are known inhibitors of glucuronyltransferase in vitro. The inhibition of glucuronide conjugation in certain infants has led to high levels of unconjugated bilirubin in the blood of breast-fed infants, leading to jaundice. This inhibition is associated with the presence of pregnane-3α-20β-diol in the mother's milk. A similar effect on sulfate conjugation has been found in pregnant rats and guinea pigs.

The metabolism of certain xenobiotics by liver microsomal monooxygenases in vitro is also decreased during pregnancy. The hydroxylation of aniline, biphenyl, and coumarin is decreased, and the concentration of cytochrome P-450 is decreased by 25%. Cytochrome P-450 is not inducible by pretreatment of pregnant rats with phenobarbital. With pregnant rabbits no change in cytochrome P-450, biphenyl-4-hydroxylase or nitroreductase at full term is observed. However, glucuronyltransferase and coumarin hydroxylase activity decrease.

7.6. Diet

Dietary factors can have a marked influence on the metabolism of xenobiotics. Starvation of mice results in a decrease in microsomal hydroxylation, whereas reduction of p-nitrobenzoic acid is not altered. Starvation of male rats decreases the activity of hexobarbital hydroxylase, pentobarbital hydroxylase, and aminopyrine N-demethylase 35–40%, whereas aniline hydroxylase, activity increases. In female rats, starvation stimulated hexobarbital hydroxylase, aminopyrine N-demethylase, and aniline hydroxylase. In castrated male rats, no decrease in hexobarbital hydroxylase or aminopyrine N-demethylase is observed. It appears that starvation impairs microsomal enzymes that are sex dependent, but not those that are less sex dependent. Treatment of castrated male rats with methyltestosterone restores enzyme activity in starved animals. It has been suggested that starvation causes an impairment of xenobiotic-metabolizing enzymes by interfering with the stimulatory effects of androgen-type steroids.

Low-protein or protein-free diets also decrease the microsomal metabolizing enzymes in rats; the effect is greater in males than females for aminopyrine N-demethylase and hexobarbital hydroxylase. No sex difference is observed for aniline hydroxylase. The content of cytochrome P-450, NADPH oxidase, and NADPH–cytochrome c reductase decrease with low-protein or protein-free diets in male and female rats.

The toxicity of xenobiotics is influenced by whether the principal microsomal reaction is an intoxication or a detoxication reaction. The toxicity of strychnine is increased in protein-deficient male and female rats, whereas the toxicity of octamethylpyrophosphamide (OMPA), CCl_4, and heptachlor decrease in protein-deficient rats. Metabolic activation is required to display the toxicity of the latter three compounds.

Conjugation of xenobiotics may also be influenced by dietary proteins. Glucuronidation of chloramphenicol in protein-deficient guinea pigs is decreased. No difference in activity of a sulphotransferase with p-nitrophenol as a substrate is observed in protein-deficient rats.

The feeding of a high-carbohydrate diet (sucrose) to rats for 2 days instead of a standard diet results in a marked decrease in the activities of aminopyrine N-demethylase, pentobarbital oxidase, and p-nitrobenzoic acid reductase. This

Table 7.2 Effect of CoCl₂ on Levels of Glutathione in Tissues of the Rat

Tissue	Pretreatment	Glutathione (μmoles/g tissue)
Liver	Saline	8.04
	CoCl₂	14.36
Kidney	Saline	3.33
	CoCl₂	5.74
Lung	Saline	2.41
	CoCl₂	3.00
Ileum	Saline	1.20
	CoCl₂	2.13

Source: Sasame and Boyd, J. Pharmacol. Exp. Ther. 205 (1978), 718. © 1978 American Society for Pharmacology and Experimental Therapeutics.

Note: Four doses of 20 mg CoCl₂/kg in saline were administered at 12-hr intervals.

decreased activity is associated with a reduced amount of cytochromes P-450 and b₅, as well as a decrease in NADPH oxidase and NADPH–cytochrome c reductase activity.

Lipids are an important component of hepatic endoplasmic reticulum, and it has been demonstrated that phosphatidylcholine is an essential component in the reconstituted liver microsomal enzyme system. With regard to essential fatty acids, a diet deficient in linoleic acid results in low hexobarbital and aniline hydroxylase activity in rats. Feeding of a diet deficient in unsaturated fatty acids to rats also results in decreased aniline hydroxylase activity as well as a decreased level of cytochrome P-450. NADPH–cytochrome c reductase activity is not altered by a fatty acid deficiency.

The effects of vitamin deficiencies on the metabolism of foreign compounds appear to result in a decrease in monooxygenase activity. A deficiency of vitamin A results in reduced microsomal metabolism, whereas in thiamine-deficient male rats the monooxygenase activity in liver microsomes is enhanced. Riboflavin deficiency in rats results in a decrease in NADPH–cytochrome c reductase and benzo[a]pyrene hydroxylase activity and an increase in cytochrome P-450 content and aniline hydroxylase activity. Liver microsomes from vitamin c–deficient guinea pigs show decreased rates of metabolism of a number of xenobiotics. This effect is associated with a decrease in cytochrome P-450. Asorbic acid deficiencies have been shown to affect the hydrolysis of procaine by microsomal hydrolases.

Vitamin E–deficient male rats have lower hepatic microsomal aminopyrine N-demethylase activity than controls. Lower aminopyrine N-demethylase activity is also found in vitamin E–deficient female rats.

Calcium-deficient diets cause a decrease in monooxygenase activity in immature male rats. A similar reduction in activity also occurs with magnesium deficiency. However, a much earlier depression of enzyme activity occurs in liver microsomes obtained from rats fed a magnesium-deficient diet than those fed a calcium-deficient diet. Since iron is an integral component of cytochrome

P-450, one would expect that a decrease in monooxygenase activity would occur in animals maintained on an iron-deficient diet. No significant change in cytochrome P-450 content has been observed. However, monooxygenase activity increases rather than decreases. Administration of salts of cobalt, cadmium, manganese, and lead result in an increase in liver glutathione 24 hr after a single treatment, with an accompanying decrease in cytochrome P-450. The effect of four doses of cobalt on reduced glutathione levels is shown in Table 7.2. With most nutritional and mineral deficiencies, the specific biochemical basis for alterations in the microsomal xenobiotic-metabolizing enzyme system remains obscure.

Water deprivation in gerbils results in an increase in the in vitro metabolism of hexobarbital and an increase in cytochrome P-450 content in liver microsomes. Hexobarbital sleeping time was also shorter in water-deprived gerbils.

7.7. Disease

The most important site of xenobiotic metabolism is the liver, and any disease or damage to this organ would be expected to have a pronounced effect on the metabolism of foreign compounds. Patients with acute hepatitis have impaired ability to metabolize a variety of foreign compounds via the monooxygenase system, i.e., there is a decrease in hexobarbital hydroxylase and pentobarbital oxidase activity. In general, an increase in xenobiotic plasma half-life in vivo is also found in cases of acute hepatitis. This effect is not due to a decrease in hepatic blood flow, but is the result of reduced extraction of the xenobiotic, resulting in decreased xenobiotic plasma clearance. Decreased acetylation of isoniazid has also been found with acute viral hepatitis.

Metabolic studies of various drugs have shown impaired metabolism in patients with chronic liver diseases, such as chronic hepatitis and cirrhosis. Cytochrome P-450, aminopyrine N-demethylase, and p-nitroanisole O-demethylase are significantly decreased in liver biopsy specimens from patients with hepatitis and cirrhosis, whereas NADPH–cytochrome c reductase activity is not altered. Hepatic microsomes from animals with obstructive jaundice or cholestasis have decreased drug-metabolizing ability. This decrease is probably due to the accumulation of bile salts, which are known inhibitors of the microsomal drug-metabolizing enzymes.

There are limited studies of the effect of liver disease on other phase I and II reactions. Dimethylaniline N-oxidase activity (non-cytochrome P-450–requiring enzyme) is reduced in liver biopsy specimens from cirrhotic patients. Decreased acetylation of p-aminobenzoic acid as well as decreased glucuronidation of N-acetyl-p-aminophenol has been found with chronic liver disease. Monoamine oxidase activity was decreased to 30% of the normal value in patients with liver cirrhosis. A decrease in hydrolase activity, i.e., serum cholinesterase, phenyl acetate esterase, serum procaine esterase, and serum aspirin esterase, has been found in patients with liver disease. Liver alcohol dehydrogenase activity has been found to be generally lower in biopsy samples from cirrhotic patients than in samples from normal controls.

Diseases of the heart may alter the flow of blood to the liver and thus would be an important factor in controlling the rate of in vivo metabolism of a foreign compound. Plasma clearance of lidocaine is reduced in patients with myocardial infarction as well as in those with cardiac failure, and this is attributed to reduced liver blood flow. Cardiac failure also has some deleterious effect on liver function, probably due to a decreased availability of nutrients for the organ as well as generalized congestion.

Diseases of the kidney also affect metabolism since the kidney is the main organ for excretion of water-soluble metabolites into urine. One would expect patients with poor renal function to excrete water-soluble metabolites at a slower rate. This should result in retention of the drug in the body, especially compounds with low hepatic extraction ratios, as well as prolongation of action. The half-lives of tolbutamide, thiopental, hexobarbital and chloramphenicol are prolonged in patients with renal impairment.

The ability of the liver to metabolize xenobiotics is affected in tumor-bearing animals according to the cell line of the hepatoma. With certain hepatoma lines, there is a decrease in the activity of microsomal drug-metabolizing enzymes in the liver, while in other types the enzyme activity is the same as controls. However, hepatic tumors generally exhibit lower activity in xenobiotic-metabolizing enzymes compared to that in normal tissue. Primary hepatic hepatomas have little or no detectable oxidative activity, whereas azo- and nitroreductase activity are in the normal range.

Suggested Reading

Brodie, B. B., Gillette, J. R., Ackerman, H. S. (Eds.). Handbook of Experimental Pharmacology, Vol. 28, part 2, Concepts in Biochemical Pharmacology. Berlin: Springer, 1971. The following chapter is of particular relevance: Dutton, G. J. Glucuronide-forming enzymes. Chapter 45, p. 38.

Casarett, L. J., Doull, J. (Eds.). Toxicology: The Basic Science of Poisons. New York: Macmillan, 1975.

Kato, R. Drug metabolism under pathological and abnormal physiological states in animals and man. Xenobiotica 7 (1977), 25.

Neims, A. H., Warner, M., Loughman, P. M., Aranda, J. V. Developmental aspects of the hepatic cytochrome P-450 monooxygenase system. Ann. Rev. Pharmacol. Toxicol. 16 (1970), 427.

Parke, D. V. The Biochemistry of Foreign Compounds. London: Pergamon Press, 1968.

Ernest Hodgson

8

Chemical and Environmental Factors Affecting Metabolism of Xenobiotics

8.1. Chemical Factors

From the point of view of both logistics and scientific philosophy, the study of the metabolism and toxicity of xenobiotics must be initiated by considering single compounds. Unfortunately, man and other living organisms are not exposed in this way, but rather they are exposed to many xenobiotics simultaneously that involve different portals of entry, modes of action, and metabolic pathways. For this reason, the effect of chemicals on the metabolism of other exogenous compounds is rapidly becoming one of the most important areas of biochemical toxicology because it bears directly on the problem of toxicity-related interactions between different xenobiotics.

Only a very small number of toxicants have been studied extensively in several organisms or have had all of their principal metabolic intermediates and end products characterized; for only very few toxicants have the enzymes involved been identified, purified, and characterized. It is not surprising, therefore, that our knowledge of the mechanism of their chemical interactions is at rudimentary stage. The magnitude of the problem can be appreciated by considering the following estimates of the number of chemical additives in use today (the source of the estimates is given in parenthesis):

  1,500 active ingredients of pesticides (Environmental Protection Agency, EPA)
  4,000 active ingredients of drugs (Food and Drug Administration, FDA)
  2,000 drug additives to improve stability, inhibit bacterial growth, etc. (FDA)
  2,500 food additives with nutritional value (FDA)
  3,000 food additives to promote product life (FDA)
50,000 additional chemicals in common use (EPA)

As documented below, xenobiotics, in addition to serving as substrates for a number of enzymes, may also serve as inhibitors or inducers of these or other enzymes. In fact, many examples are known of compounds that first inhibit and subsequently induce enzymes such as the microsomal mixed-function oxidases. The situation is even further complicated by the fact that while some substances have an inherent toxicity and are detoxified in the body, others without inherent toxicity can be metabolically activated to potent toxicants. The following examples are illustrative of the situations that might occur involving two compounds.

1. Compound A, without inherent toxicity, is metabolized to a potent toxicant. In the presence of an inhibitor of its metabolism there would be a reduction in toxic effect.
2. Compound A, in the presence of an inducer of the activating enzymes, would appear more toxic.
3. Compound B, a toxicant, is metabolically detoxified. In the presence of an inhibitor of the detoxifying enzymes there would be an increase in the toxic effect.
4. Compound B, in the presence of an inducer of the detoxifying enzymes, would appear less toxic.

In addition to the above cases, the toxicity of the inhibitor or inducer as well as the time dependence of the effect must also be considered since, as mentioned above, many xenobiotics that are initially enzyme inhibitors ultimately become inducers.

8.1.1. Inhibition

As indicated above, inhibition of xenobiotic-metabolizing enzymes can cause either an increase or a decrease in toxicity. Several well-known inhibitors of such enzymes are shown in Figure 8.1. Inhibitory effects can be demonstrated in a number of ways at different organizational levels.

8.1.1a. Types of Inhibition: Experimental Demonstration

In vivo symptoms. The measurement of the effect of an inhibitor on the duration of action of a drug in vivo is the commonest method of demonstrating its action. These methods are open to criticism, however, since effects on duration of action can be mediated by systems other than those involved in the metabolism of the drug. Furthermore, they cannot be used for inhibitors that have pharmacological activity similar or opposite to the compound being used. The most used and most reliable of these tests involve the measurement of effects on the hexobarbital sleeping time and the zoxazolamine paralysis time. Both of these drugs are fairly rapidly deactivated by the hepatic microsomal mixed-function oxidase system and thus inhibitors of this system prolong their action.

For example, treatment of mice with chloroamphenicol 0.5–1.0 hr before pentobarbital treatment prolongs the duration of the pentobarbital sleeping time in a dose-related manner; it is effective at low doses (< 5 mg/kg) and has greater than a tenfold effect at high doses (100–200 mg/kg). The well-known inhibitor of drug metabolism SKF-525A causes an increase in both hexobarbital sleeping time and zoxazolamine paralysis time in rats and mice, as do the insecticide synergists piperonyl butoxide and tropital, the optimum pretreatment time being about 0.5 hr before the narcotic is given. Similar results have been ob-

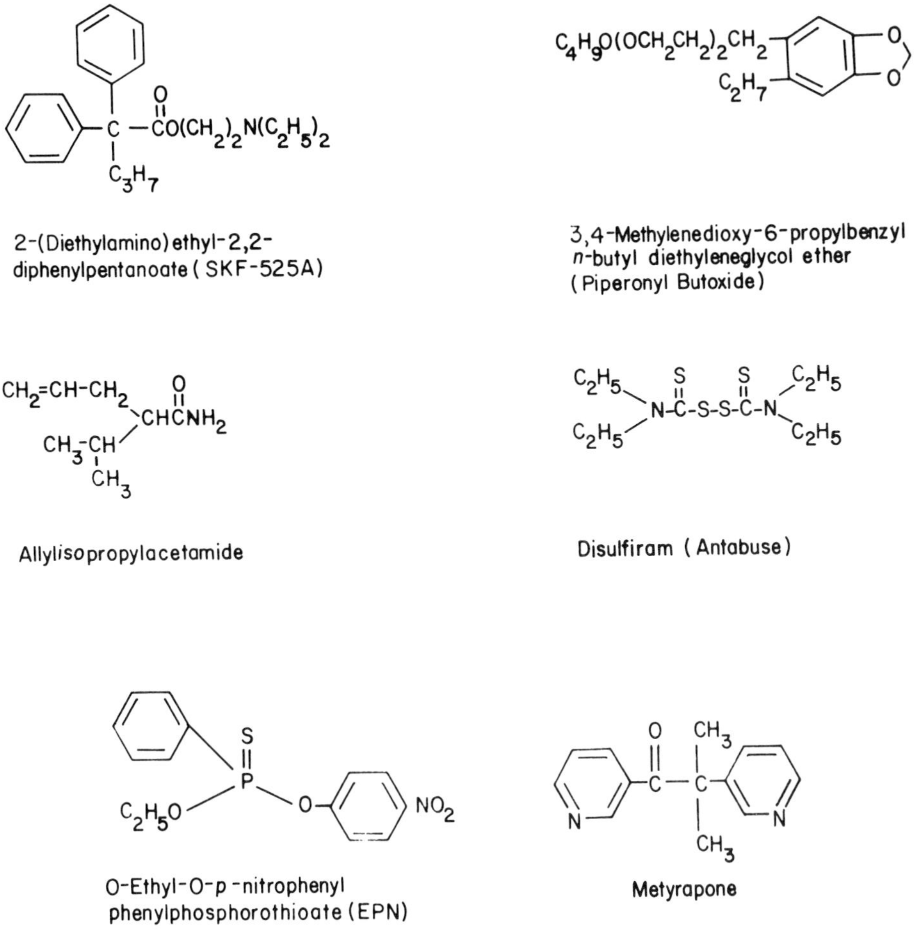

2-(Diethylamino)ethyl-2,2-
diphenylpentanoate (SKF-525A)

3,4-Methylenedioxy-6-propylbenzyl
n-butyl diethyleneglycol ether
(Piperonyl Butoxide)

Allylisopropylacetamide

Disulfiram (Antabuse)

O-Ethyl-O-p-nitrophenyl
phenylphosphorothioate (EPN)

Metyrapone

Figure 8.1 Some common inhibitors of xenobiotic metabolizing enzymes.

tained with many other methylenedioxyphenyl compounds, including the natural product safrole and some of its derivatives.

In the case of activation reactions, such as the activation of the insecticide azinphosmethyl to its potent anticholinesterase oxon derivative, a decrease in toxicity is apparent when rats are pretreated with SKF-525A.

Cocarcinogenicity may also be an expression of inhibition of a detoxication reaction, as in the case of the cocarcinogenicity of piperonyl butoxide and freon-112 and -113.

Distribution and blood levels. Treatment of an animal with an inhibitor of foreign compound metabolism may cause changes in the blood levels of an unmetabolized toxicant and/or its metabolites. This procedure may be utilized in the investigation of the inhibition of detoxication pathways; it has the advantage over in vitro methods that it yields results of direct physiological or toxicological interest since it is carried out on the intact animal. Moreover, the time sequence of the effects can be followed in individual animals, a factor of importance when inhibition is followed by induction—a not uncommon event.

For example, if animals are first treated with either SKF-525A, glutethimide, or chlorcyclizine, followed in 1 hr or less by pentobarbital, it can be shown that the serum level of pentobarbital is considerably higher than in controls within 1 hr of its injection.

Effects on metabolism in vivo. A further refinement of the previous technique is to determine the effect of an inhibitor on the overall metabolism of a xenobiotic in vivo, usually by following the appearance of metabolites in the urine and/or feces. In some cases the appearance of metabolites in the blood or tissues may also be followed. Again, the use of the intact animal has practical advantages over in vitro methods, although little is revealed about the mechanisms involved.

Studies of antipyrine metabolism may be used to illustrate the effect of inhibition or metabolism in vivo; in addition, these studies have demonstrated variation between species in the inhibition of the metabolism of xenobiotics. In the rat a dose of piperonyl butoxide of at least 100 mg/kg was necessary to inhibit antipyrine metabolism, while in the mouse a single ip or oral dose of only 1 mg/kg produced a significant inhibition. An oral dose of 0.71 mg/kg had no discernible effect on the metabolism of antipyrine in humans.

Effects on in vitro metabolism following in vivo treatment. This method of demonstrating inhibition is of variable utility. The preparation of enzymes from animal tissues usually involves considerable dilution with the preparative medium during homogenization, centrifugation, and resuspension. As a result, inhibitors not tightly bound to the enzyme in question are lost, either in whole or in part, during the preparative processes. Therefore, negative results can have little utility since failure to inhibit and loss of the inhibitor give identical results. Positive results, on the other hand, not only indicate that the compound administered is an inhibitor but also provide a clear indication of excellent binding to the enzyme, most probably due to the formation of an inhibitory complex. The inhibition of esterases following treatment of the animal with phosphates such as paraxon is a good example since the phosphorylated enzyme is stable and it still inhibited after the preparative procedures. Inhibition by carbamates is greatly reduced by the same procedures, however, since the carbamylated enzyme is unstable and, in addition, residual carbamate is highly diluted.

Microsomal mixed-function oxidase inhibitors that form stable inhibitory complexes with cytochrome P-450, such as SKF-525A, piperonyl butoxide and other methylenedioxyphenyl compounds, and amphetamine and its derivatives, can be readily investigated in this way since the microsomes isolated from pretreated animals have a reduced capacity to oxidize many xenobiotics.

Another form of chemical interaction resulting from inhibition in vivo that can then be demonstrated in vitro involves those xenobiotics that function by causing destruction of the enzyme in question. Exposure of rats to vinyl chloride results in a loss of cytochrome P-450 and a corresponding reduction in the capacity of microsomes subsequently isolated to metabolize foreign compounds. Allyl isopropylacetamide and other allyl compounds have long been known to have a similar effect.

In vitro effects. In vitro measurement of the effect of one xenobiotic on the metabolism of another is by far the commonest type of investigation of interactions involving inhibition. Although it is the most useful method for the study of an inhibitory mechanism, particularly when purified enzymes are used, it is of more limited utility in assessing the toxicological implications for the intact animal. The principal reason for this is that it does not assess the effects of factors that affect absorption, distribution, and prior metabolism, all of which occur before the inhibitory event under consideration.

Although the kinetics of inhibition of xenobiotic-metabolizing enzymes can be investigated in the same ways as any other enzyme mechanism, a number of problems arise that may decrease the value of this type of investigation. They include the following:

1. Many investigations have been carried out on a particulate enzyme system, the mixed-function oxidase system, using methods developed for single soluble enzymes. As a result, Lineweaver-Burke or other reciprocal plots are frequently curvilinear, and the same reaction may appear to have quite different characteristics from laboratory to laboratory, species to species, and organ to organ.
2. The nonspecific binding of substrate and/or inhibitor to membrane components is a further complicating factor affecting inhibition kinetics.
3. Substrates and inhibitors are frequently lipophilic with low solubility in aqueous media.
4. Xenobiotic-metabolizing enzymes commonly exist in multiple forms (e.g., glutathione S-transferases and cytochromes P-450) that are all relatively nonspecific but differ from one another in the relative affinities of the different substrates.

The primary considerations in studies of inhibition mechanisms are reversibility and selectivity. The inhibition kinetics of reversible inhibition give considerable insight into the reaction mechanisms of enzymes and, for that reason, have been well studied. Generally speaking, reversible inhibition involves no covalent binding, occurs rapidly, and can be reversed by dialysis or, more rapidly, by dilution. Reversible inhibition is usually divided into competitive inhibition, uncompetitive inhibition, and noncompetitive inhibition, although these are not rigidly separated types, and many intermediate classes have been described.

Competitive inhibition is usually due to two substrates competing for the same active site. Following classical enzyme kinetics, there should be a change in the apparent K_m but not in V_{max}. In microsomal mixed-function oxidase reactions, type I ligands, which often appear to bind as substrates but do not bind to the heme iron, might be expected to be competitive inhibitors, and this frequently appears to be the case. Examples are the inhibition of the O-demethylation of p-nitroanisole by aminopyrene, aldrin epoxidation by dihydroaldrin, and N-demethylation of aminopyrene by nicotinamide. More recently, some of the polychlorinated biphenyls, notably dichlorobiphenyl, but also, less effectively, tetrachlorobiphenyl, and hexachlorobiphenyl, have been shown to have a high affinity as type I ligands for rabbit liver cytochrome P-450 and to be competitive inhibitors of the O-demethylation of p-nitroanisole.

Pilocarpine, which potentiates nicotine-induced convulsions and hexobarbital hypnosis, has been shown to be a potent competitive inhibitor of the microsomal metabolism of these two compounds. Since pilocarpine and nicotine are type II ligands, while hexobarbital is type I, it is clear that inferences about the type of inhibition developed from a consideration of the ligand binding spectra must be regarded as highly tentative.

Competitive inhibition may also result from an inhibitor binding to a site on the enzyme other than the active site, which, nevertheless, blocks the active site to the substrate by bringing about a conformational change.

Uncompetitive inhibition has seldom been reported in studies of xenobiotic metabolism. It is seen when an inhibitor interacts with an enzyme–substrate complex but cannot interact with free enzyme. Both K_m and V_{max} change by the same ratio, giving rise to a family of parallel lines in a Lineweaver-Burke plot.

Simple noncompetitive inhibitors can bind to both the enzyme and enzyme–substrate complex to form either an enzyme–inhibitor complex or an enzyme–inhibitor–substrate complex. The net result is a decrease in V_{max} but no change in K_m.

Metyrapone, a well-known inhibitor of mixed-function oxidase reactions, can also, under some circumstances, stimulate metabolism in vitro. In either case the effect is noncompetitive, in that the K_m does not change while V_{max} does, decreasing in the case of inhibition and increasing in the case of stimulation. The characteristics of the three principle types of reversible inhibition are shown in Table 8.1.

Irreversible inhibition can arise from a variety of causes, some of which are extremely important toxicologically. In the vast majority of cases, either covalent binding or disruption of the enzyme structure are involved. In neither case can the effect be reversed in vitro by either dialysis or dilution.

Covalent binding may involve the prior formation of a metabolic intermediate that then interacts with the enzyme. An excellent example of this type of inhibition is the effect of the insecticide synergist piperonyl butoxide on hepatic microsomal mixed-function oxidase activity. This compound can form a stable inhibitory complex that blocks CO binding to cytochrome P-450 and also prevents substrate oxidation. This complex causes the appearance of a characteristic difference spectrum that has two pH-dependent peaks in the Soret region and, apart from its stability, resembles that of ethyl isocyanide. This complex is the result of metabolite formation, which is shown by the fact that the type of inhibition changes from competitive to irreversible as metabolism, in the pres-

Table 8.1 Comparison of Three Types of Reversible Inhibition

Type of inhibition	Interaction	V_{max}	K_m	Lineweaver-Burke plot[a]
Competitive	I and E	±	+	Lines converge on y axis
Noncompetitive (simple)	I, ES, and E	−	±	Lines converge on x axis
Uncompetitive	I and ES	−	−	Parallel lines

Abbreviations: I, inhibitor; E, enzyme; ES, enzyme–substrate complex; ±, unchanged; −, decreased; +, increased.

[a] Each line referred to is a plot of $1/v$ versus $1/S$ in which v is the initial velocity and S the substrate concentration in the presence of a given amount of inhibitor. By varying the amount of inhibitor in separate experiments a family of such lines is generated.

ence of NADPH and oxygen, proceeds. Piperonyl butoxide inhibits the in vitro metabolism of many substrates of the mixed-function oxidase system, including aldrin, ethylmorphine, aniline, aminopyrene, carbaryl, biphenyl, hexobarbital, p-nitroanisole, and many others. Although most of the studies carried out on piperonyl butoxide have involved rat or mouse liver microsomes, they have also been carried out on pig, rabbit, and carp liver microsomes and in a variety of preparations from houseflies, cockroaches, and other insects.

A number of classes of mixed-function oxidase inhibition, in addition to methylenedioxyphenyl compounds, are now known to form "metabolic–intermediate complexes" including amphetamine and its derivatives, and SKF-525A and its derivatives.

Disulfiram (Antabuse) inhibits aldehyde dehydrogenase irreversibly, causing an increase in the level of acetaldehyde, which has been formed from ethanol by the enzyme alcohol dehydrogenase. This results in nausea, vomiting, and other symptoms in the human—hence its use as an alcohol deterrent in alcoholism. The inhibition by disulfiram appears to be irreversible, the level returning to normal only as a result of protein synthesis.

The inhibition by other organophosphate compounds of the carboxylesterase which hydrolyzes malathion is a further example of xenobiotic interaction resulting from irreversible inhibition since in this case the enzyme is phosphorylated by the inhibitor.

Another class of irreversible inhibitors of toxicological significance consists of those compounds that bring about the destruction of the xenobiotic-metabolizing enzyme. The drug allyl*iso*propylacetamide, as well as a number of other allyl compounds, has long been known to cause the breakdown of cytochrome P-450 and resultant release of heme. More recently, the hepatocarcinogen vinyl chloride has also been shown to have a similar effect, probably also mediated through the generation of a highly reactive metabolic intermediate. A great deal of information, discussed in detail in Chapter 18, has accumulated in the past decade on the mode of action of the hepatotoxin carbon tetrachloride, which effects a number of irreversible changes in both liver proteins and lipids, such changes being generated by active intermediates formed during its metabolism.

The less specific disruptors of protein structure, such as urea, detergents, strong acids, etc., are probably of significance only in in vitro experiments.

Activation in vitro. There are several examples of activation of xenobiotic-metabolizing enzymes by compounds other than the substrate. This differs from induction (described in Section 8.1.2) in that it is an immediate effect on a preexisting enzyme, occurring in an enzyme preparation in vitro, that does not involve de novo protein synthesis. The significance, or even the occurrence, of such stimulation in vivo is not apparent.

Cytochrome P-450–mediated microsomal oxidations are stimulated by the addition of any of a rather heterogeneous group of compounds, including ethyl isocyanide, acetone, 2,2'-bipyridyl, and, under certain conditions, the inhibitor metyrapone. The effect is not uniform, however, since acetone, for example, stimulates aniline hydroxylation but has no effect on the N-demethylation of N-methylaniline, N,N-dimethylaniline, or ethylmorphine, or the O-demethylation of p-nitroanisole. 2,2'-Bipyridine, on the other hand, stimulates both aniline hydroxylation and N-demethylation of N-methyl- and N,N-dimethylaniline but, at the same time, inhibits the N-dealkylation of ethylmorphine and aminopyrine. Variations may be due, at least in part, to the activity of the flavoprotein amine oxidase present in the microsomes.

The mechanism of this stimulation is unclear, and a number of suggestions have been advanced. For example, ethyl isocyanide may act via stimulation of cytochrome P-450 reduction. Acetone and 2,2-bipyridine do not appear to have a common mode of action with ethyl isocyanide and may exert their effect on the microsomal membrane, thus changing the availability of enzyme and/or substrate.

The activation of another membrane-bound enzyme of interest in biochemical toxicology, UDP glucuronyltransferase, is probably also due to effects on the membrane. Significant stimulation is brought about by "aging" the enzyme preparation, by sonication, and by such agents as dilute detergents, proteolytic enzymes, etc.

8.1.1b. Synergism and Potentiation

These terms have been variously used and defined but, in any case, involve a toxicity that is greater when two compounds are given simultaneously or sequentially than would be expected from a consideration of the toxicities of the compounds given alone.

Some toxicologists have used the term synergism for cases that fit the above definition but only when one compound is toxic alone while the other has little or no intrinsic toxicity. This is the case with the toxicity of insecticides to insects and mammals and the effects on this toxicity of methylenedioxyphenyl synergists such as piperonyl butoxide, sesamex, and tropital. The term potentiation is then reserved for those cases in which both compounds have appreciable intrinsic toxicity, such as in the case of malathion and EPN. Unfortunately, other toxicologists have used the terms in precisely the opposite manner, while even more use the terms interchangeably, without definition, leading to such statements as "potentiation of the toxicity of X by the synergist Y." Historically, pharmacologists used the term synergism to refer to simple additive toxicity and potentiation either as a synonym, or for examples of greater than additive toxicity or efficacy. Attempts to define synergism, such as the boloform and/or bologram presentation of Black, have been useful, although his proposed mechanism, involving sequential inhibition, is probably of little general significance, as subsequently shown by Rubin and others. Although these attempts to define synergism clearly involve the concept of greater than additive toxicity they do not differentiate synergism from potentiation.

In an attempt to make the use of these terms uniform, it is suggested that insofar as toxic effects are concerned, they be used as defined above, i.e., both involve toxicity greater than would be expected from the toxicities of the compounds administered separately, but in the case of synergism one compound has little or no intrinisic toxicity administered alone, while in the case of potentiation both compounds have appreciable toxicity when administered alone. It is further suggested that no special term is needed for simple additive toxicity of two or more compounds.

Although examples are known in which synergistic interactions take place at the receptor site, the majority of such interactions appear to involve the inhibition of xenobiotic-metabolizing enzymes. Two of the best known examples in toxicology involve the insecticide synergists, particularly the methylenedioxyphenyl synergists, and the potentiation of the insecticide malathion by a large number of other organophosphate compounds.

The first example has already been mentioned. Piperonyl butoxide, sesamex, and related compounds increase the toxicity of insecticides to insects by inhibition of the insect mixed-function oxidase system. They are of commercial importance in household aerosol formulations containing pyrethrum. This inhibition, which appears to be the same in mammals and insects, involves the formation of a metabolic–inhibitory complex with cytochrome P-450. The complex probably results from the formation of a carbene, as follows:

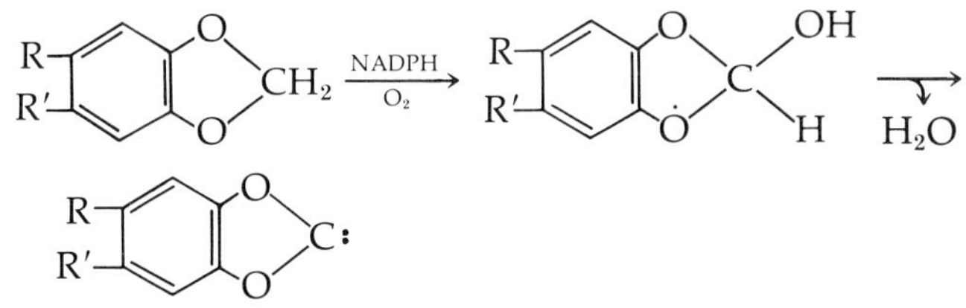

This carbene then reacts with the heme iron in a reaction involving π-bonding, as well as the dative σ bond formed by the free pair of electrons, to form a complex that blocks CO (and presumably O_2) binding and inhibits the metabolism of xenobiotics.

Other insecticide synergists that interact with the mixed-function oxidase system include aryloxyalkylamines such as SKF-525A, Lilly 18947, and their derivatives, compounds containing acetylenic bonds such as aryl-2-propynyl ethers and oxime ethers, organothiocyanates, N-(5-pentynyl)phthalimides, phosphate esters containing propynyl functions, phosphorothionates, benzothiadiazoles, and some imidazole derivatives.

The general nature of this mode of action raises important questions concerning the effects on nontarget species. The question of whether piperonyl butoxide or other methylenedioxyphenyl compounds can increase the toxicity of environmental or medicinal xenobiotics has often been asked but not yet definitely answered. It is of interest that two members of another class of insecticide synergists, 3-bromophenyl-4(5)-imidazole and 1-naphthal-4(5)-imidazole, are potent inhibitors of the metabolism of estradiol and ethynylestradiol by rat liver microsomes.

The best known example of potentiation involving insecticides and an enzyme other than the mixed-function oxidase system is the increase in the toxicity of malathion to mammals brought about by certain other organophosphates. Malathion has a low mammalian toxicity due primarily to its rapid hydrolysis by a carboxylesterase (Chapter 4). EPN, a phosphonate insecticide, was shown to cause a dramatic increase in malathion toxicity to mammals at dose levels which, given alone, caused essentially no inhibition of cholinesterase. In vitro studies further established the fact that the oxygen analog of

EPN, as well as many other organophosphate compounds, increases the toxicity of malathion by inhibiting the carboxylesterase responsible for its degradation.

In a similar way, EPN and tri-o-tolyl phosphate increase the toxicity of dimethoate by inhibiting the carboxylamidase necessary for its detoxication.

Synergistic action is often seen with drugs. Almost all cases of increased hexobarbital sleeping time or zoxazolamine paralysis time by other chemicals could be described as synergism or potentiation.

Synergism may also result from competition for binding sites on plasma proteins (Chapter 2) or for the active secretion mechanism in the renal tubule.

8.1.1c. Antagonism

In toxicology antagonism may be defined as that situation in which the toxicity of two or more compounds administered together, or sequentially, is less than would be expected from a consideration of their toxicities when administered individually. Strictly speaking, this definition includes those cases in which the lowered toxicity results from induction of detoxifying enzymes; they are considered in Section 8.12. Apart from the convenience of treating such antagonistic phenomena together with the other aspects of induction, they are frequently considered separately because of the significant time span that must elapse between treatment with the inducer and subsequent treatment with the toxicant. The reduction of hexobarbital sleeping time and the reduction of zoxazolamine paralysis time by prior treatment with phenobarbital are obvious examples of such induction effects at the level of drug action, while protection from the carcinogenic action of benzpyrene, aflatoxin, and diethylnitrosamine by phenobarbital are examples at the level of chronic toxicity.

Antagonism not involving induction is a phenomenon often seen at a marginal level of detection and is consequently both difficult to explain and of marginal significance. In addition, several different types of antagonism of importance to toxicology that do not involve xenobiotic metabolism are known but are not appropriate to discuss in this chapter. These include competition for receptor sites, such as the competition between CO and O_2 in CO poisoning, or situations in which one toxicant combines nonenzymatically with another to reduce its toxic effects, such as in the chelation of metal ions. Physiological antagonism, in which two agonists act on the same physiological system but produce opposite effects, is also of importance.

Carbaryl and carbofuran metabolism is enhanced by pretreatment with chlordane and decreased by pretreatment with methyl mercury hydroxide. Simultaneous treatment with chlordane and methyl mercury results in rates of carbaryl and carbofuron metabolism similar to those in controls, indicating an antagonism between the two compounds.

Parathion is known to inhibit mixed-function oxidase activity, while DDT, aldrin, and dieldrin are all inducers. In experiments with separate and combined treatments, pretreatment of the animal with parathion inhibited O-demethylation, O-dearylation, N-demethylation, azo-reduction, and nitro-reduction in the microsomes subsequently isolated, while the organochlorine compounds caused a stimulation of some or all of these parameters. Combined pretreatment with parathion and any one of the organochlorine compounds gave results that ranged from inhibition to induction, depending upon the particular organochlorine compound used and/or the parameter being measured. It was apparent that the results were largely antagonistic although highly unpredictable.

8.1.2. Induction

Some 25 years ago, during investigations on the N-demethylation of aminoazo dyes, it was observed that pretreatment of mammals with the substrate or, more remarkably, with other xenobiotics, caused an increase in the ability of the animal to metabolize these dyes. It was subsequently shown that this effect is due to an increase in the microsomal enzymes involved. Since that time it has become clear that this phenomenon is widespread and quite nonspecific. Several hundred compounds of diverse chemical structure have been shown to induce mixed-function oxidase and other enzymes. These compounds include drugs, insecticides, polycyclic hydrocarbons, and many others; the only obvious common denominator is that they are all organic and lipophilic.

A symposium in 1965 and a landmark review in 1967 summarized the early work. It was already clear by that time that enzymes of the mixed-function oxidase pathway other than cytochrome P-450 were also increased in these situations (Figure 8.2). It was also apparent that, even though all inducers did not have the same effects, the effects tended to be nonspecific to the extent that any single inducer induced more than one enzymatic activity.

8.1.2a. Specificity of Mixed-Function Oxidase Induction

The many inducers of mixed-function oxidase activity fall into two principal classes, one exemplified by phenobarbital and containing many drugs, insecticides, etc., of diverse chemical classes, and the other exemplified by 3-methylcholanthrene and benzpyrene and containing primarily polycyclic hydrocarbons. Many inducers require either fairly high dose levels or repeated dosing to be effective, frequently greater than 10 mg/kg and some as high as 100–200 mg/kg. However, some insecticides, such as mirex, can induce at dose levels as low as 1 mg/kg, and the most potent inducer known, 2,3,7,8-tetrachlorodibenzo-p-dioxin (TCDD), is effective at 1 μg/kg in some species.

In the liver, phenobarbital-type inducers cause a marked proliferation of the smooth endoplasmic reticulum and induction of cytochrome P-450 with approximately the same spectral characteristics as that of the liver of uninduced mammals. A wide range of oxidative activities is induced, including O-demethylation of p-nitroanisole, N-demethylation of benzphetamine, pentobarbital hydroxylation, aldrin epoxidation, and many others, but increases in aryl hydrocarbon hydroxylase activity are minimal.

Induction by polycyclic hydrocarbons, on the other hand, causes no increase in smooth endoplasmic reticulum and results in the appearance of cytochrome P-448, characterized by a shift in the λ_{max} of the reduced cytochrome–CO complex to 448 nm. This cytochrome also shows a shift in the pH equilibrium point of the reduced cytochrome–ethyl isocyanide complex. Unlike phenobarbital-

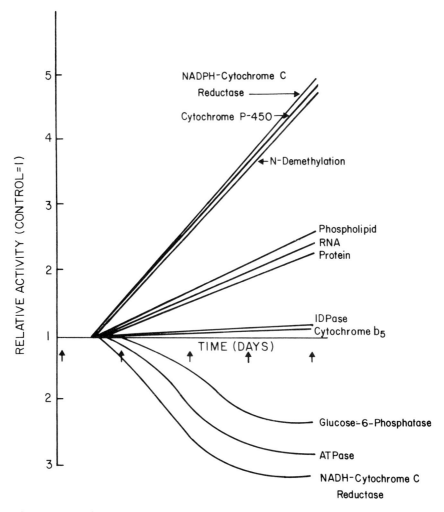

Figure 8.2 Changes in hepatic enzyme activities following daily injections of phenobarbital. Arrows indicate sequence of injections.
SOURCE: *Adapted from Ernster and Orrenius, Fed. Proc. 24 (1965), 1190.*

type induction, there is no increase in the type I binding of hexobarbital concomitant with the increase in cytochrome level. The appearance of a type I optical difference spectrum with benzpyrene or 3-methylcholanthrene and a marked drop in the K_m values for aryl hydrocarbon hydroxylase substrates is further evidence of the formation of a cytochrome P-450 (P-448 or P_1-450) of different physical and substrate-binding characteristics. A relatively narrow range of oxidative activities, primarily aryl hydrocarbon hydroxylase, is induced by polycyclic hydrocarbons. The extremely potent inducer TCDD, referred to above, appears to fall in this class.

All inducers do not fall readily into one or the other of these two classes. Some oxidative processes can be induced by either type of inducer, such as the hydroxylation of aniline and the N-demethylation of chlorcyclizine. There are also many variations in the relative stimulation of different oxidative activities within the same class of inducer, particularly of the phenobarbital type.

Pregnenolone-16α-carbonitrile (PCN) may represent a third type of inducer in that the substrate specificity of the microsomes from treated animals differs from that of the microsomes from either phenobarbital- or 3-methyl-cholanthrene–treated animals. The amount of cytochrome P-450 is increased, but there is no shift in the absorption maximum of the CO optical difference spectrum; that is, there is not discernible appearance of cytochrome P-448. It has also been suggested that another type of cytochrome P-450 may be induced by ethanol, although this finding may still be considered controversial.

Although polychlorinated and polybrominated biphenyls appear to have the characteristics of both types of inducer at the same time, more recent findings demonstrate that this observation is probably due to the presence of inducers of both types in the complex mixtures of biphenyls used.

It appears reasonable that, since there are several types of cytochrome P-450 associated with the hepatic endoplasmic reticulum, various inducers may induce one or more of them. Since each of these types has a relatively broad substrate specificity, differences may be caused by variations in the extent of induction of different cytochromes. Phenobarbital has been shown to induce two of the three forms of cytochrome P-450 that have been identified in the microsomal fraction from mouse liver by polyacrylamide gel electrophoresis in the presence of sodium dodecyl sulfate (SDS-PAGE), while the third was induced by 3-methylcholanthrene. Now that methods are available for SDS-PAGE of microsomes and for solubilization and characterization of different forms of cytochrome P-450, it is possible that the complex array of inductive phenomena will be more logically explained.

Although the bulk of published investigations of the induction of mixed-function oxidase enzymes have dealt with mammalian liver, it should be pointed out that induction has been observed in other mammalian tissues and in nonmammalian species, both vertebrate and invertebrate.

Other anomalies of the induction phenomenon include the marked induction of aryl hydrocarbon hydroxylase activity in the placenta of human mothers who smoke cigarettes, an induction which is not accompanied by a discernible increase or qualitative change in the placental cytochrome P-450. Although feeding of chlordane to rats gives rise to an initial increase in aldrin epoxidase activity, there is a decline to control values in spite of continued induction of cytochrome P-450 and smooth endoplasmic reticulum, giving rise to a condition described by the investigators as "hypoactive, hypertrophic endoplasmic reticulum."

Thus it is possible to achieve an increase in oxidative activity without any increase in cytochrome P-450, or, in other cases, to achieve an increase in cytochrome P-450 without any increase in oxidative activity.

8.1.2b. Mechanism and Genetics of Induction in Mammals

Although stress can affect the level of mammalian mixed-function oxidase activity, the effect is secondary, since induction has been demonstrated following perfusion of the isolated liver with the inducer and also following treatment of isolated hepatocytes. However, it has not been duplicated in cell-free systems, presumably due to the time required for the process and the fact that several complex multienzyme processes are required simultaneously—notably the processes involved in gene expression and protein synthesis. It has been known for some time that the induction of mixed-function oxidase activity is a true induction involving synthesis of new enzyme, and not the activation of enzyme already synthesized, since it is prevented by inhibitors of protein synthesis. For example, aryl hydrocarbon hydroxylase induction is inhibited by puromycin, ethionine, and cycloheximide. A simplified scheme for gene expression and protein synthesis is shown in Figure 8.3.

The use of suitable inhibitors of RNA and DNA metabolism has shown that inhibitors of RNA synthesis such as actinomycin D and mercapto-(pyridethyl)-benzimidazole block aryl hydrocarbon hydroxylase induction, whereas hydroxyurea, at levels that completely block the incorporation of thymidine into DNA, has no effect. Thus it appears that the inductive effect is at the level of transcription and that DNA synthesis is not required. Induction by phenobarbital appears to take place by essentially the same mechanisms as induction of aryl hydrocarbon hydroxylase by aromatic hydrocarbons.

These findings imply that compounds that induce xenobiotic-metabolizing enzymes play a role as derepressors of regulator or other genes, but this has not been clearly demonstrated. The involvement of regulator and operator genes is even more speculative; in view of the extremely variable results obtained with regard to the ratio of different enzymes induced by different inducers, it should be regarded with caution, particularly with inducers of the phenobarbital type.

The case is better argued with polycyclic hydrocarbon inducers, at least in the

Figure 8.3 Simplified scheme for gene expression in animals.

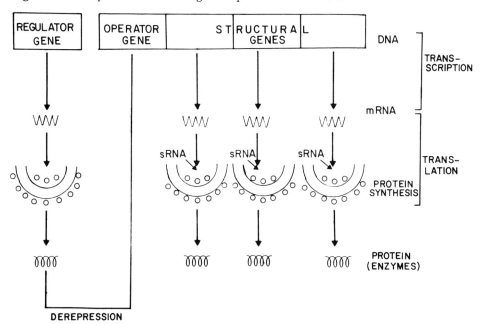

mouse, since much genetic work has been done using "aromatic hydrocarbon–responsive" strains and "nonresponsive" strains. Thus it has been demonstrated that facile inducibility of aryl hydrocarbon hydroxylase activity is due to a single dominant gene locus, Ah, even though it can be induced in so-called nonresponsive strains by potent inducers as TCDD.

8.1.2c. Effect of Induction

The effects of inducers are usually the opposite of those of inhibitors, and thus their effects can be demonstrated by much the same methods; that is, by their effects on pharmacological or toxicological properties in vivo, or by the effects on enzymes in vitro following prior treatment of the animal with the inducer.

In vivo effects are frequently reported, the most common being the reduction of the hexobarbital sleeping time or zoxazolamine paralysis time. These effects have been reported for numerous inducers and can be quite dramatic. For example, in the rat the paralysis time resulting from a high dose of zoxazolamine can be reduced from 11 hr to 17 min by treatment of the animal with benzpyrene 24 hr before the administration of zoxazolamine.

The induction of mixed-function oxidase activity may also protect an animal from the effect of carcinogens by increasing the rate of detoxication. This has been demonstrated in the rat with a number of carcinogens including benzpyrene, N-2-fluorenylacetamide, and aflatoxin. Effects on carcinogenesis may be expected to be complex since some carcinogens are both activated and detoxified by mixed-function oxidase enzymes while, at the same time, epoxide hydrase, which can also be involved in both activation and detoxication, may also be induced. For example, the toxicity of the carcinogen 2-naphthylamine, the hepatotoxic alkaloid monocrotaline, and the cytotoxic cyclophosphamide are all increased by phenobarbital induction—an effect mediated via the increased production of active intermediates.

Organochlorine insecticides are also well-known inducers. Treatment of rats with either DDT or chlordane, for example, will decrease hexobarbital sleeping time and offer protection from the toxic effect of warfarin.

Effects on xenobiotic metabolism in vivo are also widely known in both man and animals. Cigarette smoke, as well as several of its constituent polycyclic hydrocarbons, is a potent inducer of aryl hydrocarbon hydroxylase in the rat placenta, liver, and other organs. Examination of the term placentas of smoking human mothers revealed a marked stimulation of aryl hydrocarbon hydroxylase and related activities—remarkable in an organ which, in the uninduced state, is almost inactive toward foreign chemicals. Similarly, cigarette smoking lowers the plasma levels of phenacetin by induction of the enzymes responsible for its oxidation to N-acetyl-p-aminophenol. People exposed to DDT and lindane metabolized antipyrine twice as fast as a group not exposed, while those exposed to DDT alone had a reduced half-life for phenylbutazone and increased excretion of 6-hydroxycortisol.

The effects of inducers on the metabolic activity of hepatic microsomes subsequently isolated from treated animals have been reported many times. Whereas the polycyclic hydrocarbons primarily induce aryl hydrocarbon hydroxylase activity and a few related activities that are probably all catalyzed by cytochrome

P-448, the more general inducers such as phenobarbital, DDT, etc. have been shown to induce many oxidative reactions, including benzphetamine N-demethylation, p-nitroanisole O-demethylation, N-demethylation of ethylmorphine, aldrin expoxidation, and many others.

Some enzyme activities, such as zoxazolamine hydroxylase, chlorpromazine N-demethylation, and aniline hydroxylation, are induced by both types of inducers.

8.1.2d. Induction of Xenobiotic-Metabolizing Enzymes Other Than Mixed-Function Oxidases

Although less well studied, xenobiotic-metabolizing enzymes other than the microsomal mixed-function oxidases are also known to be induced, frequently by the same inducers that induce the oxidases. These include glutathione S-transferases, epoxide hydrase, and UDP glucuronyltransferase.

8.1.3. Biphasic Effects: Inhibition and Induction

Many inhibitors of mammalian mixed-function oxidase activity can also act as inducers. Inhibition of microsomal mixed-function oxidase activity is fairly rapid and involves a direct interaction with the cytochrome, whereas induction is a slower process. Therefore, following a single injection of a suitable compound, an initial decrease due to inhibition would be followed by an inductive phase. As the compound and its metabolites are eliminated, the levels would be expected to return to control values. Some of the best examples of such compounds are the methylenedioxyphenyl synergists (Figure 8.4). Since cytochrome P-450 combined with methylenedioxyphenyl compounds in the type III inhibitory complex cannot interact with CO, the cytochrome P-450 titer, as determined by the method of Omura and Sato, would appear to follow the same curve. Investigations have in general supported this concept, although in many cases the time course studied is not comprehensive enough to fully document the curve. The nature of the induced cytochrome P-450 has been less intensively investigated. The type I, II, and III substrate difference spectra, the ethyl isocyanide spectra, and the ethyl isocyanide pH equilibrium point of the cytochrome from animals treated with a single dose of piperonyl butoxide or propyl isome have been compared with those of cytochrome from control mice. Changes in liver weight and microsomal protein were also examined. The biphasic effect on the magnitude of its CO spectrum was confirmed in the cases of both synergists, the initial lowering reaching a minimum after 2–12 hr and the subsequent induction reaching a maximum after 36–48 hr. This biphasic effect, when produced by piperonyl butoxide, is accompanied by specific changes in the levels of the cytochrome P-450 difference spectra produced by hexobarbital, a type I compound, and pyridine, a type II compound. In addition, the ethyl isocyanide equilibrium point, calculated from the pH effect on the 455- and 430-nm peaks of the ethyl isocyanide difference spectrum, undergoes a biphasic shift. In contrast, propyl isome has the same effect on the substrate difference spectra as it does on the cytochrome level and produces no change in the ethyl isocyanide equilibrium point with time. It is of interest that two methylenedioxyphenyl compounds that have essentially identical interactions with both oxidized and reduced microsomes both in vivo and in vitro have

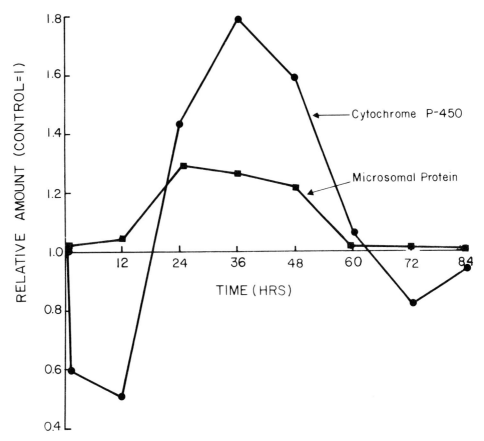

Figure 8.4 Effect of a single injection of piperonyl butoxide on cytochrome P-450 and microsomal protein in mouse liver.
SOURCE: *Adapted from Philpot and Hodgson, Chem.-Biol. Inter. 4 (1971), 185.*

different inductive effects: piperonyl butoxide apparently gives rise to a qualitative as well as a quantitative change, whereas propyl isome gives rise only to a quantitative change. The difference also extends to more general effects: piperonyl butoxide causes a significant increase in liver weight and microsomal protein, whereas propyl isome has no such effect. In both cases, however, the biphasic effect is apparent.

It is apparent from extensive reviews of the induction of mixed-function oxidase activity by xenobiotics that many compounds other than methylenedioxyphenyl compounds have the same effect. It might be expected that any synergist that functions by inhibiting microsomal mixed-function oxidase activity could also induce this activity on longer exposure. This would result in a biphasic curve as described above for methylenedioxyphenyl compounds. This curve has been demonstrated for NIA 16824 (2-methylpropyl-2-propynyl phenylphosphonate) and WL 19255 (5,6-dichloro-1,2,3-benzothiadiazole), although the results were less marked with R05-8019 [2-(2,4,5-trichlorophenyl)-propynyl ether] and MGK 264] [*N*-(2-ethylhexyl)-5-norbornene-2,3-dicarboximide].

8.2. Environmental Factors

Because the in vitro effects of light, temperature, etc. on xenobiotic-metabolizing enzymes are not different from their effects on other enzymes or enzyme systems, we are not concerned with them at this point. Sections 8.2.1–8.2.4 deal with the effects of environmental factors on the intact animal as they relate to the in vivo metabolism of foreign compounds or to the metabolism of such compounds by enzymes subsequently isolated.

8.2.1. Temperature

Although it might be expected that variations in ambient temperature would not affect the metabolism of xenobiotics in animals with homeothermic control, this is not the case. Temperature variations can be a form of stress and, thereby, produce changes mediated by hormonal interactions. Such effects of stress require an intact pituitary–adrenal axis and are eliminated by either hypothysectomy or adrenalectomy. There appear to be two basic types of temperature effect on toxicity: either an increase in toxicity at both high and low temperatures or an increase in toxicity with an increase in temperature. For example, both warming and cooling increases the toxicity of caffeine to mice, whereas the toxicity of d-amphetamine is lower at reduced temperatures and shows a regular increase with increases in temperature.

In many studies it is unclear whether the effects of temperature are mediated through metabolism of the toxicant or via some other physiological mechanisms. In other cases, however, temperature clearly affects metabolism. For example, in cold-stressed rats there is an increase in microsomal hydroxylation of acetanilide, whereas in mice there is an increase in the metabolism of 2-naphthylamine to 2-amino-1-napthol.

8.2.2. Ionizing Radiation

In general, ionizing radiation reduces the rate of metabolism of xeniobiotics both in vivo and in enzyme preparations subsequently isolated. This has been seen in the case of the hydroxylation of steroids and the development of desulfuration activity toward azinphosmethyl in young rats and in the case of glucuronide formation in mice. Pseudocholinesterase activity is reduced by ionizing radiation in the ileum of both rats and mice.

8.2.3. Light

Because many enzymes, including some of those involved with xenobiotic metabolism, show a diurnal pattern that can be keyed to the light cycle, light cycles rather than light intensity would be expected to affect these enzymes. In the case of hydroxyindole-O-methyltransferase in the pineal gland, there is a diurnal rhythm with the greatest activity at night, and continuous darkness causes maintenance of the high level. Cytochrome P-450 and the microsomal mixed-function oxidase system show a diurnal rhythm in both the rat and the mouse, with the greatest activity occurring at the beginning of the dark phase.

8.2.4. Moisture

No moisture effect has been shown in vertebrates, but in insects it has been noted that housefly larvae reared on diets containing 40% moisture have four times more activity for the epoxidation of heptachlor than larvae reared in a similar medium saturated with water.

8.2.5. Altitude

Altitude can either increase or decrease toxicity. It has been suggested that these effects are related to metabolism of the toxicant rather than to a physiological mechanism involving the receptor system, but this is not clearly demonstrated in the majority of examples.

Examples of altitude effects include the observations that at altitudes of 5000 ft or higher the lethality of digitalis or strychinine to mice is decreased, whereas that of d-amphetamine is increased.

8.2.6. Other Stress Factors

Noise has been shown to affect the rate of metabolism of 2-napthylamine, causing a slight increase in the rat. This increase is additive with that caused by cold stress.

Suggested Reading

Conney, A. H. Pharmacological implications of microsomal enzyme induction. Pharmacol. Rev. 19 (1967), 317.

Conney, A. H., Pantuck, E. J., Hsiao, K. -C., Kuntzman, R., Alvares, A. P., Kappas, A. Regulation of drug metabolism in man by environmental chemicals and diet. Fed. Proc. 36 (1977), 1647.

Engel, P. C. Enzyme Kinetics. New York: Wiley, 1977.

Franklin, M. R. Inhibition of mixed-function oxidations by substrates forming reduced cytochrome P-450 metabolic-intermediate complexes. Pharmacol. Ther. [A] 2 (1977), 227.

Gelboin, H. V. Mechanisms of induction of drug metabolism enzymes. In Brodie, B. B., Gillette, J. R., Ackerman, H. S. (Eds.). Handbook of Experimental Pharmacology, Vol. 28, Part 2, Concepts in Biochemical Pharmacology. Berlin: Springer, 1971, Chapter 48.

Hodgson, E., Philpot, R. M. Interaction of methylenedioxyphenyl (1,3-benzodioxole) compounds with enzymes and their effects on mammals. Drug Metab. Rev. 3 (1974), 231.

Mannering, G. J. Inhibition of drug metabolism. In Brodie, B. B., Gillette, J. R., Ackerman, H. S. (Eds.). Handbook of Experimental Pharmacology, Vol. 28, Part 2, Concepts in Biochemical Pharmacology. Berlin: Springer, 1971, Chapter 49.

Parke, D. V. (Ed). Enzyme Induction. London: Plenum Press, 1975.

Sanvordeker, D. R. Lambert, H. J. Environmental modification of mammalian drug metabolism and biological response. Drug Metab. Rev. 3 (1974), 201.

Schenkman, J. B., Robie, K. M., Jansson, I. Aryl hydrocarbon hydroxylase: Induction. In Jollow, D. J., Kocsis, J. J., Snyder, R., Vainio, H. (Eds.). Biological Reactive Intermediates, Formation, Toxicity and Inactivation. New York: Plenum Press, 1977, Chapter 8.

Wilkinson, C. F. Insecticide interactions. In Wilkinson, C. F. (Ed.). Insecticide Biochemistry and Physiology. New York: Plenum Press, 1976, Chapter 15.

H. B. Matthews

9

Elimination of Toxicants and Their Metabolites

9.1. Introduction

The existence of a variety of toxic compounds as natural constituents of the environment predates the existence of life. The original single-celled forms of life existed in equilibrium with toxic compounds in their aquatic environment and thrived or perished according to the prevailing conditions. In the simple forms of life endogenous wastes and toxic xenobiotics ingested with the food moved with a favorable concentration gradient and passively diffused from the organism into the aquatic environment. However, the evolution of more complex forms of life necessitated the development of specialized mechanisms to eliminate the endogenous wastes and the accumulations of toxic xenobiotics. Whereas excretion by the earlier forms of aquatic life was largely passive and involved large volumes of water, conservation of water is necessary for terrestrial life and conservation of minerals and nutrients is necessary for all larger forms of life. Therefore, the evolution of more complex mechanisms for the elimination of both endogenous and exogenous toxins paralleled the evolution of more complex forms of life.

It may seem surprising that higher organisms are able to eliminate efficiently such a large and diverse number of compounds, many of which were first synthesized within the past century. Among these new compounds are food additives, drugs, pesticides, and industrial chemicals that may be deliberately ingested or inadvertently encountered as a result of food contamination or environmental exposure. Other toxic compounds such as toxic elements and mycotoxins, which existed in the environment prior to the existence of the more complex forms of life, may not have previously been encountered at the high concentrations that occasionally occur in isolated areas today. However, with further study it becomes obvious that xenobiotics are not readily excreted until they are in a form similar to that of endogenous compounds that are eliminated by the same routes and for which evolution has necessarily provided adequate mechanisms of elimination. Therefore, in the case of those toxic xenobiotics that are readily absorbed but not readily excreted, their metabolic conversion to more polar and thus more readily excreted compounds is often an important determinant of their rate of excretion. Descriptions of the absorption and metabolism of xenobiotics are presented in some detail in other chapters. In this chapter the physiological mechanisms that account for the excretion of most toxic xenobiotics, the significance of the minor routes of excretion, and the possible adverse effects of toxic xenobiotic excretion via the sex-related routes of elimination are discussed.

9.2. Renal Excretion

The kidneys are the only organs that are primarily and most perfectly designed for excretion. The function of these organs accounts for the elimination of most of the by-products of normal metabolism and most of the polar xenobiotics and hydrophilic metabolites of lipophilic xenobiotics that an animal encounters in its environment. The functional unit of the kidney is the nephron. The components of a single nephron are shown diagrammatically in Figure 9.1.

9.2.1. Glomerular Filtration

Renal excretion is the product of numerous complex processes that occur in the kidney. They are simplistically and briefly described as follows. Glomerular

Figure 9.1 Diagrammatic illustration of the major components of a typical nephron in a mammalian kidney.

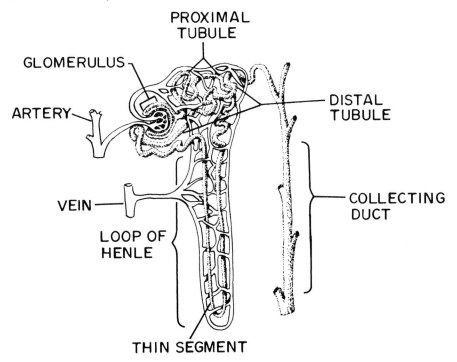

filtration, the initial step in urine formation, is the passive filtering of the plasma as a result of its passage through myriad glomerular pores, 70–100 Å in diameter, under hydrostatic pressure (i.e., blood pressure) generated by the heart. The average rate of glomerular filtration in a 70-kg man is 125 ml/min or 180 liters/day. Glomerular filtration shows no specificity other than molecular size, and any free solute in the plasma that is small enough to pass through the glomerular pores will appear in this ultrafiltrate. Small molecules that are bound to or nonspecifically absorbed onto molecules that are too large to pass through the glomerular pores do not appear in the filtrate. Since the glomerular filtrate is the product of ultrafiltration under hydrostatic pressure, it is logical that any factor that affects the hydrostatic pressure or integrity of the glomerulus will also affect the rate of filtration and thus may result in elevated plasma concentrations of excretory products and toxicants.

9.2.2. Tubular Reabsorption

Because the daily volume of the glomerular filtrate is approximately four times that of the total body water and contains many solutes such as glucose, amino acids, and salt that are necessary to the normal physiology of the organism, it is obvious that most of the glomerular filtrate and its contents must be recovered. Thus, the second major process occurring in the kidney is tubular reabsorption. A number of discrete mechanisms, both active and passive and of varying degrees of specificity, are involved in tubular reabsorption. Many of these reabsorptive mechanisms reside in the cells that make up the proximal segments of the tubules. This portion of the tubules accounts for the reabsorption of 65–90% of the glomerular filtrate. Glucose, certain cations, proteins, amino acids, and a number of other organic acids are actively reabsorbed. Water and the chloride ion are passively reabsorbed as a result of the osmotic and electrochemical gradients generated by the active transport of sodium and potassium. The function of Henle's loop is to establish a mechanism whereby the osmolarity of the fluid in the collecting duct can be regulated. The remainder of the water and ion reabsorption occurs in the distal tubule and collecting ducts, where the rate of reabsorption is regulated to maintain the osmolar concentration of the blood.

The reabsorption of xenobiotics is in most instances passive and is governed by the same principles that control the passage of all molecules across cellular membranes. Lipophilic compounds pass across cell walls much more readily than polar compounds. Therefore, the passive tubular reabsorption of lipophilic xenobiotics is greater than the reabsorption of polar xenobiotics or endogenous wastes, and the renal excretion of lipophilic xenobiotics is proportionately less.

9.2.3. Tubular Secretion

Tubular secretion is a second process by which solutes may be excreted by the kidney. The tubular secretory mechanisms transport solutes from the peritubular fluid to the lumen of the tubule. As with tubular reabsorption, tubular secretion is selective and may be either active or passive. One active mechanism accounts for the secretion of a number of organic acids, including glucuronide and sulfate conjugates, and a second active mechanism secretes strong organic bases. The secretion of weak bases and at least two weak acids occurs by a passive mechanism that takes advantage of the fact that these compounds are much more lipophilic in the un-ionized form and thus more readily diffuse across the cell membranes of the tubule walls. The pH of the tubular lumen is such that these compounds become ionized in the tubular lumen and are thus unable to diffuse back across the cell wall. This mechanism is referred to as diffusion trapping, and, as might be expected, it is very sensitive to fluctuations in the pH of the urine.

9.2.4. Factors Affecting Renal Excretion of Xenobiotics

Xenobiotics are excreted via the same mechanisms by which endogenous wastes are eliminated; that is, polar xenobiotics that are freely soluble in the plasma water are removed from the plasma primarily by glomerular filtration and are concentrated in the tubules and excreted in the urine with minimal involvement of tubular reabsorption or secretion. The rate of renal elimination of most xenobiotics is largely dependent upon the rate of glomerular filtration. The rate of glomerular filtration is dependent upon the blood supply to the kidney, a relatively constant value in a healthy animal, and the concentration of the un-bound xenobiotic in plasma. The concentration of the xenobiotic in plasma available for glomerular filtration is dependent upon the dose, the rate of absorption, the binding to plasma proteins, and the polarity of the compound in question. Since lipophilic compounds cross cell membranes more readily, they distribute into a much larger tissue volume than polar compounds, which are more likely to be restricted to the vascular volume. However, lipophilic compounds that are metabolized to more polar compounds are usually rapidly returned to the circulation and are readily excreted. Therefore, the rate of metabolism of a xenobiotic may also play an important role in its rate of excretion.

Xenobiotics that are bound to plasma proteins are not removed by glomerular filtration but may be subject to tubular secretion as long as the binding is reversible. If xenobiotic binding to plasma proteins is reversible, and if the xenobiotic in question is subject to tubular secretion, it will be excreted by the kidney. The key to this excretion is reversible binding, because as the free fraction of a xenobiotic in plasma (no matter how small that fraction) is removed from the plasma and secreted by the tubular cells, more of the xenobiotic will disassociate from the binding site to maintain the bound/free equilibrium in plasma. The newly freed fraction then becomes available for tubular secretion and so on until the compound is removed from the plasma. On the other hand, certain nonpolar compounds, such as some halogenated hydrocarbons that may be present in the plasma in significant concentrations, may not be irreversibly bound but only absorbed onto plasma proteins and still not excreted at an appreciable rate. This lack of excretion is due to the fact that these compounds are quite lipophilic. Therefore, even if they are subject to glomerular filtration, since they readily cross cell membranes they will be passively reabsorbed as a result of the concentration gradient generated by the tubular reabsorption of the glomerular filtrate.

9.3. Hepatic Excretion

The primary blood supply to the liver arrives via the portal vein, which collects venous blood from the intestines. Therefore, the liver is interposed between the intestinal tract and the general circulation and is ideally located to play its role in the metabolism of nutrients taken into the body and the detoxication of xenobiotics that may be absorbed with the nutrients. The epithelial hepatic cell is the smallest unit of the liver and accounts for most of the varied functions of this organ, including storage, secretion, metabolism, and excretion, most of which are discussed in some detail in any biochemistry text. The metabolism of xenobiotics by the liver is discussed in some detail in chapters 4 and 5 of this text. Metabolic products formed by hepatic metabolism of either nutrient or toxic compounds may be released into the circulating blood or excreted in the bile. Nonnutritive waste products released by the liver into the blood may be removed from the blood by the kidneys and excreted in the urine, or by the liver on subsequent circulations of the blood and excreted in the bile. The end result is that the liver plays a role second only to that of the kidney in excretion, and the liver plays the most important role of all the tissues in the formation of the xenobiotic metabolites that are excreted. However, since hepatic excretion is considerably less conspicuous than renal excretion and is considerably more difficult to measure, hepatic excretion was largely neglected until the second half of the twentieth century and is still not nearly so well defined as renal excretion.

9.3.1. Liver Morphology

The bulk of the liver is made up of hepatic cells arranged in plates two cells thick (Figure 9.2). These plates are in turn arranged radially around the terminal branches of the hepatic veins and are exposed to blood from the portal vein and hepatic artery flowing through interconnecting spaces referred to as hepatic sinusoids. The sinusoidal walls are freely permeable to relatively large particles, but the uptake of certain anions from the blood may also be facilitated by special transport proteins. The mechanism by which nonionic compounds are concentrated in the liver is not well understood. Solutes may be transferred from the hepatic cells to the bile or blood by active or passive processes, but for most lipophilic xenobiotics there is very little transfer prior to metabolism to more

Figure 9.2 Diagrammatic illustration of the relationship of the hepatic cell plates, sinusoids, and canaliculi to blood and bile flow.
SOURCE: *Redrawn from Ham, Textbook of Histology (Philadelphia, J. B. Lippincott Co.).*

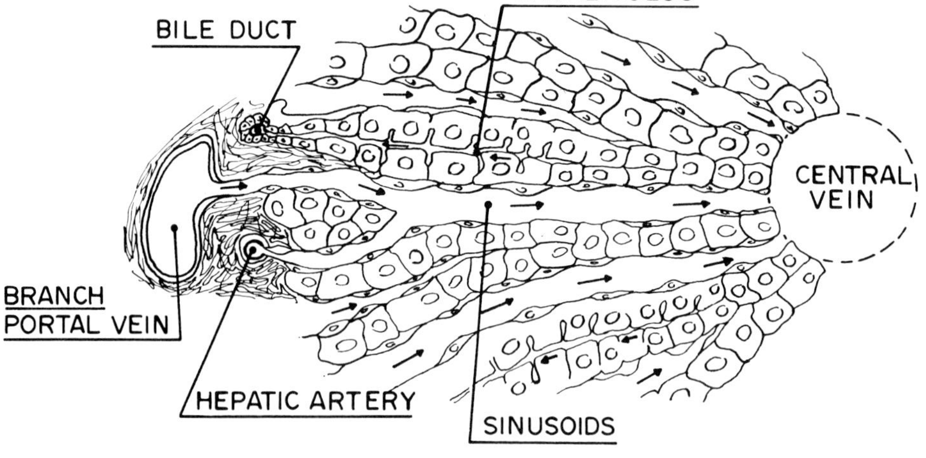

polar compounds. Metabolism of these compounds is often affected by mixed-function oxidase enzymes located in the endoplasmic reticulum of these hepatic cells. Xenobiotic metabolism by liver mixed-function oxidases (Chapter 4) is often the rate-limiting factor in both hepatic and renal excretion of lipophilic xenobiotics.

9.3.2. Bile Formation and Secretion

Bile formation is less well understood than the formation of urine, but the secretion of bile by the hepatic cells into the bile canaliculi, which lie on the inside of the bilayer plates of cells, is thought to be a product of the active transport of certain ionized compounds and the passive transport of other solutes and water which follow a concentration or electrochemical gradient. Active secretion of anions and cations appears to be controlled by different mechanisms, but the compounds actively excreted are usually amphipathic molecules, that is, they have both a polar and a nonpolar portion in their molecular structure. Bile acids are the classical example of endogenous amphipathic molecules. Conjugates of lipophilic xenobiotics are examples of amphipathic molecules that have an exogenous origin. The pKa of most conjugates excreted in bile is in the range of 3–4; therefore, the conjugates are more than 99% ionized at physiological pH, a fact that facilitates active transport.

As a result of both active and passive secretion into the bile, the contents of bile may be classified into different groups. Brauer has divided the solutes found in bile into three classes, A, B, and C, according to their concentration in bile versus blood. Class A includes compounds such as Na^+, K^+, Cl^-, and glucose, for which the bile/blood ratio is close to unity and excretion is thought to be passive. Class B consists of those compounds for which the bile/blood ratio is greater than 10 and includes those compounds that are thought to be actively excreted, such as conjugates of xenobiotics and bile acids. The bile/blood ratio may be as high as 1000 for bile acids. Class C compounds have a bile/blood ratio less than unity; this class includes such compounds as proteins, inulin, sucrose, and phosphates. Factors such as pore size, concentration gradients, and/or selective reabsorption may act to limit or conserve the secretion of class C compounds, but these factors have not yet been defined.

Bile secreted by the liver cells into the bile canaliculi flows into the finest branches of the bile duct, the cholangioles, which in turn empty into the hepatic duct, which carries the bile to the gallbladder. The gallbladder acts as a reservoir where bile is held until an animal ingests a meal. When an animal ingests a meal, hormonal secretions cause the gallbladder to release its contents into the duodenum via the common bile duct, where the bile acids facilitate the absorption of lipids from the small intestine. Some species (the rat, whale, and deer) have no gallbladder and bile flows into the duodenum as it is formed. Thus, for practical purposes the rat is often the species of choice in laboratory studies of biliary excretion.

9.3.3. Enterohepatic Circulation

Lipophilic compounds may appear in bile at low concentrations prior to metabolism. However, as might be expected, a compound that was absorbed from the intestine upon ingestion is likely to be reabsorbed from the intestine if it is secreted in bile prior to any alteration in its molecular structure. In addition, conjugates excreted in the bile may be hydrolyzed by intestinal microflora and the aglycone may be reabsorbed. Most of the material reabsorbed from the intestine is returned to the liver via the portal circulation; however, a portion may also escape into the general circulation. A compound that is excreted in the bile, reabsorbed from the intestine, and returned to the liver is said to have undergone enterohepatic circulation. Enterohepatic circulation serves as an efficient physiological mechanism for the conservation of bile acids and certain hormones. It is estimated that bile acid molecules average ten cycles of enterohepatic recirculation prior to being excreted in the feces. However, when xenobiotics are caught up in this cycle, their biological half-lives and effect on the liver may be significantly increased.

9.4. Examples of Renal and Hepatic Excretion of Organic Xenobiotics

Renal and hepatic excretion account for most of the excretion of endogenous wastes, as well as for the excretion of most of the xenobiotics that the organism may ingest, inhale, or absorb through the skin. The kidney is the only organ that functions almost exclusively as an organ of excretion. The hepatic cells are much less specialized than those found in the kidney and their functions are many and varied. Nevertheless, hepatic cells perform an invaluable function as a complement to renal excretion and in the excretion of compounds that are not so effectively eliminated by the kidney. Many other organs and tissues are also involved in the elimination of toxic xenobiotics, as will be discussed later in this chapter, but in most cases the elimination of xenobiotics by organs other than the liver and kidney is incidental to another function of that organ. The liver and kidney are the only organs involved in excretion in which a major portion of the excretion is active excretion; that is, excretion against a concentration or electrochemical gradient mediated by a specific physiological mechanism. Since hepatic and renal excretion are in many ways similar and oftentimes complementary to one another, and since most toxic xenobiotics are excreted to some degree via both routes, hepatic and renal excretion of toxic xenobiotics are discussed together in this section.

9.4.1. Effect of Polarity on Absorption and Excretion

Unless administered by injection for medicinal or experimental purposes, it is necessary for a toxic compound to be absorbed through the gastrointestinal tract, skin, or lungs in order to effectively enter the body. That portion of the dose of a toxicant that is not absorbed cannot reach its site of action any more than if it were not encountered. As a general rule, the more lipophilic a xenobiotic the more readily it will passively diffuse across cell membranes and the more readily it will be absorbed. Thus, it follows that nonionized compounds are usually much more efficiently absorbed than ionized compounds, and the ionic form of a toxicant, when it effects polarity, may be a critical determinant of its toxicity. There are specific physiological mechanisms that account for the intestinal absorption of mineral nutrients and numerous polar organic substances that are of nutritional value, but most toxic xenobiotics depend on passive absorption to gain entry into the body. Once in the body, polar compounds are more readily excreted in the aqueous media of urine and bile than are nonpolar compounds. Examples of toxic polar xenobiotics that are poorly absorbed but rapidly excreted are the strongly ionized herbicides diquat and paraquat. Due to poor absorption, an oral dose of these herbicides is eliminated primarily in the feces, whereas an injected dose is rapidly eliminated in the urine. Unfortunatley, paraquat is so toxic that even with poor absorption a relatively small oral dose can have dire consequences for the exposed individual.

Even though lipophilicity facilitates absorption, a xenobiotic need not be highly lipophilic to be passively absorbed from the gastrointestinal tract. Many compounds that are readily absorbed are polar enough to be rapidly excreted in the urine prior to any metabolic conversion to a more polar compound. Examples of compounds that are readily absorbed and rapidly excreted are a number of nonnutritive food additives such as food dyes, cyclamates, and saccharine. Saccharine is absorbed directly from the stomach of laboratory rats, very rapidly cleared from the blood by the kidney, and may be detected in urine taken from the bladder as the unaltered parent compound less than 5 min after an oral administration. Other, more toxic, compounds that are readily absorbed from the gastrointestinal tract and are polar enough to be eliminated in the urine prior to any metabolic conversion are the phenoxyacetic acid herbicides, 2,4-D and 3,4,5-T, numerous drugs, and the halogenated phenols.

9.4.2. Metabolic Facilitation of Excretion

Many toxic xenobiotics, such as most insecticides, certain drugs, plasticizers, fire retardents, and other industrial chemicals, as well as the toxic by-products of industrial processes, are quite lipophilic compounds. These compounds are usually readily absorbed from the gastrointestinal tract and lungs and may be readily absorbed from the skin. The lipophilicity that facilitates absorption of these compounds also facilitates their passive diffusion across other cell membranes and results in their wide dispersion throughout the body tissues. However, since these compounds are quite lipophilic they have very little water solubility and are only sparingly excreted in the aqueous media of urine and bile prior to metabolic conversion to more polar products. Even when lipophilic compounds are subject to glomerular filtration or elimination in the bile, they are largely reabsorbed in the renal tubules or by the intestine.

The traces of unaltered lipophilic xenobiotics that are eliminated in urine and feces represent the passive equilibration of these compounds between the renal and intestinal tissues and their contents. Since the contents of the renal and intestinal excretions are constantly renewed, an unaltered toxic xenobiotic may be slowly eliminated over an extended period of time. This rate of passive elimination will depend upon the concentration of the xenobiotic in renal or intestinal tissue and the excreta/tissue ratios, both of which decrease as the lipophilicity of a given xenobiotic increases. Highly lipophilic xenobiotics are usually much more concentrated in adipose tissue than in hepatic, renal, or intestinal tissue.

9.4.2a. Degradative Metabolism

Many toxic lipophilic xenobiotics, including the carbamate and phosphate insecticides, phthalate plasticizers, phytotoxins, mycotoxins, and certain drugs that must be metabolized prior to excretion, are degraded to smaller, more polar molecules that may be excreted directly or may be conjugated with another polar group prior to excretion. Much, ,if not most, of this metabolism occurs in the liver and is discussed in Chapters 4 and 5 of this text. The products of these degradative reactions are more polar and more readily excreted than the parent compounds, and the rates of excretion are often a reflection of the rates of metabolism. The products of degradative metabolism are relatively small molecules and are usually excreted primarily in the urine; however, a portion of these metabolites may also be excreted in the bile, and volatile metabolites and carbon dioxide may be expired by the lungs.

9.4.2b. Oxidative Metabolism

Cyclic and polycyclic hydrocarbons are usually not subject to degradative metabolism. Cyclic xenobiotics are metabolized to more polar compounds by oxidative processes that introduce a hydroxyl group into the ring structure. The hepatic mixed-function oxidases account for most of the metabolism of cyclic xenobiotics. The products of these enzymatic reactions may be polar enough to be excreted to some degree prior to conjugation with more polar groups such as glucuronic acid, but more frequently a hydroxylated xenobiotic is excreted as a conjugate. When conjugates are excreted in bile they may be hydrolized in the intestine prior to being excreted in feces, but conjugates are usually excreted intact in the urine.

9.4.3. Excretion of Poorly Metabolized Xenobiotics

Halogenation is a very effective method of inhibiting both the physical and biological degradation of cyclic and polycyclic hydrocarbons while at the same time increasing the lipophilicity and molecular weight and reducing the volatility of these compounds. Thus, halogenated hydrocarbons have found wide use in industry and agriculture, and consequently halogenated hydrocarbons are widely dispersed in the environment. Compounds such as polyhalogenated benzenes, biphenyls, and naphthalenes are widely used in industry, and chlorinated insecticides such as DDT, dieldrin, mirex, and kepone have been widely used in agriculture in the past. Due to their resistance to metabolism, a significant portion of a dose of these compounds may be stored in the adipose tissue or liver, depending upon the lipophilicity of the compound. Certain of these compounds which are completely halogenated, such as mirex and hexachlorobenzene or on which the halogen atoms are ideally placed to prevent metabolism, such as certain polychlorinated or polybrominated biphenyls, are never effectively excreted and are stored in the adipose tissue and skin for the lifetime of the exposed animal. The more poorly metabolized polar xenobiotics are stored at higher concentrations in the liver and other lean tissues and are eventually excreted in the feces due to their passive equilibration with the bile and intestinal contents. There is very little excretion of these compounds in urine.

9.4.4. Effect of Molecular Weight on Excretion

Whereas it is the polarity of nonvolatile organic xenobiotics that determines whether or not they will be excreted, it is the molecular weight of nonvolatile organic xenobiotics that determines the primary route by which they will be

Table 9.1 Effect of Molecular Weight on Route of Xenobiotic Excretion by the Rat

Xenobiotic	Molecular weight	Percent of total excretion detected in	
		Urine	Feces
Biphenyl	154	80	20
4-Monochlorobiphenyl	188	50	50
4,4'-Dichlorobiphenyl	223	34	66
2,4,5,2',5'-Pentachlorobiphenyl	326	11	89
2,3,6,2',3',6'-Hexachlorobiphenyl	361	1	99

Source: Data from the laboratory of H. B. Matthews.

excreted. The molecular weight referred to is the molecular weight of the excreted product; that is, if a xenobiotic or metabolite of a xenobiotic is conjugated prior to excretion, it is the molecular weight of the entire conjugate that determines the major route of excretion. Conjugation with glucuronic or sulfuric acids increases the molecular weight by 193 or 96, respectively, conjugation with glycine or taurine adds 74 or 124, respectively, and conjugation with glutathione increases the molecular weight by 306. The critical molecular weight for a significant amount of organic xenobiotic excretion in bile is approximately 325 ± 50 for the rat and varies with species up to 475 ± 50 for the rabbit. The critical molecular weight for excretion of organic molecules in the bile of most other species lies within this range. For man, the critical molecular weight for excretion in bile is generally thought to lie near the high end of this range. In all species, biliary excretion of organic xenobiotics with molecular weights less than 300 is universally low, and biliary excretion of those with molecular weights greater than 500 is universally high.

The effect of increasing molecular weight on renal versus hepatic excretion of chlorinated biphenyls is illustrated in Table 9.1. Each of these chlorinated biphenyls is readily metabolized, and in each case the major metabolites are hydroxylated biphenyls conjugated with glucuronic acid. The only factor affecting the relative importance of renal versus hepatic excretion is the molecular weight of the metabolite excreted. It should be pointed out that the less chlorinated biphenyls shown in Table 9.1 are subject to more biliary excretion than the excretion in feces would imply. All of these biphenyl–glucuronide conjugates are subject to hydrolysis in the intestine, and the aglycones, the hydroxylated biphenyls, undergo enterohepatic circulation. On reabsorption from the intestine, much of the reabsorbed, less chlorinated biphenyls are excreted by the kidney, whereas the more highly chlorinated biphenyls are still preferentially excreted in the bile. The end result is an even more dramatic effect of molecular weight on the ultimate route of excretion. The mechanisms that determine the molecular weight effect on the route of excretion and the reasons for variation with species are not yet well understood.

9.5. Xenobiotic Elimination by Lungs

The lungs contain myriads of small, pocketlike structures, the alveoli, which are the functional units in the transfer of gases between the inhaled air and blood. Gas exchange takes place at the very thin, but highly vasculated alveolar membrane and is facilitated by a total alveolar surface area that exceeds that of the skin by approximately 50-fold. The two most important gases exchanged, oxygen and carbon dioxide, have specific transport mechanisms in blood, but most transport across the alveolar membranes is passive. Therefore, any compound in the blood that has sufficient volatility will pass from the blood to the air in the lungs and will be expired.

9.5.1. Factors Affecting Xenobiotic Expiration

Most gaseous xenobiotics are eliminated principally by the lungs. The rate of elimination of a gaseous xenobiotic is dependent upon the solubility of the gas in blood, the rate of respiration, and the rate of blood flow to the lung for elimination. For example, ether, a highly soluble volatile solvent, is more rapidly eliminated by hyperventilation, whereas the elimination of sulfur hexafluoride, a poorly soluble gas, is almost unaffected by hyperventilation. The proportionality among xenobiotic volatility, blood solubility, and the concentration of a volatile xenobiotic in the blood is the principle utilized to measure blood alcohol content and thus estimate sobriety with a breathalyzer.

9.5.2. Examples of Volatile Xenobiotics Expired by the Lungs

Because any compound in blood that has sufficient volatility will pass from the blood across the alveolar membrane into the lung and be exhaled, the list of xenobiotics and xenobiotic metabolites that have been detected in the exhaled air is extensive. Among the xenobiotics that are eliminated primarily in exhaled air are anesthetic gases, pesticide fumigants, some volatile organic solvents, and volatile metabolites of some nonvolatile xenobiotics.

In studies of the metabolism and disposition of radiolabeled xenobiotics, the portion of the radiolabel that is eliminated by the lungs can vary considerably according to the position of the radiolabel in the molecule. This is due to the fact that one portion of the xenobiotic molecule may be metabolized to carbon dioxide or another volatile metabolite and expired while another portion of the molecule that is not so extensively degraded is excreted via another route. For example, the carbonyl portion of many carbamate insecticides is degraded to carbon dioxide. When the radiolabel is in the carbonyl portion of a carbamate insecticide, a disposition study may show that greater than 60% of the radiolabel is eliminated in the expired air. However, when the radiolabel is in another portion of the same compound, a similar study may show that greater than 70% of the radiolabel is eliminated in the urine and that elimination via the lung is negligible.

9.5.3. Alveolobronchiolar Transport Mechanisms

A second, less obvious group of mechanisms for xenobiotic elimination by the lungs are the alveolobronchiolar transport mechanisms. These mechanisms include the fluids secreted by the bronchi and trachea, the lipoprotein surfactant layer secreted by cells in the alveolar structures, and the material ingested by macrophages. These secretions may contain a variety of dissolved xenobiotics, and the macrophages often contain particulates. A number of drugs that are known to have an affinity for the lungs are known to be eliminated at least in part via the fluids secreted by the respiratory surfaces.

As discussed in Chapter 2, most of the inhaled particulate matter is deposited in the upper respiratory tract and is moved up and out by the mucociliary bronchotracheal escalator. The mucociliary bronchotracheal escalator is a term used to describe the ciliated surfaces of the upper respiratory tract which are in constant movement to carry the mucus generated by the lung cells and any associated xenobiotics and/or particulate material into the pharynx. Greater than 90% of inhaled particulate matter is delivered to the pharynx by the mucociliary bronchotracheal escalator within 1 hr after it is inhaled. Once in the pharynx this material is usually swallowed and may occasionally be eliminated by expectoration.

9.6. Elimination of Toxic Inorganic Xenobiotics

Many elemental poisons mediate their toxic action by replacing another element of the same chemical series from its normal physiological role, thus disrupting that physiological function. Examples of such toxic elements are fluorine, arsenic, and strontium, which displace chlorine, phosphorus, and calcium, respectively; and at least a portion of the toxic action of cadmium is thought to be due to its displacement of zinc from a number of metaloproteins. Zinc ranks second behind iron as the most common metal found in the body.

The elimination of individual toxic inorganic xenobiotics is discussed in more detail than the elimination of organic xenobiotics because there are fewer inorganic xenobiotics and because their elimination can less easily be generalized.

9.6.1. Fluorine and Strontium

Most toxic elements are subject to the same storage, excretion, and conservation mechanisms as the elements that they displace. The major portion of a dose of fluorine, arsenic, or strontium is rapidly eliminated by renal excretion; however, a fraction of the fluorine and strontium is retained in the hard tissues, bone, and teeth. It is well established that low doses of inorganic fluorine have a beneficial effect in the prevention of dental caries. It has also been shown that low dietary levels of strontium stimulate the growth of guinea pigs, but this effect is less well established for other species. The most widespread interest in strontium has been a result of atomic testing and the resulting fallout of strontium-90, which is, like calcium, eliminated in milk that is consumed primarily by the younger segment of the population, who then store a larger portion of the strontium in their hard tissues.

9.6.2. Cadmium

As opposed to fluorine and strontium, only negligible amounts of cadmium are eliminated by renal excretion. This may be due to a renal mechanism that has evolved for the conservation of zinc or to an affinity of cadmium for kidney tissue. In laboratory studies of the disposition of cadmium, the highest tissue concentrations are found in the kidney. The second highest tissue concentration and the largest total depot of cadmium are found in the other major organ of excretion, the liver. Animals that receive a chronic exposure to cadmium excrete cadmium very sparingly in the urine for an extended period of time, 6–7 weeks; however, if exposure is continued, cadmium excretion in urine may show a sharp increase of up to 100 times the previous levels. A sharp increase in cadmium excretion in urine is often associated with kidney damage induced by the chronic exposure. Chronic exposure to cadmium results in renal tubular damage in humans.

The primary route of cadmium elimination is by the gastrointestinal tract. Cadmium is eliminated by the gastric and intestinal mucosa and by excretion in bile. Biliary excretion of cadmium by laboratory animals is subject to manipulation by the size of the dose administered and the temperature at which the animal is maintained. The percentage of the cadmium dose excreted in bile increases as the dose and temperature increase. Biliary excretion of cadmium also varies with species and is much greater in the laboratory rat than in the rabbit or dog.

9.6.3. Mercury

Unlike many toxic elements, mercury is readily absorbed from the gastrointestinal tract and from the lungs. Mercury is a general protoplasmic poison because of its affinity for the thiol groups of all proteins. Mercury is concentrated and eliminated by the kidney, which is thus particularly susceptible to its toxic action. Up to 85–90% of a dose of mercury may be found in the kidneys as late as 2 weeks after administration. Mercury accumulates in the collecting tubules, the distal parts of the proximal convoluted tubules, and the wide parts of Henle's loop, but not in the glomeruli. Two-thirds of the mercury stored in the kidney is eventually excreted in the urine. As opposed to some other heavy metals, mercury is not concentrated in the liver and is only very slowly excreted in the bile. However, the rate and route of mercury excretion is highly dependent upon the form administered—that is, elemental mercury or any one of several organic or inorganic mercury compounds.

9.6.4. Selenium and Beryllium

Selenium and beryllium are two other toxic elements that are absorbed from the lungs as well as the gastrointestinal tract. Beryllium is only partially absorbed from the gastrointestinal tract but is more readily absorbed from the lungs. On inhalation, beryllium is toxic to the lungs, whereas intravenous injection of beryllium produces a necrosis of the renal tubular epithelial cells, especially in the distal third of the proximal tubules. Up to 30% of a dose of volatile selenium may be expired by the lungs, and a portion of the dose may be excreted in the feces. However, most of a dose of selenium or beryllium is excreted in the urine. Selenium is excreted the more rapidly of the two, the excretion of beryllium being prolonged by an affinity of this toxic element for the lungs and bone.

9.6.5. Lead

Lead is still one of the more commonly used toxic heavy metals, but its modern use is not nearly so diverse as during the seventeenth through the nineteenth centuries. The gastrointestinal absorption of lead varies with age; adults absorb 5–10% of an oral dose, whereas children may absorb up to 50% of an oral dose. Lead is stored in the liver and bone, particularly bone, where it accumulates over a period of many years if not throughout the lifetime. Analysis of bone samples indicates that consumption of lead by the general population was 10–15 times greater during the seventeenth to nineteenth centuries than it is today.

However, there has been at least one recently documented case of lead poisoning that resulted from the consumption of bone meal as a dietary supplement. In all species most of the absorbed lead is excreted in the feces due to elimination in the bile and by passage from the intestinal mucosa into the intestinal contents. Renal excretion accounts for a very minor portion of excreted lead.

9.7. Minor Routes of Toxic Xenobiotic Elimination

Elimination of xenobiotics via the so-called minor routes is usually the result of passive diffusion of xenobiotics across cell walls and equilibration with material that is subsequently eliminated. In most instances, toxic xenobiotic elimination via the minor routes is incidental to the major function of the organ or tissue concerned. Therefore, any secretion, excretion, or other elimination of matter from the body may serve as a route of xenobiotic elimination. The rate of xenobiotic elimination via the minor routes is dependent upon the concentration of the xenobiotic in the blood, the ability of the given xenobiotic to cross cell membranes, the affinity of the xenobiotic for the substance eliminated, and the volume eliminated. In most cases no active processes are involved, but a favorable gradient for the passive transport of xenobiotics via the minor routes is maintained by cellular secretory mechanisms, by cellular growth and division, or in some cases by the passive diffusion of a xenobiotic from a tissue into a medium that is constantly renewed, such as the air in the lungs or the intestinal contents. The range of compounds eliminated by the minor routes is as diverse as the range of the physiological media that are eliminated. Any xenobiotic that is in solution in or is bound to any substance that is eliminated from the body will be eliminated with that substance.

9.7.1. Sex-Linked Routes of Elimination

Certain minor routes of toxic xenobiotic elimination—milk, eggs, and fetus—are restricted to the female of the species. In most instances these routes of elimination afford minimal benefit to the mother but may affect the health or survival of the offspring. For obvious reasons, the sex-linked routes of xenobiotic elimination have elicited considerably more scientific interest than the other minor routes of xenobiotic elimination combined.

9.7.1a. Milk

Because milk is an emulsion of lipid in an aqueous solution of protein it may contain virtually any compound that is in solution in the mother's body water, absorbed onto her blood proteins, or in solution in her blood lipids that can also cross the mammary cell membrane. Therefore, of the minor routes of xenobiotic elimination, milk may contain the widest range of foreign compounds. The list of xenobiotics reported to be eliminated in human milk contains more than 40 compounds and ranges from polar compounds such as alcohol and caffeine, to less polar compounds such as drugs, vitamins, and some hormones, to quite lipophilic compounds such as halogenated insecticides and industrial chemicals.

Elimination of toxic xenobiotics in milk is highly dependent upon the half-life of the xenobiotic in question. The half-lives of most polar substances and the more rapidly metabolized lipophilic substances in milk are usually relatively short because these compounds are rapidly excreted via the major routes of excretion. Therefore, the percentage of the total dose of such compounds that is eliminated in milk is usually small and the consequences of a single maternal exposure are usually negligible unless the dose is great enough to be toxic to the mother. However, repetitive or chronic maternal exposure to a polar toxic xenobiotic, such as certain drugs, may have an effect on the nursing young. As mentioned earlier in this chapter, lipophilic xenobiotics are not eliminated by the major routes of excretion prior to metabolism to more polar compounds. Therefore, it is the lipophilic xenobiotics that have long biological half-lives that are most frequently detected in milk at the highest concentrations and for the longest periods of time. For example, it has been demonstrated that under experimental conditions of steady-state administration, greater than 25% of the intake of the halogenated insecticides β-hexachlorocyclohexane and dieldrin is eliminated in the milk of cows. Certain other halogenated compounds such as polybrominated biphenyls and certain halogenated insecticides may be eliminated primarily in the milk of actively nursing females.

Intoxication of the young as a result of nursing mothers that were exposed to a toxic compound has been demonstrated in laboratory rats exposed to hexachlorobenzene, DDT, and tetrachlorodibenzodioxin as well as other highly toxic or slowly metabolized lipophilic compounds. However, well-documented evidence of such intoxications requires carefully controlled experimental conditions in order to differentiate intoxication via the milk from transplacental intoxication. The mothers must either be treated immediately after parturition, or if the compound to be tested is too toxic for an acute dose or requires time to accumulate in the maternal tissues, the newborn experimental animals must be fostered from unexposed mothers to preexposed nursing mothers immediately after birth.

There are at least two documented incidents of human infant intoxication that resulted when nursing mothers were exposed to a toxic xenobiotic. These instances occurred in Turkey and Japan, where large numbers of people were exposed to hexachlorobenzene and polychlorinated biphenyls, respectively. A large number of infants and children showed signs of intoxication in each incident. However, many of the mothers were exposed while pregnant and many of the children were old enough to eat the same food as the mothers. Cases in which the timing of the incident was such that infant intoxication could be attributed solely to toxic xenobiotic received in mother's milk were limited but were documented in each incident.

9.7.1b. Eggs

The physiological conditions affecting the elimination of xenobiotics in eggs are in many respects similar to those described for milk, the major difference being the more discrete separation of the lipid portion, the yolk of the egg, from the aqueous solution of protein, the egg white. Studies of xenobiotic elimination in eggs have been less extensive than similar studies of xenobiotic elimination in milk. Chickens and domestic quail have been the species of choice for laboratory studies of xenobiotic elimination in eggs, and studies of xenobiotics in the eggs of wild species have been largely restricted to other species of birds. Nevertheless, the limited data available indicate that xenobiotics, particularly lipophilic xenobiotics and mercury, are eliminated in the eggs of all classes of egg-laying animals.

As a rule, the elimination of polar xenobiotics in eggs is a transient phenomenon and polar xenobiotics may be more concentrated in the egg white. More commonly the xenobiotics detected in eggs are lipophilic and are more concentrated in the egg yolk. Egg-laying animals are often less able to degrade toxic xenobiotics than are mammals. Therefore, exposure to lipophilic xenobiotics can have a greater effect on the young of egg-laying animals because these species may accumulate higher concentrations of toxic xenobiotics in their bodies. Liopohilic xenobiotics concentrate in the more lipophilic portions of the mother's body and equilibrate with the egg yolk during the period of its formation.

A few lipophilic compounds such as mirex and certain polybrominated biphenyls are not metabolized by birds and are thus not eliminated by renal or hepatic excretion. These compounds have been shown to be eliminated primarily in the eggs of chickens and quail, and the tissue levels of these compounds in female birds are significantly lower than those of male birds that have been similarly exposed. Thus, toxic xenobiotic elimination in eggs may have limited beneficial effects for the mother, but xenobiotic elimination in eggs may also endanger the survival of the young and possibly even the survival of the species when environmental contamination is widespread.

9.7.1c. Fetus

Accumulation of xenobiotics in, and elimination with, the fetus may be the result of maternal exposure during pregnancy or the redistribution of a preexisting store of xenobiotics from the maternal tissues to the developing fetus. However, in order to reach the fetus a xenobiotic must cross the placenta. The placenta actively transports amino acids, glucose, vitamins, and certain inorganic ions that are required by the developing fetus, but it may act as a barrier to the transport of certain xenobiotics. However, the selectivity of the placental barrier is somewhat restricted to the more polar xenobiotics. Lipophilic xenobiotics passively diffuse across the placenta and the concentrations of lipophilic xenobiotics in fetal tissues are similar to those in maternal tissues. Under experimental conditions lipophilic halogenated hydrocarbons have been shown to concentrate in fetal liver, adipose tissue, and intestines of the laboratory rat. However, because lipophilic xenobiotics readily cross the placenta in both directions, the greatest protection afforded the fetus is by the much greater volume of maternal tissues, particularly adipose tissue and liver, into which lipophilic xenobiotics may partition for storage or metabolism and excretion. Nevertheless, tragic examples in which maternal exposure to toxic xenobiotics resulted in human fetal intoxication have been observed in incidents involving the teratogenic effects of thalidomide, the carcinogenic effects of diethylstilbesterol, and the toxicity of mercury.

9.7.2. Alimentary Elimination

It has been stressed throughout this chapter that xenobiotics equilibrate with all biological fluids, and this is not less true of those fluids that are secreted by the alimentary tract. The plasma/fluid ratio and the total amount of a xenobiotic that may be eliminated in a secretion is dependent upon a number of factors, including the polarity, molecular size, and degree of ionization of the xenobiotic, as well as the volume and pH of the biological fluid. There is some evidence that penicillin may be actively excreted by the salivary glands and that some quaternary ammonium compounds may be actively secreted into the intestine, but most xenobiotic elimination by the alimentary tract is passive and is highly dependent upon the factors mentioned above.

Unless favored by a pH gradient, the concentration of a xenobiotic in a biological fluid seldom exceeds that in plasma. It is the volume of fluid secreted that, more than any other factor, accounts for the passive elimination of xenobiotics by the alimentary tract. The volumes of the secretions into the alimentary tract are considerable. The adult human secretes approximately 0.5–1.5 liters of saliva, 2–3 liters of gastric juice, and about 3 liters of intestinal secretions per day, in addition to fluids secreted by the lungs and pancreas. Most of this approximately 2 gallons of fluid secreted each day is reabsorbed, as is much of its associated xenobiotics, but this volume of fluid carries an appreciable concentration of xenobiotics and provides the opportunity for these compounds to mix and equilibrate with the gastric and intestinal contents and to be excreted with the unabsorbed material.

Of all the alimentary secretions, the largest number of xenobiotics have been isolated from saliva, no doubt due because of the ease with which saliva is obtained for assay rather than to any special property of saliva. Xenobiotics that have been detected in saliva include the following: antibiotics such as penicillin and streptomycin; drugs of abuse such as cannabinols, opiate narcotics, nicotine, and alcohol; halogenated pesticides such as DDT and dieldrin; and toxic inorganic compounds such as mercury, cadmium, and strontium. Urea, usually considered a waste product, is a natural component of saliva.

The list of toxic xenobiotics eliminated in the other alimentary secretions is probably similar to that listed for saliva. A few alimentary secretions have special properties that may increase the range or concentration of xenobiotics they may contain. Gastric juice, due to its low pH, contains higher concentrations of basic drugs, and secretions from the respiratory tract contain more lipoproteins and may contain more lipophilic compounds. As mentioned previously, the mucociliary bronchotracheal escalator removes particulate matter from the respiratory tree and delivers it into the pharynx, where most of it is swallowed and eliminated by passage through the gastrointestinal tract.

The intestines not only secrete the largest volume of alimentary secretions, approximately 3 liters/day, the gastric and intestinal mucosa also play a critical if not the major role in the elimination of several toxic inorganic xenobiotics, including cadmium, lead, and mercury. The mechanism by which these toxic elements are eliminated is not well understood, but intestinal cell shedding has been proposed to be the major source of fecal mercury.

Finally, lipophilic xenobiotics are slowly eliminated by the intestines by a mechanism that has not been clearly defined, but it is assumed that lipophilic xenobiotics passively diffuse across the intestinal walls and equilibrate with the intestinal contents. The end effect is that lipophilic xenobiotics are slowly eliminated by the constant renewal of the intestinal contents and the renewal of the intestine wall/content equilibrium. Xenobiotics that have been shown to be eliminated by this mechanism are diphenylhydantoin, kepone, and tetrachlorodibenzodioxin.

9.7.3. Obscure Routes of Xenobiotic Elimination

As mentioned previously, any xenobiotic that can passively diffuse across a cell membrane will establish a concentration equilibrium between the contents of that cell and plasma. If the contents of that cell are excreted, secreted, or lost from the body in some other fashion, then any associated xenobiotic will also be eliminated. Therefore, it should not be surprising that toxic xenobiotics have been reported to be eliminated in sweat and skin oil as well as in hair, feathers, and nails, and they will probably be reported to be in the cells of the epidermis that are sloughed off as soon as a method for their collection and analysis is devised.

In those cells that have a secretory function, a favorable gradient for the passive elimination of xenobiotics is maintained by the constant renewal of the cell contents. The sweat glands have been shown to eliminate a large number of metal ions and a smaller number of polar xenobiotics. Sebaceous glands in the skin secrete the oils that keep the skin and hair soft and pliable. These oily secretions are, of course, much more lipophilic than sweat and are probably responsible for the lipophilic compounds, halogenated insecticides, and polychlorinated biphenyls that have been detected in human hair samples taken from the general population as well as in the hair of laboratory animals that were treated with these compounds.

In those cells responsible for the growth of hair, feathers, and nails, a favorable gradient for xenobiotic elimination is maintained by new growth. Many toxic elements, including selenium, mercury, and arsenic, have a particular affinity for hair at concentrations that are proportional to the dose received. However, certain organic xenobiotics, bromobenzene for example, have also been shown to be incorporated into hair.

Even though certain toxic xenobiotics that are extremely resistant to metabolism and excretion may be eliminated in hair, skin oil, or sweat at rates equal to those for all other routes of elimination, the benefit to the individual derived from xenobiotic elimination via the obscure routes is, in all known cases, negligible. Nevertheless, one or more of these routes of elimination may, with more quantitative data than are currently available, eventually be used as a nonintrusive assay sample to provide an estimate of the total body burden of certain toxic xenobiotics.

Suggested Reading

Bidstrup, P. L. Toxicity of Mercury and Its Compounds. Amsterdam: Elsevier, 1964.

Comar, C. L., Bronner, F. Mineral Metabolism, Vol. 2, Part A. New York: Academic Press, 1964.

Fribert, L., Piscator, M., Nordberg, G. F., Kjellstrom, T. Cadmium in the Environment, Second Edition, Cleveland: CRC Press, 1974.

Lee, D. K., Falk, H. L., Murphy, S. D., Geiger, S. R. Handbook of Physiology, Section 9, Reactions to Environmental Agents. Baltimore: American Physiological Society, 1977.

Pitts, R. F. Physiology of the Kidney and Body Fluids, third edition. Chicago: Year Book, 1974.

Popper, H., Schaffner, F. Liver: Structure and Function. New York: McGraw-Hill, 1957.

Smith, R. L. The Excretory Function of Bile. London: Chapman and Hall, 1973.

A. Russell Main

10

Toxicant–Receptor Interactions
Fundamental Principles

10.1. Introduction

The concept of toxicant receptors is based on the closely related concept of drug receptors. A drug receptor is defined as "a macromolecule with which a drug interacts to produce its characteristic effect."[1] The rationale underlying this definition is readily understood when it is realized that the "receptors" for a great many drugs are unknown. The above definition may therefore include enzymes, polynucleotides, and other macromolecules that would lie outside the biochemical definition of a receptor. In these circumstances the putative (assumed) receptors are often named after drugs; thus, the "morphine receptor." Since there are many thousands of drugs, the unwary might conclude that there are thousands of corresponding receptors, but this is not true. Drugs are designed for receptors, not receptors for drugs. Most drugs are foreign to the body, and it would indeed be puzzling if the body contained hosts of receptors waiting to bind the latest drug synthesized by pharmaceutical chemists.

In the view of a pharmacologist, a poison (toxicant) is merely a drug that has been administered at a dose level that results in detrimental effects, including death. A drug that has beneficial effects when administered at one dose level may then become toxic and even lethal as the dose level increases. Pharmacologists have quantified these observations in the form of a therapeutic index:

$$\text{Therapeutic index} = LD_{50}/ED_{50}$$

The LD_{50} is the dose of given drug that kills one-half of a given animal population, and the ED_{50}, called the median effective dose, is the dose that produces the

---

[1] Goldstein, A., Aranow, L., Kalman, S. M. Principles of Drug Action. New York: Wiley, 1974.

beneficial effect in one-half of a comparable animal population. The therapeutic index is of interest when developing guidelines for the safe use of drugs.

Although drugs are of considerable interest, the toxicologist must also deal with industrial and agricultural compounds that are not drugs, such as herbicides, fungicides, insecticides, industrial solvents, fuels, gases, and wastes. In the case of such compounds, as with drugs, the existence of a receptor may be assumed to explain the toxic action. In these circumstances the operational definition of a drug receptor can be extended to a toxicant receptor: a toxicant receptor is then a macromolecule with which a toxicant interacts to produce its toxic effect. This definition may include macromolecules such as enzymes, which clearly are not receptors from the biochemical point of view. From the biochemical point of view receptors constitute a fairly distinct class of compounds that have unique and characteristic functions and modes of action. A biochemical receptor is not, for example, an enzyme; and toxicants that inhibit enzymes or are themselves enzymes would by definition be excluded from the principles described in this chapter. Thus, the action of organophosphate and carbamate insecticides and the diptheria toxin (an enzyme) would not be of concern here. A number of toxins act by binding to polynucleotides (e.g., actinomycin D); the term receptor is applied to sites on polynucleotides. The degree to which the principles described here would apply to the direct interaction of toxicants with polynucleotides is uncertain and so is beyond the scope of this chapter. However, a number of toxicants, including some steroids, act by binding to receptors that are involved in protein synthesis at the transcriptional and translational level, and the principles described here would apply to them.

We begin then by considering what is meant by the term receptor.

10.2. Receptors

10.2.1. Origins of the Receptor Concept

Paul Ehrlich (1845–1915) and J. N. Langley (1852–1926) are credited with independently introducing the concept of receptors. With Ehrlich, the concept appeared to originate from his studies on antibody–antigen interactions. The high degree of specificity that an antibody has for the antigen that induces its production led Ehrlich to postulate the existence of stereospecific complementary sites on the two molecules. The antigen and antibody bound at these sites tightly interlock because they have complementary structures. The lock-and-key fit between enzymes and substrates postulated by Emil Fisher is based on the same principle. Ehrlich later became involved in chemotherapy studies which included the arsenicals that proved effective against syphilis and trypanosomes. Ehrlich noticed that a relatively slight modification in the structure of a chemical compound could convert it from an ineffective to a potent therapeutic agent. This suggested a high degree of stereospecificity in the action of drugs and led Ehrlich to extend his receptor theory to drug interactions. At the same time, Ehrlich introduced the concept of structure–activity relationships, which depends on the use of closely related series of chemical compounds. It is important to note that in extending his receptor theory, Ehrlich had to postulate the existence of receptors, so that at first drug receptors were purely an invention whose existence was predicted on the basis of the observed stereospecificity of drug effects. That such receptors were eventually identified as discrete molecules is a tribute to the insight of Ehrlich.

Langley studied the effects of drugs and other stimuli on nerve action. The key experiments involved the motor neurons of certain skeletal muscles of the frog. When he cut the nerve, Langley observed that he could still stimulate the muscles to contract by applying nicotine at the junction between the muscle and nerve. However, if he applied curare to the junction, nicotine no longer stimulated the muscle. Langley then postulated the existence of a substance at the neuromuscular junction which could bind both nicotine and curare. If nicotine was bound, the muscle contracted; but if curare was bound, the action of nicotine was blocked. Curare by itself did nothing. The material to which nicotine and curare bound was called by Langley, "the receptive substance," and the concept of neural receptors was born.

10.2.2. Identification of Real Receptors

These early studies initiated the concept that drugs act by binding to specific receptors in the organism. With the discovery of hormones and neurotransmitters, a rational biological basis for the existence of receptors to which drugs could bind began to emerge. The receptors that normally interact with hormones and neurotransmitters could also interact with drugs. Hence, it is currently accepted that drugs do not create actions but simply modulate rates of ongoing functions. However, the location of a number of receptors in particular types of cells and tissues has been determined, and the isolation and characterization of a few receptors by the use of radioactively labeled ligands and specific ligand affinity columns has been achieved. The reason receptors are difficult to isolate and purify is that the effects by which receptors are identified depend on their location in the organism. Once removed from the organism, the identity of the receptor by its effect is lost. In contrast, enzymes are readily identified by the reactions they catalyze. Consequently, enzymes were purified and characterized as proteins many years before the same was done for receptors. Enzymes have many properties in common with those attributed to receptors, and it is therefore not surprising that early receptor theory borrowed heavily from enzymology. Analogies between the two classes of macromolecules will be made in the description of receptors which follows.

The susceptibility of both enzymes and receptors to poisoning by foreign compounds and the role that these poisons have had in the discovery of new members of both classes of macromolecules deserve special mention. We have already seen how nicotine and curare, both powerful poisons, led to the discovery of the synaptic receptor at the neuromuscular junction of somatic nerves. Many years passed before it was discovered in 1926 that acetylcholine was the natural messenger or transmitter substance for these particular receptors. Similarly, atropine, tetrodotoxin, muscarine, and morphine have been instrumental in identifying receptors whose natural ligands or messengers were unknown and, in some instances, continue to be unknown. Thus, toxicant–receptor interactions have been of fundamental significance in the discovery and elucidation of many receptors.

10.2.3. Nature of Receptors

With the discovery first of hormones and neurotransmitters and later of the receptors to which these messengers bind, it has become possible to narrow and more closely define the term receptor as it applies to chemical messengers of one sort or another. Although enzymes have much in common with receptors, their action with substrates following initial binding appears to be quite different from the action of a hormone or transmitter on a receptor. These differences are sufficiently great and significant to warrant treating enzymes and receptors separately. The definition here would also exclude the receptors on antibodies and the sensory receptors such as those involved in sight, feel, hearing, and balance. Here the "messengers" are physical phenomena such as light and sound waves and the force of gravity. It is conceivable that chemical toxicants could directly affect these receptors, but it seems doubtful that the interaction would be at a site with the stereospecific properties envisaged for receptors. The same could be said about the receptor sites on polynucleotides, although the context is quite different.

The term receptor adopted here applies to protein molecules that interact with messengers by binding to them at a special receptor site. The shape of the site and the messsenger are complementary, so that binding in many instances is quite tight. The formation of the receptor–messenger complex triggers an action that leads to the biochemical, physiological, or neurological effect characteristic of the messenger. The receptor–messenger complex is held by noncovalent bonds only, and neither the binding nor the action it triggers alters the chemical structure of the messenger. The noncovalent bonds include ion–ion attractions by coulombic forces, ion–dipole attraction, dipole–dipole interaction (hydrogen bonding), and Van der Waal forces.

10.3. Messengers

10.3.1. Messengers: Neurotransmitters and Hormones

The definition of a receptor given above depends to a considerable extent on the meaning of the word messenger. In endocrinology a messenger is a hormone, but the meaning here has been extended to include neurotransmitters and any other endogenous molecule that reacts with a protein molecule in the manner described in the above definition.

Hormones act in at least three ways: they regulate enzyme and protein synthesis; they regulate enzyme activity, largely through actions that lead to the activation or inactivation of the enzyme in question; and they influence membrane permeability.

Neurotransmitters are, of course, a link in the transmission of nerve impulses, and the system at the synaptic junction in which they operate ensures that the impulses travel in only one direction. However, transmitters and the receptors with which they react are only one of a number of messenger–receptor systems that operate within nerves. Whether the messengers that interact with receptors on axonic membranes, for example, should be classified as hormones or whether they deserve some other name is a moot point. Whatever the name given these messengers, it is clear that they react with receptors and that these receptors are vulnerable to poisoning. Indeed, the number of receptors involved in nerve action makes the nervous system one of the most vulnerable to poisoning.

The essential role of nerves in the operation of many vital functions in turn makes poisons that affect receptors involved in nerve action among the most lethal known. Many of the messengers and receptors operating in nerves are similar to those operating in other cells. For example, cyclic adenosine monophosphate (cAMP) operates in nerve cells as it does in many other cells. Toxins that affect the receptors controlling adenylate cyclase, which produces cAMP, or that would compete with cAMP for its receptor site on protein kinase, would be expected to interfere with the normal functioning of the nerve. This in turn could lead to failure of the function controlled by the nerve and to poisoning. The point here is that while nerve cells are highly specialized, they have certain messenger–receptor systems in common with other cells. cAMP also appears to be involved in regulatory mechanisms concerned with the specialized role of nerves in addition to its more general role in metabolic regulation. For example, the β-adrenergic receptors of sympathetic ganglia activate adenylate cylase when occupied by norepinephrine or dopamine. The cAMP produced by the activated adenylate cyclase then acts by phosphorylating certain membrane proteins, which results in hyperpolarization of the membrane. This action is part of a neural inhibitory mechanism:

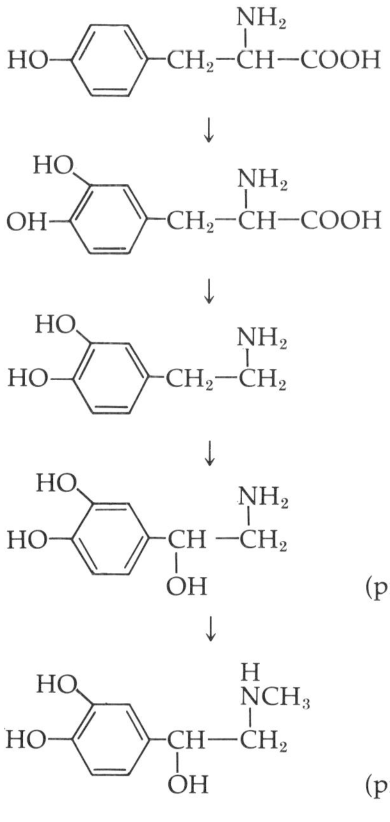

HO—⟨ ⟩—CH$_2$—CH—COOH   Tyrosine
with NH$_2$

↓

L-Dopa

↓

Dopamine

↓

Norepinephrine
(preferred by β-adrenergic receptors)

↓

Epinephrine (adrenaline)
(preferred by α-adrenergic receptors)

10.3.2. Structural Classification of Messengers

Hormones and neurotransmitters tend to bind tightly to their receptors, and it is believed that such binding reflects in part a structural complementarity between messenger and receptor site. Potent toxicants would also be expected to have structures that complement the sites of the receptors since they owe their potency in part to tight binding. It is therefore of interest to examine the range of structures of natural or endogenous messengers since toxicants might be expected, in many instances, to resemble them.

Hormone messengers vary greatly in structure. A relatively large class of hormones are peptides and proteins. The dividing line between peptides and proteins is about 5000 daltons or 40 residues. Molecules below 5000 daltons are peptides, while those above are proteins. Thus, glucagon, with 29 amino acid residues, is a peptide hormone, whereas insulin, with 51 residues, is a protein. There are at least 25 known peptide hormones, including ACTH, growth hormone or somatotropin (GH), thyrotropin (TSH), follitropin or follicle-stimulating hormone (FSH), luteinizing hormone (LH), prolactin, oxytocin, vasopressin, melanotropins, calcitonin, secretin, gastrin, etc. Evidently, the receptor sites on many receptors accept fairly large and complex molecules.

The steroid hormones include the sex hormones, such as testosterone, estrogen, and progesterone:

Testosterone   Progesterone

Other steroids, such as cortisone, have a more generalized effect.

A number of hormones are derived from amino acids. As already mentioned, some, such as epinephrine, act not only as hormones but also as neurotransmitters, depending on the location of the receptor and the site at which the epinephrine is generated. In mammals norepinephrine is a nerve transmitter. These so-called catecholamines are derived from tyrosine, as are the thyroid hormones, thyroxine, triiodothyronine, and L-dopa. Serotonin (5-hydroxytryptamine) and tryptamine are derived from tryptophan. The prostaglandins are derived from the 20-carbon fatty acid, arachidonic acid.

Some of the more common neurotransmitters have already been mentioned (e.g., epinephrine and serotonin), but there are others, including acetycholine, glutamic acid, γ-aminobutyric acid, glycine, and dopamine. Although these transmitters are relatively small molecules, curiously enough this does not necessarily mean that their receptors will bind only small toxicant molecules. For example, the cholinoreceptor, which accepts acetylcholine, binds the large (71-residue) toxicant protein molecule α-bungarotoxin very tightly. However, the cholinoreceptor is also bound by smaller molecules, such as muscarine, which resembles acetylcholine and is about the same size. Thus, while the structure of a messenger may give some idea of the types of molecules that could act as toxicants, it is by no means an unfailing guide.

The number of messengers and corresponding receptors, putative or identified, appears to be less than 100 at this writing. The number of receptors would therefore be many times less than the number of enzymes identified, of which there are thousands. Nevertheless, from the standpoint of toxicants and intoxication, receptors appear to be far more important than their numbers would suggest, relative to enzymes. The reason may be that receptors tend to occupy central and vulnerable positions in the regulation of life processes, whereas many enzymes operate, as it were, on the periphery of the system. This is not meant to imply that enzyme toxicants are not of great significance, but only that the number of enzymes does not give a true reflection of their significance in comparison with receptors.

10.4. Enzymes as Receptors

Some enzymes appear to possess receptor sites in addition to their active site. A notable example is protein kinase, which contains two subunits: one is a regulatory subunit, which contains a receptor site for cAMP; the other subunit contains the catalytic or enzymic active site. Occupation of the receptor site by cAMP causes the regulatory subunit to separate from the enzymic subunit, which then becomes active. When joined to the regulatory subunit, the enzymic subunit is inactive. In addition to situations such as this, it is quite conceivable that enzymes of unknown function will be discovered to act functionally as receptors.

Many enzymes contain allosteric sites that regulate the activity of the enzyme by feedback and other mechanisms. The molecules that occupy the allosteric sites may be the substrate or the end products of a metabolic pathway. Normally, such molecules are not considered to be messengers nor are the allosteric sites equated to receptor sites. Nevertheless, enzyme allosteric sites probably operate by mechanisms that are closely related if not identical to those of receptors. Moreover, poisoning by occupation of allosteric sites is a very real possibility. Evidently, this is one of those gray areas where the definitions of receptor sites and enzyme allosteric sites have so much in common that they could easily overlap. However, enzyme allosteric site mechanisms of toxicity are not included here, largely on the somewhat questionable ground that receptors and enzymes operate at different levels of metabolic and neural regulation.

10.5. Theory of Toxicant–Receptor Interactions

The key elements of the theory are the receptor site and the assumption that occupation of the site by the appropriate messenger initiates the action that leads to the characteristic biochemical, neurological, or physiological effect. On this basis it is reasonable to assume that the intensity of the effect must be related to the fraction of receptor sites bound at a particular locale. The treatment that follows is based on this assumption, but it may not always be adequate. The frequency of occupation may also be of importance in some systems, such as in the operation of cholinoreceptors. If it is assumed that each time a messenger molecule occupies a receptor a characteristic action is triggered, then the intensity of the action may be related to the number of occupations per unit time as well as to the fraction of available receptors occupied. If a messenger binds tightly, as indicated by a low dissociation constant, this may indicate that it occupies the receptor site for a relatively long time. This in turn means that the frequency of occupation is quite low. In certain types of nerves, the impulses repeat on the order of every millisecond. Occupational frequency of the cholinoreceptor by acetylcholine would then have to be quite high, and the duration of occupancy correspondingly low. Tight binding would then be detrimental to the action of the receptor, which is perhaps one reason that the messenger acetylcholine is quite small. Smaller molecules will tend not to bind with the same energy as larger molecules because binding energy is a function of the number of atoms or groups on a molecule as well as of how well they fit the receptor.

A receptor site, once occupied by a messenger or agonist, produces the action that triggers the effect. For example, glucagon is considered to react with a cell membrane receptor which, once occupied, interacts with adenylate cyclase in such a way as to activate this enzyme. Having triggered the action, the messenger or agonist must then dissociate from the receptor site; and the receptor site must in turn be restored to its original condition before action can occur again. An agonist may act as a toxicant by failing to dissociate readily enough, thereby preventing further action.

An antagonist is considered to act by competing with the messenger for the site and blocking the messenger from the site, thus preventing the effect. All these reactions involve reversible binding of messengers, agonists, or antagonists to the receptor site. The following scheme summarizes the concept:

$$
\begin{array}{c}
\mathrm{RT} \underset{}{\overset{+\mathrm{T}}{\rightleftharpoons}} \mathrm{R} \underset{}{\overset{+\mathrm{M}}{\rightleftharpoons}} \mathrm{RM} \cdots\cdots\!\!\rightarrow \text{ effect} \\
{\scriptstyle +\mathrm{A}} \updownarrow \\
\mathrm{RA} \cdots\cdots\!\!\rightarrow \text{ effect}
\end{array}
\tag{10.I}
$$

where R is a receptor, M a messenger, A an agonist, and T an antagonist. The messenger–receptor complex is RM, the antagonist–receptor complex is RT, and the agonist–receptor complex is RA. Both RA and RM lead to effects. The light arrow leading to effect is meant to indicate that the effect does not result from a chemical reaction. Binding is considered to be on the receptor site only and is therefore purely competitive for the three types of ligands. While T blocks, the effect produced by A may be of a different intensity than that produced by M, so the effects may not be qualitatively identical. Assuming the effect can be measured, the scheme

$$
\mathrm{R} + \mathrm{M} \overset{K_d}{\rightleftharpoons} \mathrm{RM} \cdots\cdots\!\!\rightarrow \text{ effect}
\tag{10.II}
$$

leads to the equation

$$
\text{Effect} = \frac{[\mathrm{M}]}{[\mathrm{M}] + K_d} \cdot E_{\max}
\tag{10.1}
$$

where $K_d = [R][M]/[RM]$, and E_{max} is the maximum effect. The maximum effect will be reached when all the receptor sites are occupied by M. The plot of effect against [M] will then lead to the rectangular hyperbola type of curve shown below, if conditions are arranged so that $[M]_T \gg [R]_T$, where T indicates total concentrations:

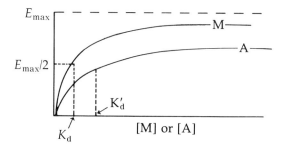

If A were used, an analogous equation and plot would be obtained. K_d would then be given by $K'_d = [A][R]/[RA]$. The schemes, equations, and plots given here unfortunately are not realistic from an experimental point of view. Since the effects in almost all cases must be measured in the intact organism, the difficulties of obtaining reliable values for [M] or [A] are almost insurmountable. Nevertheless, it should be noted that dose–effect curves are typically of the same form as shown above and the underlying reason is the formation of receptor–messenger or receptor–toxicant complexes.

If the "effect" produced by a toxicant were death, or the raising or lowering of some measurable physiological parameter such as blood pressure or blood sugar, brought about by blocking of a receptor, then a toxicant–effect plot analogous to the curve shown above would result.

The principal theoretical criteria for determining the extent to which a receptor would be occupied by a messenger, agonist, or toxicant, are the equilibrium constants, K_d and K'_d, characterizing their binding to the receptor site.

We now digress to point out again that a messenger or an agonist may become a toxicant if its concentration at some vital receptor site becomes too high. As with drugs, the actions of messengers tend to be very complex, and there are many reasons for this. One is the distribution of the receptors in many different kinds of specialized cells. Although the basic action of the messenger may be the same in each cell, namely the formation of a receptor–messenger complex, the final effect may depend on the function of the cell. Thus, the same receptor may cause the skin to perspire, the iris to constrict, the diaphragm to contract, the intestines to evacuate, and the skeletal muscles to quiver—and you may get a headache, too. An oversupply of a messenger at one of these locales may then become fatal, whereas at some others it would be relatively harmless. The cholinoreceptors are a case in point. They occur in peripheral nerves that control a wide variety of muscle and organ functions (e.g., salivation). Blocking of the cholinoreceptor may affect any or all of the functions controlled by these nerves, but death may occur primarily by blocking of the vital breathing or cardiac function. Sometimes control centers in the brain are affected by such agents as morphine, and this results in a loss of vital function.

It should also be mentioned that receptors tend to be localized in cell membranes or organelles, although at times they may be in the cytosol of special cells (e.g., reproductive cells of the ovaries have steroid receptors). Insulin receptors are, for example, located in the membrane of fat cells; and cholinoreceptors are located in the postsynaptic membranes of neuromuscular junctions.

In vivo effects can then be very complex. In order to obtain useful predictive information such as the K_d values, the situation has to be simplified by setting up more closely controlled in vitro experiments. To do this, the location of the receptor in particular tissues, and, further, in particular components of the cells making up the tissues, is determined. The use of radioactive labels on messengers or toxicants has proven to be indispensable for this purpose. Once the receptor is located, the tissue cells are removed and minced, and the receptor molecule is solubilized by a variety of treatments, including nonionic detergents such as Triton X-100, sonication, tryptic digestion, or sometimes suitable adjustment of the ionic strength.

Once in solution, the binding of the receptor by various ligands, including labeled messengers and toxicants, can be studied, assuming that a ligand concentration of the same order as the receptor concentration can be employed. This usually means that ligand and receptor bind very tightly; for receptors are, in general, present at very low concentrations in tissues.

The scheme is

$$R + L \overset{K_d}{\rightleftharpoons} RL$$

where R is the receptor, L is the ligand (messenger, toxicant, etc.), and RL is the receptor–ligand complex. K_d is the dissociation constant and is given by

$$K_d = \frac{[R][L]}{[RL]} \tag{10.2}$$

where [R][L] and [RL] are the concentrations at equilibrium.

The concentration of L must be measured independently of the concentration of RL, and this can be accomplished by equilibrium dialysis experiments or by taking advantage of the different emission spectra of L and RL if L is fluorescent. Equation (10.2) can be rewritten

$$K_d = \frac{([R]_T - [RL])[L]}{[RL]} \tag{10.3}$$

since $[R]_T = [R] + [RL]$, where $[R]_T$ is the total concentration of R. Similarly, $[L]_T = [L] + [RL]$.

Equation (10.3) can then be rearranged as follows:

$$\frac{1}{[RL]} = \frac{K_d}{[L][R]_T} + \frac{1}{[R]_T} . \tag{10.4}$$

The plot of 1/[RL] against 1/[L] gives a straight line with an intercept on the 1/[L] axis of $1/K_d$ and an intercept on the 1/[RL] axis of $1/[R]_T$:

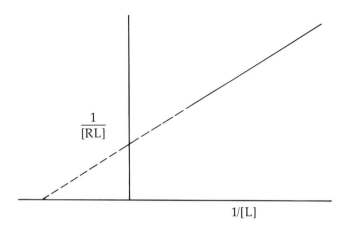

K_d and $[R]_T$ can then be calculated. $[RL]$ and $[L]$ must, of course, be determined for various values of $[L]$. Since $[L]$ is measured and $[L]_T$ is known, $[RL]$ can be calculated from $[RL] = [L]_T - [L]$.

Equation (10.2) can be written in the Hill form to test whether or not the ligand is binding to more than one kind of site:

$$R + nL \overset{K_d}{\rightleftharpoons} RL_n \tag{10.III}$$

where

$$K_d = [R][L]^n/[RL_n] \tag{10.5}$$

where n is the slope. Taking logarithms of Equation (10.5) and rearranging gives

$$\log ([RL_n]/[R]_T - [RL_T]) = n \log [L] - \log K_d. \tag{10.6}$$

If the slope n is greater than one, more than one type of binding site is indicated.

If there is reason to believe that the receptor molecule contains more than one site and the concentration of the receptor molecule is known, then the number of sites can be calculated from a Scatchard plot. It is assumed that these sites bind equally well, so the reaction scheme is

$$R + L \overset{K_d}{\rightleftharpoons} RL.$$

$[R]$ is now the concentration of receptor sites. The total concentration of sites is $[R] + [RL]$. If the concentration of the receptor molecule containing more than one site is $[Q]$, then it follows that the concentration of sites in terms of $[Q]$ must be $n[Q]$, where n is the number of sites per Q.

Then $n[Q] = [RL] + [R]$ and

$$[Q] = ([RL] + [R])/n. \tag{10.7}$$

Since [RL] can be determined and [Q] is known, the ratio [RL]/[Q] can be calculated. Let this ratio be r,

$$r = [RL]/[Q]. \tag{10.8}$$

Substituting Equation (10.7) into Equation (10.8) gives

$$r = n[RL]/([R] + [RL])$$

and

$$1/r = \frac{[R]}{n[RL]} + \frac{1}{n}. \tag{10.9}$$

From Equation (10.2), $[R]/[RL] = K_d/[L]$. Substituting this into Equation (10.9) gives

$$1/r = \frac{K_d}{n[L]} + \frac{1}{n} = \frac{K_d + [L]}{n[L]} \tag{10.10}$$

from which

$$r = \frac{n[L]}{K_d + [L]} \tag{10.11}$$

Equation (10.11) is rearranged into a linear form as follows: cross-multiplying gives

$$K_d r + r[L] = n[L]$$

and multiplying thru by $1/K_d[L]$ gives

$$\frac{r}{[L]} = -\frac{r}{K_d} + \frac{n}{K_d}. \tag{10.12}$$

The plot of $r/[L]$ against r will give a straight line with a slope of $-K_d$. On the r axis, when $r/[L] = 0$, on extrapolation the intercept gives the number of binding sites (Scatchard plot):

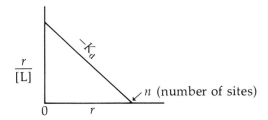

10.6. Receptors and Toxicants

Toxicologists tend to be interested primarily in toxicants of social and economic significance such as pesticides, industrial chemicals, and drugs. Many of these are synthetic chemicals, and they are rarely endogenous. Pesticides may exploit a wide variety of receptors, depending on the nature of the pest. For example, many weed killers are designed to exploit the receptors associated with the indoleacetic acid type of plant hormone, while others interfere with receptors involved in photosynthesis. The widely used and now generally banned chlorinated hydrocarbon insecticide DDT is believed to operate by binding to receptor sites on the axons of nerves and, possibly, on receptors at the synaptic junction. In addition, it has other effects that may involve receptor interactions. The problem here is that the receptors have never been identified or isolated, nor has the action of DDT been correlated with that of some known messenger. This is true of the whole family of chlorinated hydrocarbons, and it means that we do not know their mode of action at the molecular level. This ignorance has been costly since it has led in part to the banning of these useful insecticides, and it has made uncertain approaches to the problem of insect resistance to them.

In general, it can be said that toxicologists are forced to use the term receptor in the same way as do pharmacologists since the receptors for most toxicants are hypothetical. However, with the emergence of methods for locating and purifying receptors and with increasing knowledge of the role of receptors in the regulation of body functions, the possibilities of gaining an understanding of the mode of action of toxicants that may bind to receptors has improved greatly. It therefore seems prudent for the toxicologist to maintain an active interest in the dramatic progress currently being made in the field of receptors and receptor theory. A case in point is the second-messenger concept of cAMP, i.e., that it transmits and amplifies the action of a primary messenger. The primary messenger alerts the cell by acting on a receptor located on the membrane facing the cell exterior. The alert takes the form of activating adenylate cyclase, which in turn catalyzes the production of cAMP. The cAMP in turn communicates the message to the machinery within the cell by a variety of mechanisms, two of which were mentioned in Section 10.3.1. It has become evident then that cAMP and the cyclic nucleotides in general are involved in a number of regulatory mechanisms, not all of which are fully understood at present. Such advances serve to reinforce the continuing and increasing emphasis that the toxicologist must place on the biochemical concept of receptors.

Suggested Reading

Cuatrecasas, P. Membrane receptors. Ann. Rev. Biochem. 43 (1974), 169.

Goldstein, A., Aronow L. Kalman, S. M. Principles of Drug Action. New York: Wiley, 1974.

Goodman, L. S., Gilman, A. The Pharmacological Basis of Therapeutics, fifth edition. New York: Macmillan, 1975.

Metzler, D. E. Biochemistry. New York: Academic Press, 1977, Chapters 4, 5, and 16.

Pasqualini, J. R. Receptors and Mechanism of Action of Steroid Hormones. Modern Pharmacology—Toxicology, Vol. 8 (Part 1). New York: Marcel Dekker, 1976.

Tolkovsky, A. M., Levitzki, A. Mode of coupling between the β-adrenergic receptor and adenylate cyclase in turkey erythrocytes. Biochem. 17 (1978), 3795.

A. Russell Main

11

Cholinesterase Inhibitors

11.1. Introduction

Inhibitors of cholinesterases (ChE) are divided into two groups depending on their modes of action. In one group are the reversible inhibitors that bind to the enzyme by noncovalent bonds to form a reversible enzyme–inhibitor complex (EI). When the inhibitor (I) is mixed with enzyme (E) an equilibrium with EI is quickly established. The minimal reaction scheme for this type of inhibitor is then

$$E + I \rightleftharpoons EI. \tag{11.I}$$

The second group consists of the irreversible inhibitors, which include the organophosphate and carbamate compounds of special interest in this chapter. Irreversible inhibitors react with ChE to form two types of complexes. The first is a reversible complex such as the EI complex in Scheme (11.I). The reversible complex leads to the second complex, in which part of the inhibitor is covalently bound to the enzyme active site. The covalently bound complex is relatively stable, and this stability accounts for the "irreversible" nature of inhibition. The minimal reaction scheme for this type of inhibitor is then

$$E + I \rightleftharpoons EI \rightarrow E' \dashrightarrow E + products \tag{11.II}$$

EI is the reversible complex, and E' is the stable covalently bound complex. E' may break down slowly to regenerate free enzyme, as indicated by the light arrow. The rate of regeneration varies and depends on the particular inhibitor and ChE involved.

Organophosphate and carbamate compounds poison by inhibiting ChE in the nervous systems of most members of the animal kingdom. The particular ChE involved are essential to the operation of nerves which, in turn, control functions vital to the animal. Thus, inhibition of ChE by these compounds leads directly to death. Because of their high toxicity, the organophosphate and carbamate compounds are widely used as insecticides; and in this capacity they present both a benefit and a hazard to mammals, including man. Hence they are of particular interest to toxicologists.

A number of other highly poisonous compounds that inhibit ChE will also be mentioned, but the toxicity of these compounds is not due to their ability to inhibit ChE. For example, tubocurarine is a deadly poison and inhibits ChE. However, tubocurarine poisons by blocking the cholinoreceptor of certain motor neurons, not by inhibiting ChE. Compounds such as tubocurarine inhibit ChE reversibly; and while reversible inhibitors are not the main focus here, there are a number of reasons for considering them. Perhaps the best is that by studying the effect of reversible inhibitors on ChE activity we have learned some useful things about the active site. This knowledge has, in turn, been applied to the design of new organophosphate and carbamate inhibitors and to the development of compounds that are used to treat people who have been accidentally poisoned.

The substrate reactions of ChE are also worth considering in connection with organophosphate and carbamate inhibitors. The most compelling reason is that organophosphates and carbamates react by exactly the same mechanism as the substrates. Replace the I with an S (for substrate) in reaction Scheme (11.II), darken the light arrow, and you have the reaction scheme for substrates of ChE. While Scheme (11.II), with the modifications just mentioned, describes the substrate reaction, it is not complete. An additional scheme must be added; and this, too, is relevant to irreversible inhibitors. The substrate reactions also provide the basic criteria used to characterize ChE and to distinguish between the two main types of ChE. Finally, the function of ChE, insofar as a function can be assigned, is to catalyze the hydrolysis of acetylcholine (ACh). It is this hydrolysis that inhibition by organophosphate and carbamate compounds prevents. We begin then by considering the substrate reactions and the classification and distribution of ChE.

11.2. Substrate Specificity and Classification of Cholinesterases

ChE catalyze the hydrolysis of a wide variety of aliphatic and aromatic carboxylic esters of the general formula

$$R_1-\overset{\overset{\displaystyle O}{\|}}{C}-O-R_2 \quad \text{and} \quad R_1-\overset{\overset{\displaystyle O}{\|}}{C}-S-R_2$$

However, the property that distinguishes ChE from other esterases is their ability to hydrolyze choline esters and other esters in which the R_2 group contains a positively charged nitrogen function. While it is true that the best substrates are often choline esters, some choline esters are not good substrates. For example, acetylcholinesterase (AChE) from human erythrocytes hydrolyzes ACh as rapidly or more rapidly than any other substrate, but the hydrolysis of butyrylcholine (BuCh) and benzoylcholine is negligible. On the other hand, AChE hydrolyzes 3:3 dimethylbutyl acetate, the carbon isostere of ACh, at 60% the rate of ACh, while phenyl acetate is hydrolyzed as rapidly as ACh at saturation substrate concentrations:

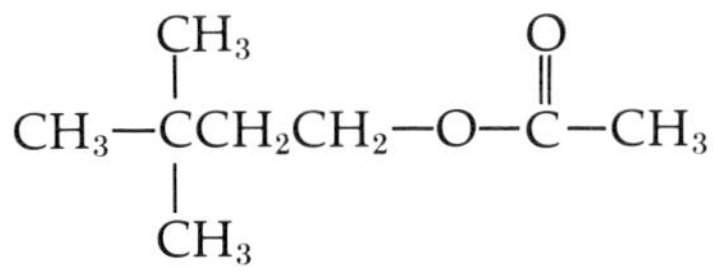

$$CH_3-\overset{\overset{\displaystyle CH_3}{|}}{\underset{\underset{\displaystyle CH_3}{|}}{C}}CH_2CH_2-O-\overset{\overset{\displaystyle O}{\|}}{C}-CH_3 \qquad CH_3-\overset{\overset{\displaystyle CH_3}{|}}{\underset{\underset{\displaystyle CH_3}{|}}{N^+}}-CH_2CH_2-O-\overset{\overset{\displaystyle O}{\|}}{C}-CH_3$$

3:3-Dimethyl butylacetate 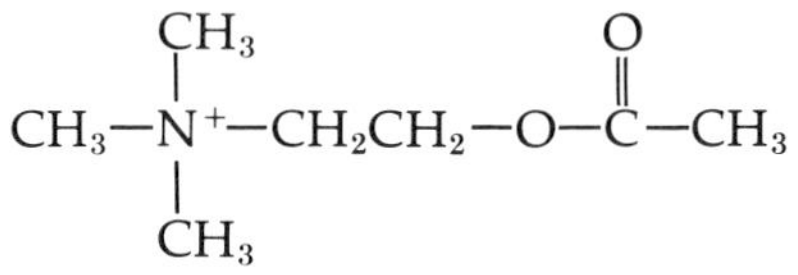   Acetylcholine

Some authors have questioned the use of the term cholinesterase to apply to esterases that hydrolyze aliphatic or aromatic esters more readily than choline esters; but in view of the specificites just mentioned, such a distinction seems unwarranted. What is apparent is that esterases that hydrolyze choline esters, whatever the degree of their specificity in this regard, can readily be distinguished from the many esterases that do not hydrolyze choline esters. This brings us to the thorny question of classifying ChE.

In 1914 Dale suggested that an esterase might exist that hydrolyzed ACh, and in 1926 Leowi and Navratil demonstrated that such an enzyme did exist in the course of work which also showed ACh to be a chemical transmitter of nerve impulses. However, it was not until 1932 that Stedman, Stedman, and Easson measured the rate of hydrolysis of ACh by chemical means and showed that the enzyme responsible was distinct from other esterases known at that time. The enzyme was called "choline-esterase," and it was first found in horse serum. Soon after, ChE were located in the sera and red blood cells of other animals and in nerve tissue, including parts of the brain. In 1940 Alles and Hawes compared the substrate kinetics of the ChE in human serum with that in human red blood cells and found them to be different. In addition, they found that while the erythrocyte ChE hydrolyzed acetyl-β-methylcholine at a significant rate, the serum ChE hardly touched it:

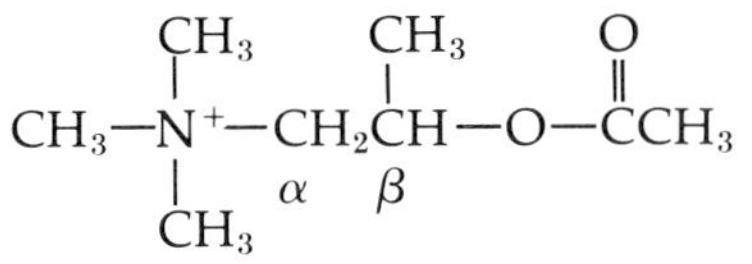

$$CH_3-\overset{\overset{\displaystyle CH_3}{|}}{\underset{\underset{\displaystyle CH_3}{|}}{N^+}}-\underset{\alpha}{CH_2}\overset{\overset{\displaystyle CH_3}{|}}{\underset{\beta}{CH}}-O-\overset{\overset{\displaystyle O}{\|}}{C}CH_3$$

Acetyl-β-methylcholine

The most interesting difference, however, was in the kinetics. With the erythrocyte ChE, the velocity (v) of the reaction increased initially as the substrate concentration [S] increased and finally reached a maximum as would be expected from Michaelis-Menten kinetics. However, as [S] was increased further, v began to decrease, a phenomenon that is variously described as inhibition by excess substrate or inhibition at high substrate concentrations. For both theoretical and practical reasons, the relationship is often shown by plotting $-\log$ [S] or p[S] against v. A typical plot is shown in Figure 11.1.

In contrast to the behavior of the erythrocyte ChE, the v against [S] plots of the serum ChE did *not* show inhibition at high values of [S] but increased faster than predicted by Michaelis-Menten kinetics at high values of [S]. Serum ChE are therefore activated by excess substrate. The erythrocyte and serum ChE v against [S] relationships are compared in Figure 11.1A and B using different functions.

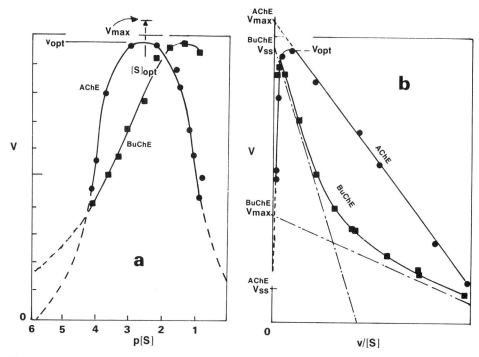

Figure 11.1   **a.** A plot of (*v*) against (*p*S), which is typical of the plots observed by many workers when determining the relationship between acetylcholine concentration (*s*) and its rate of hydrolysis by AChE (*v*). The precise shapes of the curves obtained have varied with conditions, but they have the form of the curve shown.

b.   Plots of (*v*) against (*v/s*) for AChE and BChE. Both plots follow Equation (5). With AChE V_{ss} is much less than V_{max}, but with BChE V_{ss} is more than twice V_{max}. V_{ss} is the maximum velocity attained for the breakdown of the ES_2 complex in scheme II or the equivalent EAS complex of scheme IV.

Augustinsson, in 1948, applied a kinetic analysis developed in 1930 by Haldane to the behavior of the erythrocyte ChE. Inhibition by excess substrate was assumed to involve formation of an ES_2 intermediate complex in addition to the usual ES complex of Michaelis and Menten. The reaction schemes were as follows:

$$E + S \xrightleftharpoons{K_s} ES \xrightarrow{k} E + P$$
$$ES + S \xrightleftharpoons{K_{ss}} ES_2 \tag{11.III}$$

where E is ChE, S is ACh, K_s and K_{ss} are equilibrium constants and the ES_2 complex is unreactive. The equation derived from Scheme (11.III) is

$$v = \frac{V}{1 + K_s/[S] + [S]/K_{ss}} \tag{11.1}$$

Equation (11.1) predicts that the plot of $p[S]$ against v will be symmetrical and bell shaped like that in Figure 11.1A. The maximum v at the apex of the plot is not V, the Michaelis-Menten maximum v; rather it is the optimum v (v_{opt}). At v_{opt}

there is a corresponding and particular substrate concentration ([S]$_{opt}$) that can be read off the experimental plot. V, K_s, and K_{ss} can be calculated from [S]$_{opt}$ as follows: The first derivative of the reciprocal of Equation (11.1) with respect to [S] is

$$\frac{-d(v^{-1})}{d[S]} = \frac{K_s d[S]^{-1}}{d[S]} + K_{ss}^{-1}. \tag{11.2}$$

When $v = v_{opt}$, $d(v^{-1})/d[S] = 0$, and [S]$_{opt}$ at this point is given by

$$[S]_{opt} = \sqrt{K_s K_{ss}}. \tag{11.3}$$

The relationship of V to v_{opt} is then obtained by substituting the expression for [S]$_{opt}$ in Equation (11.3) for [S] in Equation (11.1), from which

$$V/v_{opt} = 1 + 2\sqrt{K_s/K_{ss}} \tag{11.4}$$

Estimations of V, K_s, and K_{ss} are important since they characterize the substrate reaction and allow quantitative comparisons to be made with other substrates.

Following Alles and Hawes, the question arose as to the relationship of ChE found in other tissues to the two ChE of the blood. The initial findings indicated that the ChE in nerve tissue behaved like that of the erythrocyte, while the ChE found in tissues such as the pancreas behaved like the serum enzyme. In 1943 Mendel, Mundel, and Rudney observed that the erythrocyte ChE did not hydrolyze tributyrin and methyl butyrate whereas serum ChE did. From this they concluded, quite incorrectly, that the erythrocyte ChE was "specific" in the sense that it hydrolyzed only choline esters, while the serum enzyme was nonspecific. They then suggested the name pseudo-ChE for the serum enzyme, a name that others have objected to, but some authors still use, probably because no function has been found for serum ChE. The erythrocyte ChE was named the "true" or "specific" ChE; and these names, tóo, are used by some authors. Nerve and erythrocyte ChE hydrolyze BuCh very slowly. This is in marked contrast to the serum ChE, which hydrolyzed BuCh more rapidly than ACh. For this and other reasons, Augustinsson and Nachmansohn suggested in 1949 that the erythrocyte type of ChE be named "acetylcholine-esterase." Similarly, Sturge and Whittaker in the same year suggested that the erythrocyte enzyme be named "aceto-cholinesterase," and they also named the serum enzyme "butyro-cholinesterase." With slight modifications both names have been widely adopted to describe these two types of ChE. Thus, the erythrocyte type is now commonly called acetylcholinesterase (AChE) while the serum type is called butyrylcholinesterase (BuChE). The specificities are compared in Table 11.1. The three substrates following ACh in Table 11.1 are the ones chiefly used to distinguish between AChE and BuChE.

Some of these differences do not apply to insect ChE. For example, fly head ChE hydrolyzes BuCh quite readily, but in some other respects behaves like mammalian AChE. The BuChE in the sera of certain species such as rat and ducks is propionyl rather than butyryl specific. Rabbit serum contains both AChE and BuChE. Broad generalizations concerning the type of ChE in a given tissue therefore are usually not valid, and one cannot always predict the type of ChE by its location. Even nerve tissues contain both types of ChE. The end

Table 11.1 Specificities of Mammalian[a] AChE and BuChE Toward Selected Substrates

Substrate	AChE and source[b]	BuChE and source[b]
Acetylcholine	100	100
Butyrylcholine	2(a)	330(A)
Benzoylcholine	1.5(a)	35(A)
(D,L)Acetyl-β-methylcholine	33(a)	1(A)
Propionylcholine	87(a)	170(A)
Acetylthiocholine	83(b)	140(A)
(D,L)Acetyl-β-methylthiocholine	83(c)	50(B)
L-(+)Acetyl-β-methylcholine	54(?)	2(B)
D−(−)Acetyl-β-methylcholine	0(?)	0(B)
Phenyl acetate	113(b)	91(A)
3:3 Dimethylbutyl acetate	60(a)	35(A)
Triacetin	42(a)	14(A)
Tributyrin	2(a)	45(A)

Note: Velocities are relative to ACh = 100%. Values are based on saturation or optimal substrate concentrations. Interpretations should be made with reservations since K_m values are omitted. However, the table illustrates the classical specificity differences between AChE and BuChE.

[a] With one exception, electric eel AChE.

[b] ChE code: (a) human erythrocyte AChE; (b) bovine erythrocyte AChE; (c) electric eel AChE; (A) human serum BuChE; (B) horse serum BuChE.

plates of various motor neurons in a number of mammals, for example, appear to contain as much or more BuChE than AChE as judged by histochemical techniques.

11.3. Acylated Intermediate and Active Site of Cholinesterases

11.3.1. Acylated Intermediate

When ChE react with substrates, a Michaelis-Menten enzyme–substrate complex forms first. The ester substrate then acylates the active site to form an acyl-ChE intermediate. The acyl group is covalently attached by an ester bond to a seryl residue at the active site. The sequence is exactly the same as for an irreversible inhibitor, but with substrates the acyl-ChE intermediate is not stable and rapidly interacts with water to liberate the free enzyme and acid. The reaction scheme is

$$\text{EOH} + \overset{\displaystyle O}{\overset{\|}{\text{RC}}}-\text{O}-\text{R}' \underset{}{\overset{K_s}{\rightleftharpoons}} \text{EOH}(\overset{\displaystyle O}{\overset{\|}{\text{RC}}}-\text{OR}') \underset{\text{R'OH}}{\overset{k_2}{\searrow}} \overset{\displaystyle O}{\overset{\|}{\text{EOC}}}-\text{R} \underset{\text{H}_2\text{O}}{\overset{k_3}{\rightarrow}} \text{EOH} + \text{H}^+ \overset{\displaystyle O}{\overset{\|}{\text{RCO}}}{}^- \quad (11.\text{IV})$$

EOH is free enzyme. The OH on EOH belongs to a seryl residue. EOH(RC(O)—OR') is the Michaelis-Menten complex, and EOC(O)R is the acyl-enzyme intermediate. It is assumed that the Michaelis-Menten complex is formed under equilibrium conditions, and K_s is the equilibrium constant governing its concentration at equilibrium. The rate of acylation is controlled by k_2, while the deacylation or regeneration rate is controlled by k_3. Under steady-state conditions, the Michaelis-Menten equation,

$$v = \frac{V[S]}{[S] + K_m} \qquad (11.5)$$

is a model for Scheme (11.IV), where

$$V = \frac{[E]_0 k_2 k_3}{k_2 + k_3} \qquad (11.6)$$

and

$$K_m = \frac{k_{-1} + k_2}{k_1} \cdot \frac{k_3}{k_2 + k_3}.$$

If $k_{-1} > k_2$, then

$$\frac{k_{-1} + k_2}{k_1} \simeq \frac{k_{-1}}{k_1} = K_s \qquad \text{and} \qquad k_m \simeq \frac{K_s k_3}{k_2 + k_3}. \qquad (11.7)$$

If $k_3 > k_2$, then $K_m \simeq K_s$; but the condition $k_3 > k_2$ frequently does not hold.

The events that led to the discovery of an acylated intermediate are of some interest since they led directly to the phosphorylation theory of how organophosphates inhibit and to the development of dephosphorylating reagents that regenerate free enzyme. Two lines of study appear to have been followed.

One involved the use of radiolabeled organophosphates such as diisopropyl phosphorofluoridate (DFP). The phosphorous label then remained fixed on the inhibited ChE, which clearly indicated that ChE formed stable covalent bonds with the phosphorus of organophosphate inhibitors.

The other line of study followed from the use of hydroxylamine to determine the activity of AChE by the Hestrin method. Under alkaline conditions, hydroxylamine will react readily with carboxylic esters to form hydroxamic acids. The reaction is analogous to that of water hydrolyzing an ester:

$$
\overset{O}{\underset{\parallel}{RC}}-OR' + HOH \rightleftharpoons \overset{O}{\underset{\parallel}{RC}}-OH + HOR'
$$
Acyl acid

$$
\overset{O}{\underset{\parallel}{RC}}-OR' + H\overset{}{N}OH \rightleftharpoons \overset{O}{\underset{\parallel}{RC}}-\overset{H}{N}OH + HOR'
$$

Hydroxyl-   Hydroxamic
amine   acid

The hydroxamic acid formed is measured spectrophotometrically after complexing with ferric ion at low pH to produce a blue color. The essential point here is that hydroxylamine will react *only with an ester* and not with the acid and alcohol products of hydrolysis. Thus, *no* hydroxamic acid is formed when hydroxylamine is added to a solution of choline and acetate. However, it was found that when AChE was added to a solution containing only acetate and choline the further addition of hydroxylamine resulted in the formation of "acetylhy-droxamic" acid: This meant that the acetate must have formed an intermediate ester with AChE with which the hydroxylamine reacted. The reaction went to equilibrium which favors the hydrolysis products but does include significant amounts of ACh. Thus it was clear that substrate hydrolysis by ChE involves the formation of covalently linked acylated enzyme intermediate:

$$\text{EOH} + \text{HO}\overset{\overset{\text{O}}{\|}}{\text{C}}-\text{CH}_3 \rightleftharpoons \text{EO}-\overset{\overset{\text{O}}{\|}}{\text{C}}-\text{CH}_3 + \underset{\text{H}}{\text{HNOH}} \rightarrow \text{CH}_3\overset{\overset{\text{O}}{\|}}{\text{C}}\underset{\text{H}}{\text{NOH}} + \text{EOH}$$

Acetic acid   Acetylated enzyme   Acetylhydroxamic acid

Irwin Wilson, to whom much of the credit for these discoveries is given, then reasoned that if hydroxylamine could attack an acetylated enzyme intermediate, it might also attack the phosphorylated enzyme and regenerate free enzyme. To test this idea Wilson inhibited AChE with tetraethyl pyrophosphate (TEPP) to form the diethylphosphorylated enzymes (diEPAChE):

$$(\text{C}_2\text{H}_5\text{O})_2\overset{\overset{\text{O}}{\|}}{\text{P}}-\text{O}-\overset{\overset{\text{O}}{\|}}{\text{P}}(\text{OC}_2\text{H}_5)_2 + \text{EOH} \rightarrow \text{EO}\overset{\overset{\text{O}}{\|}}{\text{P}}(\text{OC}_2\text{H}_5)_2 + \text{H}^+ + {}^-\overset{\overset{\text{O}}{\|}}{\text{O}}\text{P}(\text{OC}_2\text{H}_5)_2$$

TEPP   AChE   diEPAChE

Diethylphosphorylated eel AChE is normally very stable, with a half-life of 27 days, and this accounts for the term "irreversible" inhibition. When hy-droxylamine was added to the diEPAChE, Wilson observed 87.5% recovery of activity in 5 hr, indicating that the half-life had been reduced by a factor of about 500. This experiment and others that followed clearly indicated that organophos-phates inhibit by forming a stable phosphorylated enzyme, and they lead to the development of effective regenerating compounds (described in Section 11.6.3).

11.3.2. Active Site of Cholinesterases

The structure of ACh and the point of hydrolytic cleavage might suggest to anyone who thought about it that the active site of ChE would contain two subsites: one corresponding to the esteratic group and the other to the positively charged quaternary N group of ACh.

The possibility that an anionic subsite does in fact exist has been explored in a number of ways. For example, the binding and activities of charged and un-charged substrates and of homologous series of positively charged reversible inhibitors have been compared. The effect of pH on inhibition of AChE by eserine is a classic example. Eserine is a tertiary amine that protonates and has a pK of about 8.0. The positively charged protonated form which exists below pH 8 is then a much better inhibitor than the uncharged form which exists above pH 8, clearly suggesting a negatively charged anionic site.

The binding of homologous series of simple aliphatic substituted amines has been examined to determine the relative contribution of coulombic as compared to Van der Waals binding at the anionic site. A series consisting of mono-, di-, tri-, and tetramethylammonium ions would then permit the contribution of each methyl group to binding to be estimated. In practice this was done by determining the K_i values of each member of the series, where K_i is an equilibrium constant governing purely competitive inhibition of the ChE by the ammonium ion in question. With the methylammonium series, K_i decreased with increasing numbers of methyl groups up to and including the tetramethylammonium ion (Table 11.2). This clearly indicated that Van der Waals forces make an important contribution to binding and, further, that all three of the methyl groups on choline are involved. By comparing the K_i values of the protonated form of dimethylaminoethanol with its carbon isostere, isoamylalcohol, the existence as well as the contribution of coulombic binding can be shown:

$$
\begin{array}{cc}
\overset{\displaystyle CH_3}{\underset{\displaystyle H}{|}} & \overset{\displaystyle CH_3}{\underset{\displaystyle H}{|}} \\
CH_3-C-CH_2CH_2OH & CH_3-\overset{+}{N}-CH_2CH_2OH \\
\text{Isoamylalcohol} & \text{Dimethylaminoethanol}
\end{array}
$$

The charged form of dimethylaminoethanol inhibited 30 times better than the uncharged isoamylalcohol, supporting the idea of a negatively charged subsite. These are only a few of many examples from the literature that strongly suggest the presence of an anionic subsite on AChE. The nature and importance of an anionic site on BuChE has been the subject of much controversy, but present evidence supports the existence of an anionic site on BuChE as well.

The esteratic site undergoes acylation, and we have already mentioned that the OH of a seryl group at the active site is the group acylated. The evidence for the seryl group on the active site of ChE comes entirely from sequence studies with ^{32}P- or ^{14}C-labeled organophosphates. ChE were inhibited with ^{32}P-labeled organophosphates and the excess inhibitor removed. The ChE were then degraded either stepwise or by complete acid hydrolysis. In either case the ^{32}P was always found attached to a seryl residue.

This finding was at first difficult to accept because the OH of seryl, by itself, is relatively unreactive, even though the O is highly nucleophilic. It is unreactive because the H is bound so tightly, as reflected by a high pK greater than 11. In seeming contradiction, pH activity studies with AChE suggested a functional group at the active site with a pK of about 7. The most likely residue is His, since the pK of its imidazole side group is about 7. In addition, the N of imidazole is sufficiently nucleophilic to undergo acylation:

$$
\begin{array}{ccc}
-CH_2-C{=\!=}CH & \quad -CH_2-C{=\!=}CH & \\
\underset{\displaystyle H}{HN}\underset{\displaystyle C}{\diagdown}\underset{}{N\!:\!H^+} & \underset{\displaystyle H}{HN}\underset{\displaystyle C}{\diagdown}\underset{}{N\!:} & +\ H^+ \\
\text{below pH 7} & \text{above pH 7} & \\
\text{Inactive ChE} & \text{Active ChE} &
\end{array}
$$

Thus, the ^{32}P-labeled seryl residues clearly implicated a Ser residue, while the pH activity curves indicated a His residue as the group undergoing acylation. The problem was resolved when the charge relay network of chymotrypsin showed how hydrogen bonding between the unprotonated N of His and the H on Ser could activate the O of Ser by pulling the H away.

Table 11.2 K_i and K_{ai} Values[a] for Various Reversible Inhibitors of AChE

Inhibitor	K_i(M)	K_{ai}(M)
$\overset{+}{H}NH_2CH_3$	6.3×10^{-2}	1.1×10^{-1}
$\overset{+}{H}NH_2CH_3$	6.3×10^{-2}	1.1×10^{-1}
$\overset{+}{H}NH(CH_3)_2$	2.6×10^{-2}	3.2×10^{-2}
$\overset{+}{H}N(CH_3)_3$	4.8×10^{-3}	4.0×10^{-3}
$\overset{+}{N}(CH_3)_4$ (TMA)	2.8×10^{-3}	2.0×10^{-2}
$\overset{+}{N}(CH_3)_3CH_2CH_2OH$	1.3×10^{-3}	6.3×10^{-3}
$\overset{+}{H}N(CH_3)_2CH_2CH_2OH$	3.7×10^{-3}	3.6×10^{-3}
$\overset{+}{N}(CH_3)_3CH_2CH_2Cl$	1.85×10^{-3}	4.3×10^{-3}
$\overset{+}{N}(C_2H_5)_4$ (TEA)	1.2×10^{-3}	7.6×10^{-3}
$\overset{+}{N}(C_3H_7)_4$	1.2×10^{-4}	2.0×10^{-4}
$\overset{+}{N}(C_4H_9)_4$	6.7×10^{-5}	1.4×10^{-4}
$\overset{+}{N}(C_5H_{11})_5$	3.8×10^{-4}	9.0×10^{-4}
$\overset{+}{N}(CH_3)_3$ phenyl (PTA)	5.3×10^{-5}	2.0×10^{-3}
	7.7×10^{-5}	5.7×10^{-4}
$\overset{+}{N}(CH_3)_3$ phenyl-OH	6.3×10^{-7}	1.4×10^{-5}
$\overset{+}{N}(CH_3)_4(CH_2)_{10}\overset{+}{N}(CH_3)_4$ (decamethonium)	5.8×10^{-6}	1.3×10^{-5}
(bis-pyridinium NH₂ compound)	5.2×10^{-8}	—
(atropine)	4.0×10^{-3}	—

[a] K_i measures binding to free enzyme; K_{ai} measures binding to the acylated enzyme.

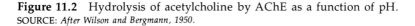

$$H-N\underset{HC=\underset{His}{C}}{\overset{\overset{\overset{H}{C}}{}}{}}N: \longleftrightarrow \cdots\cdots H \longleftrightarrow \cdots\cdots O-Ser$$

Whether the ChE network includes an Asp or Glu carboxylate is not known. The evidence for both a His and a Ser residue operating at the esteratic site is convincing. The effect of pH on the esteratic site of ChE can be summarized by the scheme in Figure 11.2. The second H of EH_2 is included because, after reaching a maximum in the region of pH 8, the activity begins to fall again, indicating a second ionizing group with a pK_2 of about 9.3. Ionization of the OH group on a Tyr residue has been suggested for this group.

$$-CH_2-\underset{}{\overset{}{\bigcirc}}-OH \rightleftharpoons H^+ + -CH_2-\underset{}{\overset{}{\bigcirc}}-O^-$$

active below pH 9   inactive above pH 9

Tyrosine

The active site of ChE may then be depicted as having two pockets: an esteratic pocket containing His, Ser, and Tyr side groups and an anionic pocket containing the ionized carboxylate side group either Asp or Glu. The active site, with a molecule of ACh on it, is shown in Figure 11.3, which might correspond to the ES reversible-binding complex.

The pH activity curve for BuChE increases in the same way as the AChE

Figure 11.2 Hydrolysis of acetylcholine by AChE as a function of pH.
SOURCE: *After Wilson and Bergmann, 1950.*

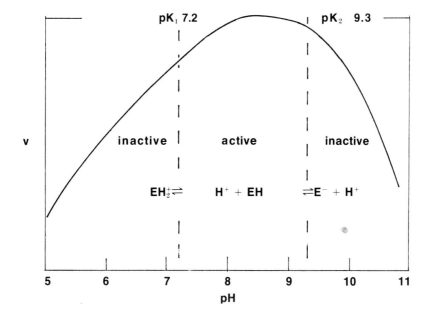

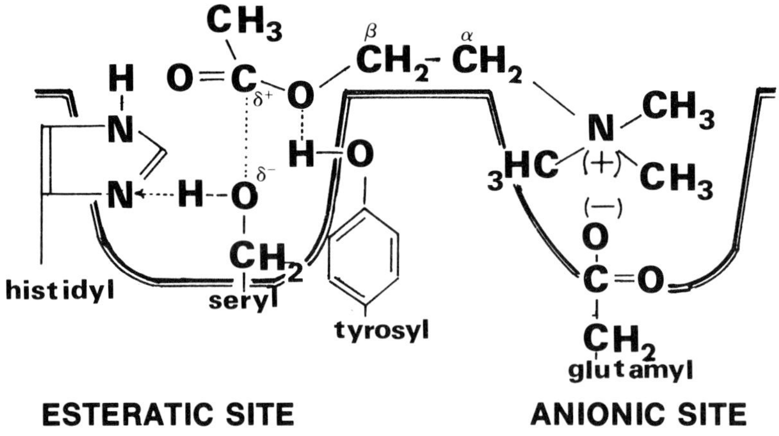

Figure 11.3 The two-pocket model of the active site of AChE. A molecule of ACh occupies the site with an orientation which allows the relatively positive carbonyl carbon (C=O) to interact with the nucleophilic oxygen on the activated hydroxyl group of serine. Activation occurs by hydrogen bonding to an imidazole nitrogen as shown. Other hydrogen bonds are conjecture. The convention of naming the carbons of the ACh ethylene bridge is also shown.

curve, but the activity does not begin to decrease until about pH 9–9.5, after which it may drop. The reports describing the behavior of BuChE at high pH are frequently contradictory.

11.3.3. Explanation of Inhibition at High Substrate Concentrations

Given an active site with an anionic subsite and a reaction scheme with an acyl intermediate, two explanations for inhibition at high substrate concentrations seem possible. The first was suggested in 1943 by Zeller and Besseger and involved binding of one molecule of substrate by only its ester group to the esteratic site, while another bound to the anionic site by only its quaternary N group. The ES_2 complex thus formed would be unreactive, as assumed in Scheme (11.III). With the advent of the concept of an acylated enzyme intermediate, another possibility became apparent. This involved binding of a second molecule of substrate by its positive quaternary N to the empty anionic pocket of the acylated enzyme to form an EAS complex. If the substrate in the following scheme is depicted as AB, where A is the acyl group and B is the alcohol leaving group, the reactions leading to the second possibility are as follows:

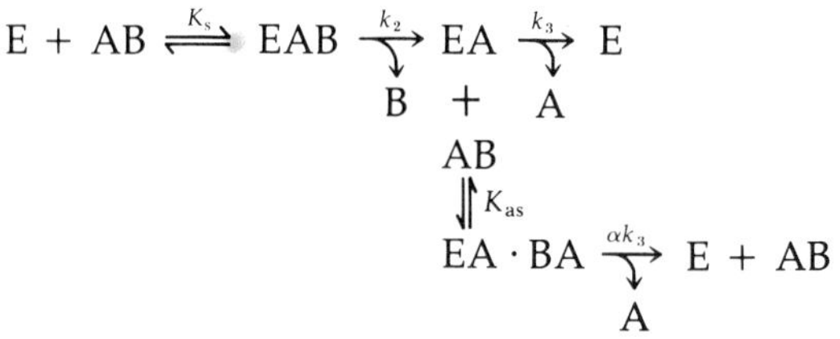

$$
\begin{array}{c}
E + AB \xrightleftharpoons{K_s} EAB \xrightarrow{k_2} EA \xrightarrow{k_3} E \\
\qquad\qquad\quad B\ +\ A \\
\qquad\qquad\quad AB \\
\qquad\qquad\quad \big\updownarrow K_{as} \\
\qquad\qquad\quad EA \cdot BA \xrightarrow{\alpha k_3} E + AB \\
\qquad\qquad\qquad\qquad A
\end{array}
$$

The formation of EA·BA is governed by K_{as}. If EA·BA is unreactive, α of αk_3 is zero. However, it is now apparent that when ACh is the substrate, $\alpha = 0.1$, and EA·BA is, in fact, reactive. This has important consequences with respect to reaction with reversible inhibitors since such inhibitors can form an EAI complex, analogous to the EAS complex, as well as an EI complex. There is no way that an ES_2 complex could be reactive, and for this and other reasons it is now generally accepted that inhibition by excess substrate involves formation of an EAS complex and that an ES_2 complex is of little significance. The equation derived from Scheme (11.V), assuming $\alpha = 0$, is of exactly the same form as Equation (11.1), except that K_{as} is substituted for K_{ss}.

11.4. Reversible Inhibitors

Almost all reversible inhibitors of interest contain at least one positively charged N group. This group attaches to the negatively charged anionic site by a combination of coulombic and Van der Waal forces. Reversible inhibitors of ChE therefore inhibit, at least in part, by occupation of the anionic site.

Reversible inhibitors range from relatively simple compounds such as protonated triethylamine and tetramethylammonium ions to such complex compounds as d-tubocurarine:

d-Tubocurarine

The best inhibitors are either tertiary amines or quaternary ammonium ions. Primary and secondary amines are not good inhibitors, largely because they are deficient in the alkyl groups which contribute a major portion of the energy-binding inhibitors to the anionic site. Among the best inhibitors are compounds containing aromatic groups in addition to a charged N function. That sites outside the anionic pocket can also contribute greatly to binding is suggested by the 3-hydroxy group on 3-hydroxyphenyl trimethylammonium, which binds 122 times better than phenyl trimethylammonium ion.

A bis- (standing for bisymmetrical) quaternary compound, decamethonium, is also included in Table 11.2. Bis-quaternary compounds were introduced in 1948 by Barlow and Ing, who became curious about the structural features of d-tubocurarine that are responsible for its potency as a neuropharmaceutical. They noted the two symmetrically disposed quaternary N groups in the isoquinolinium rings and wondered if they might be the key feature. To test this hypothesis they made a number of homologous series of bis-quaternary compounds, including a series in which the quaternary functions were separated by a straight-chain polymethylene bridge, i.e., $(CH_3)_3\overset{+}{N}-(CH_2)_n-\overset{+}{N}(CH_3)_3$.

When n was 10–12, inhibition of AChE was maximal, and the distance separating the quaternary N groups was 14–15 Å. This distance is the same as that separating the quaternary N's on tubocurarine, indicating that the potency of tubocurarine as an AChE inhibitor does depend on the bis-quaternary N groups. Some of the most powerful carbamate inhibitors and the most effective re-activators of phosphate-inhibited AChE contain bis-quaternary groups. In con-trast, bis-quaternary compounds are relatively poor inhibitors of BuChE.

Table 11.2 contains a compound with quaternary N groups in unsaturated rings, in addition to substituted N in a saturated ring structure (i.e., atropine). The N in saturated ring structures can be tertiary as well as quaternary since the N in saturated ring structures acts like the N in aliphatic amines and is proto-nated at and below pH 8. However, the tertiary N in unsaturated rings, such as the N of pyridine, are largely unprotonated at pH 7 and contain no charge. Consequently, they are poor inhibitors. However, quaternary N in unsaturated rings, such as methylpyridinium, are relatively good inhibitors:

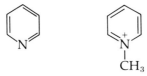

Pyridine   Methylpyridinium

We turn briefly now to the kinetics of reversible inhibition. Inhibition by reversible inhibitors is usually studied by mixing the inhibitor with substrate and measuring the velocity. The inhibitor can bind with the free enzyme:

$$E + I \underset{}{\overset{K_i}{\rightleftharpoons}} EI.$$

It can also bind to EA to form EAI. EAI in turn can yield products,

$$EA + I \underset{}{\overset{K_{ai}}{\rightleftharpoons}} EAI \xrightarrow{\beta k_3} EI + products.$$

If the reaction is carried on at high substrate concentrations, then the following additional reaction may occur if the substrate is a choline ester:

$$EA + S \underset{}{\overset{K_{as}}{\rightleftharpoons}} EAS \xrightarrow{\alpha k_3} ES' + products.$$

We assume that ES' is formed in negligible amounts, meaning that K_s^0 in the following scheme is very large. Reversible inhibition in the presence of sub-strate under steady-state conditions can then be described by the following sequence:

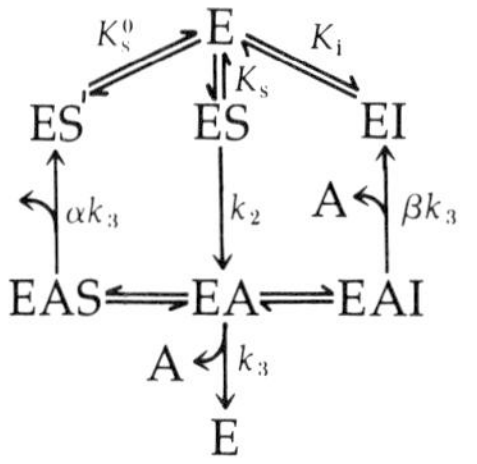

$$\tag{11.VI}$$

The equation is then

$$v = \frac{V[1 + (\alpha[I]/K_{ai}) + (\beta[S]/K_{as})]}{1 + K_m/[S])[1 + ([I]/K_i)] + ([S]/K_{as'}) + ([I]/K_{ai'}) + (K_m/K_s^0)} .$$
(11.8)

Scheme (11.VI) can be simplified by experimental manipulation. For example, at high substrate concentrations the reaction to form EI may be negligible since the concentration of free enzyme will be low. The $[I]/K_i$ term in Equation (11.8) can then be ignored. If a neutral substrate such as phenyl acetate is used, no EAS complex is formed, and so on.

Thus, by making suitable experimental provisions, K_i and K_{ai} can be evaluated, and these values are included in Table 11.2. Comparison of K_i and K_{ai} values then indicates that binding of a reversible inhibitor to the free enzyme is often significantly different from binding to the acylated enzyme. Since the irreversible inhibitors and substrates react by the same mechanism, reversible inhibitors can interact during irreversible inhibition in a manner that is precisely analogous with that just outlined. However, the kinetic treatment then differs somewhat, as will be described in the following section.

11.5. Irreversible Inhibitors of Cholinesterases

11.5.1. Kinetics of Irreversible Inhibition

Organophosphates and carbamates react with ChE by the same mechanism as do the substrates, but the kinetics of their reaction are treated differently. The reason is that the inhibited enzyme is not regenerated to any appreciable extent during the first minutes or hours, so that the reaction must proceed for a relatively long time before a steady state is approximated. Regeneration of free enzyme from carbamylated complexes is frequently fast enough to permit a steady state to be reached, but even here, the information obtained under steady-state conditions may not adequately describe the power of the inhibitor. The inhibitory power depends on the rate at which the phosphorylated or carbamylated complex is formed as well as on its stability. The rate of formation is measured during the initial period of the reaction, before steady-state conditions are approached. The rate of regeneration is usually measured by removing or diluting the inhibitor and by complexing the free enzyme with substrate so that further inhibition is effectively stopped. Rates of regeneration are then measured in the absence of further inhibition. However, rates of regeneration can be measured at steady state as well.

11.5.2. pI_{50}

The first published experiments with organophosphates were based on protocols developed earlier to study inhibition of ChE by carbamates, particularly eserine. The essential feature of this protocol, and the feature that distinguished it from protocols for reversible inhibitors, was that the inhibitor was incubated with the ChE for some convenient, measured time before substrate was added to measure residual activity. With reversible inhibitors it does not matter what order substrate, inhibitor, and enzyme are added. To determine an I_{50}, a range of inhibitor concentrations was chosen such that the lowest caused almost no inhibition and the highest almost complete inhibition after incubation with the enzyme for the constant time interval selected. The percent inhibition was then plotted against the inhibitor concentration, expressed in terms of its negative log, p[I]. A smooth curve was drawn through the points, and the pI value that intersected the curve at 50% inhibition was the pI_{50}. Inhibition is frequently reported as a pI_{50} value, but the I_{50} calculated from it is also used.

11.5.3. Bimolecular Rate Constant k_i

If an organophosphate is pictured as consisting of a phosphorylating group, P joined to a leaving group X to form PX, then the earliest accepted inhibition scheme was

$$E + PX \xrightarrow[X]{k_i} EP \qquad (11.VII)$$

Scheme (11.VII) pictures a simple bimolecular reaction between E and PX to form EP. The reaction is governed by the bimolecular rate constant k_i. Aldridge proposed this formulation in 1950 when he recognized that inhibition of AChE by the organophosphate paraoxon,

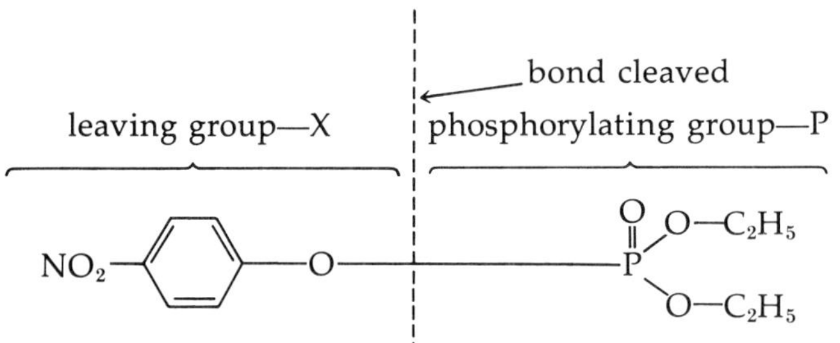

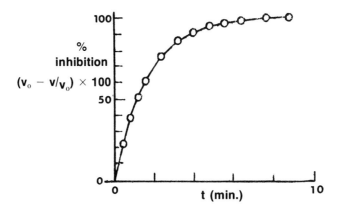

Paraoxon

(diethyl p-nitrophenyl phosphate)

was progressive with time, and, as shown below, followed an exponential curve:

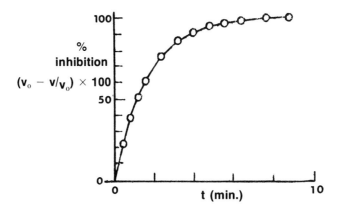

From Scheme (11.VII), the rate of the reaction is given by

$$\frac{-d[E]}{dt} = \frac{-d([E]_0 - [EP])}{dt} = \frac{d[EP]}{dt} = k_i([E]_0 - [EP])[E]_0 \qquad (11.9)$$

where the relationship $[E] = [E]_0 - [EP]$ follows from the conservation equation $[E]_0 = [E] + [EP]$. Arrangement of Equation (11.9) for integration between the limits $[EP] = 0$ when $t = 0$ and $[EP] = [EP]$ when $t = t$ gives

$$\ln \left(\frac{[E]_0}{[E]_0 - [EP]} \right) = k_i[I]t. \qquad (11.10)$$

Equation (11.10) is converted to a form that makes use of the experimentally determined values v_0 and v by substituting (v_0/v) for $[E]_0/([E]_0 - [EP])$. This can be done since $v \ \alpha([E]_0 - [EP]) = [E]$. Equation (11.10) then becomes

$$\ln (v_0/v) = k_i[I]t. \qquad (11.11)$$

$[I]$ approximates $[I]_0$ and is essentially constant over the course of inhibition because $[I]_0$ is chosen so that it is much greater than $[E]_0$. Consequently, $[I]_0 - [E_0] \simeq [I]_0$. Since $[I]$ remains constant, the reaction is essentially first order with respect to $[E]$. To determine the first-order rate constant at a given constant value of $[I]$, Equation (11.11) is written in the linear form (Figure 11.4A):

$$\ln v = -k_i[I]t + \ln v_0. \qquad (11.12)$$

The plot of $\ln v$ against t gives a straight line with a slope of $-k_i[I]$, from which k_i can be calculated since $[I]$ is known. The dimensions of k_i are $M^{-1}t^{-1}$, or $(\text{moles/liter})^{-1}t^{-1}$, and are those of a bimolecular rate constant. The k_i values of some common organophosphate inhibitors are given in Table 11.3.

The relationship of I_{50} to k_i is obtained by placing $v = 0.5v_0$ in Equation (11.11). Then $\ln 2 = 0.693 = tk_iI_{50}$. If the AChE were inhibited 50% in 15 min and the k_i were that of paraoxon, 1.1×10^{-6} $M^{-1}min^{-1}$, then $I_{50} = 0.693/tk_i = 4.2 \times 10^{-8}$ M and the pI_{50} is 7.38.

An I_{50} value of 4×10^{-8} M may be approaching the AChE concentration, so it would be possible that the inhibitor and enzyme concentration would be about equal. The reaction would then follow second-order kinetics (Figure 11.4B). For very good inhibitors the I_{50} value might approximate one-half the enzyme concentration since, in a period of 15 min, the reaction may have gone to completion. In spite of such possibilities, I_{50} values have over the years proven to give reliable indications of relative inhibitory power, and they continue to be widely used.

The first-order rate constant ρ is given by

$$\rho = \ln (v/v_0)/t = [I]k_i. \qquad (11.13)$$

ρ has an experimental meaning, $\ln (v/v_0)/t$, and a theoretical meaning, $[I]k_i$. The theoretical meaning is dictated by Scheme (11.VII), from which Equation (11.13)

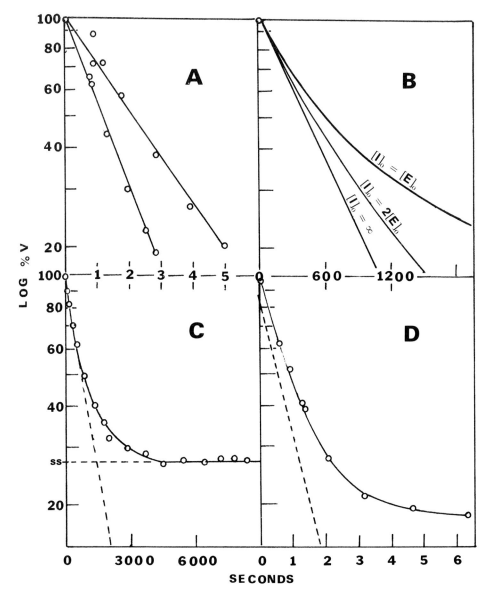

Figure 11.4 Inhibition progress curves. **A.** First-order rate plots for inhibition of bovine erythrocyte acetylcholinesterase by 2×10^{-4}M and 5×10^{-4}M di-n-propyl p-nitrophenyl phosphate (n-propyl paraoxon) at 5°C, pH 7.6. The first-order rate constants (ρ) were 20 min^{-1} and 33.6 min^{-1}. **B.** Theoretical inhibition progress curves illustrating curving as the initial inhibitor concentration, $[I_0]$, approaches the initial enzyme concentration $[E]_0$: $[I]_0 \rightarrow [E]_0$. The curves were calculated by assuming that $k_i = 1 \times 10^7$M^{-1}min^{-1}; that $i_0 = 1 \times 10^{-8}$M; and that (a) $[I]_0 = [E]_0$, (b) $[I]_0 = 2[E]_0$, (c) $[I]_0 \gg [E]_0$. **C.** Inhibition progress curve when regeneration is significant. The reaction reached a steady state at about 4500 sec. The curve is that for the inhibition of bovine erythrocyte acetylcholinesterase by 2×10^{-4}M phenyl N-methyl carbamate at 25°C, pH 7.6. $\rho = 0.056$ min^{-1}. **D.** Inhibition progress curve reflecting a multiple enzyme system. Inhibition of bovine erythrocyte acetylcholinesterase by 2×10^{-4}M tetram at 5°C, pH 7.0 is shown. The first-order rate constant of the first form (broken line) was 65.4 min^{-1}.

Table 11.3 Phosphorylation (k_2), Dissociation (K_d), and Bimolecular Rate Constants (k_i) of Some Organophosphate and Carbamate Inhibitors of Cholinesterases from Various Sources

Enzyme	Compound	k_2 (min^{-1})	K_d (M)	k_i (M^{-1}min^{-1})	Temp. (°C)
AChE (bovine)	Malaoxon	67	2.7×10^{-4}	2.4×10^5	5
BuChE (human)	Malaoxon	6.6	6.2×10^{-4}	1.1×10^4	25
AChE (bovine)	DFP	40.7	1.2×10^{-3}	3.4×10^4	25
BuChE (horse)	DFP	145	2.6×10^{-5}	5.5×10^6	25
AChE (bovine)	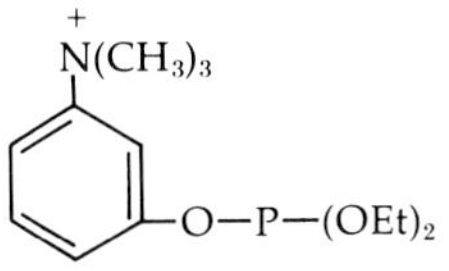 $\overset{+}{N}(CH_3)_3$ — phenyl—O—P—(OEt)$_2$ (phosphostigmine)	5.2	1.2×10^{-4}	4.3×10^4	25
AChE (bovine)	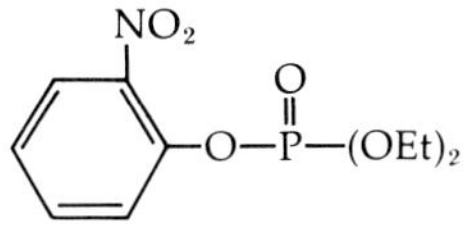 NO$_2$-phenyl—O—$\overset{O}{\underset{\parallel}{P}}$—(OEt)$_2$	3	1.44×10^{-3}	2.1×10^3	5
	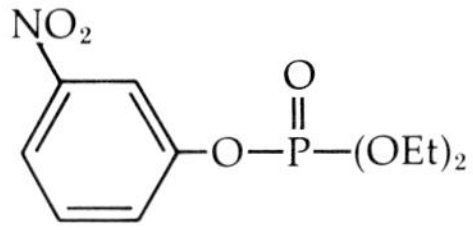 NO$_2$-phenyl—O—$\overset{O}{\underset{\parallel}{P}}$—(OEt)$_2$	0.81	2.2×10^{-4}	3.7×10^3	25
	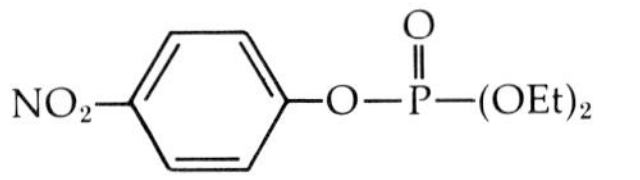 NO$_2$-phenyl—O—$\overset{O}{\underset{\parallel}{P}}$—(OEt)$_2$ (paraoxon)	43	3.6×10^{-4}	1.2×10^5	25
AChE (bovine)	(Et)$_2$N—CH$_2$CH$_2$—S—$\overset{O}{\underset{\parallel}{P}}$—(OEt)$_2$ (amiton)	157	2.8×10^{-4}	5.6×10^5	5
BuChE (human)	(Et)$_2$N—CH$_2$CH$_2$—S—$\overset{O}{\underset{\parallel}{P}}$—(OEt)$_2$	90	1.5×10^{-5}	5.8×10^6	5

Insecticidal carbamates

Enzyme	Compound	k_2 (min^{-1})	K_d (M)	k_i (M^{-1}min^{-1})	Temp. (°C)
AChE (bovine)	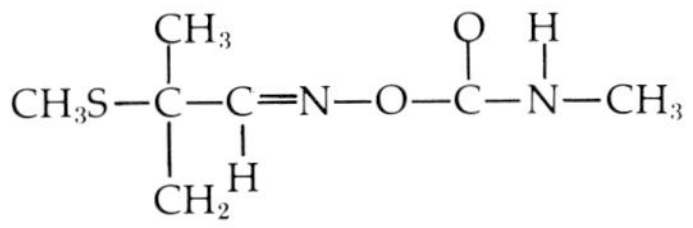 CH$_3$S—C(CH$_3$)(CH$_2$H)—C=N—O—C(=O)—N(H)—CH$_3$ Aldicarb	146	1×10^{-2}	1.6×10^4	
AChE (bovine)	Carbaryl	>20	$>5 \times 10^{-2}$	2.2×10^4	
AChE (housefly)	Carbaryl	0.8	5×10^{-7}	1.6×10^7	

Continued

Table 11.3 (*Continued*)

Enzyme	Compound	k_2 (min⁻¹)	K_d (M)	k_i (M⁻¹min⁻¹)	Temp. (°C)
	Pharmaceutical carbamates				
AChE (bovine)	Eserine	10.8	3.3×10^{-6}	3.3×10^6	
AChE (electrical)	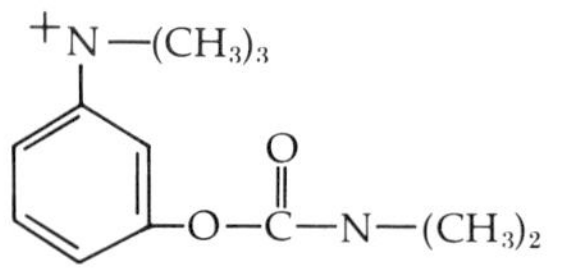 (neostigmine)	46.5	1.2×10^{-6}	4.0×10^6	

was derived. Equation (11.13) predicts that as [I] increases, ρ will increase and that the plot of ρ against [I] will be linear. It is understood that although [I] is essentially constant over the course of a single inhibition experiment, a range of [I] values can be selected and a particular value of ρ can be determined for each value of [I] selected. The experimental results first obtained gave linear [I] versus ρ plots, suggesting that Scheme (11.VII) adequately described the reaction between ChE and organophosphates. This suggested in turn that inhibitory power depended solely on the phosphorylating potential of the bond joining phosphorus to the leaving group. However, many workers felt that steric factors also contributed to inhibitory power, and, as we shall see in the next section, they were right.

11.5.4. Affinity (K_d) and Acylation (k_2) Constants

The steric factors involved the shapes or steric configurations of the organophosphate inhibitors and the possibility that they might fit into the active site of the ChE in much the same way as the substrates do. This would mean that phosphorylation of the enzyme would be preceded by the formation of a reversible binding complex. The reaction scheme would then be

$$E + PX \overset{K_d}{\rightleftharpoons} EPX \overset{k_2}{\to} EP \qquad\qquad (11.\text{VIII})$$

where EPX is the reversible binding complex and K_d (subscript d for dissociation) is the equilibrium constant governing binding. k_2 is a phosphorylation rate constant, and Scheme (11.VIII) assumes EP does not break down to regenerate free enzyme. This assumption is valid for the first minutes of the reaction, during which the rate of formation of EP is measured since the dephosphorylation rate constant k_3 is thousands to millions times less than k_2.

An equation is derived from Scheme (11.VIII) in much the same way that Equation (11.10) was derived from Scheme (11.VII). The assumption that [I] remains constant over the course of inhibition is made again. The enzyme conservation equation now includes the [EPX] term, so that $[E]_0 = [E] + [EPX] + [EP]$. The rate of formation of EP is given by

$$d[EP]/dt = k_2[EPX] \tag{11.14}$$

An expression for [EPX] is found from the equation defining K_d and the conservation equation:

$$K_d = \frac{[E] \cdot [I]}{[EPX]} = \frac{([E]_0 - [EPX] - [EP])[I]}{[EPX]} \tag{11.15}$$

Solving Equation (11.15) for [EPX],

$$[EPX] = \frac{[E_0 - EP]}{1 + K_d/[I]} \; . \tag{11.16}$$

Substitution of this expression for [EPX] into Equation (11.14), followed by integration, etc. as before, gives

$$\rho = \frac{\ln (v_0/v)}{t} = \frac{k_2}{1 + K_d/[I]} . \tag{11.17}$$

Although ρ, the first-order rate constant, has the same experimental meaning as in Equation (11.13), its theoretical meaning based on Scheme (11.VIII) is more complex. In order to interpret Equation (11.17), it is instructive to compare it with the more familiar Michaelis-Menten equation [Equation (11.5)]. By replacing ρ with v, k_2 with V, K_d with K_m, and [I] with [S], it is seen that equation (11.17) has precisely the same form as Equation (11.5). The plot of ρ against [I] would then be analogous with that of v against [S], and gives the familiar rectangular hyperbola:

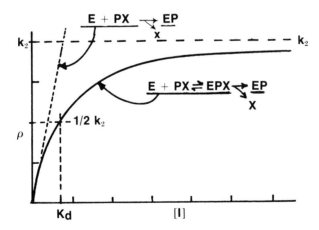

Since Equation (11.17) has the same form as the Michaelis-Menten equation, it can be transformed into analogous linear forms. For example, the double reciprocal Lineweaver-Burk form has the analogous form

$$\frac{1}{\rho} = \frac{k_2}{[I]K_d} + \frac{1}{k_2} \; . \tag{11.18}$$

The validity of Equation (11.17) and the concepts underlying it have been tested using Equation (11.18) which predicts intercepts on the $1/\rho$ and $1/[I]$ axes. A typical double reciprocal plot is shown below. The intercepts give $1/k_2$ and $-1/K_d$:

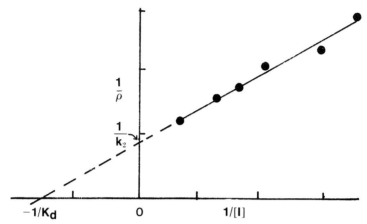

If values of [I] are used that are much less than K_d, the plot of the points will not give intercepts, but will appear to pass through the origin on extrapolation.

The inhibitory power of an organophosphate depends then both on the way it binds and the rapidity with which it phosphorylates the active site as reflected by K_d and k_2, respectively. The K_d and k_2 values of a number of organophosphates are given in Table 11.3.

The relationship between K_d and k_2 in Equation (11.17) and k_i in Equation (11.13) can be seen by considering the case when $[I] \ll K_d$. Equation (11.17) then reduces to

$$\rho = \frac{k_2}{K_d} [I]. \tag{11.19}$$

From Equation (11.13), $\rho = k_i[I]$. Therefore, when $[I] \ll K_d$,

$$k_i = \frac{k_2}{K_d} . \tag{11.20}$$

Under these conditions, k_i gives a measure of the overall rate of inhibition. Equation (11.20) also emphasizes the fact that the organophosphate inhibitory power depends on both k_2 and K_d.

A considerable body of evidence has confirmed the fact that a reversible affinity binding complex does precede phosphorylation, and this concept has been extended to include carbamates.

11.5.5. Carbamylated Active Site and Decarbamylation

Carbamates were for many years regarded as purely reversible inhibitors. However, as early as 1954, Myers and Kemp recognized that "dimethylcarbamoyl fluoride . . . inhibited esterases by the same mechanism as the dialkyl phosphoryfluoridates," that is, by acylating the active center in the same way as carboxylic ester substrates. In 1960 Wilson, Hatch, and Ginsberg confirmed the conclusions of Myers and Kemp, and in doing so proposed a scheme that is essentially the same as that describing the substrate reaction. The scheme is

$$E + CX \underset{K_d}{\rightleftharpoons} ECX \xrightarrow{k_2} EC \xrightarrow{k_3} E + C. \qquad (11.IX)$$

with k_i over the top arrow and X below ECX.

An equation is derived from Scheme (11.IX) within the context of the experimental conditions described in connection with the derivation of Equations (11.13) and (11.17). The difference is the added degree of complexity brought about by including k_3 and the deacylation step.

When k_3 is included, the rate of formation of EC is given by $d[EC]/dt = k_2[ECX] - k_3[EC]$, which leads to the experimentally useful equation

$$\ln \frac{v - v_{ss}}{v_0 - v_{ss}} = -t \left(\frac{k_2}{1 + (K_d/[I])} + k_3 \right). \qquad (11.21)$$

In Equation (11.21) v_{ss} is the velocity at the steady state. As shown in Figure 11.4C, v_{ss} is independent of time once the steady state has been reached and is constant for a given value of [I]. As before, v is the velocity at some time t before the steady state is reached. If k_3 is much less than k_2, then v_{ss} will be very small with respect to v_0 and to values of v that are even 0.1% of v_0. If v_{ss} and k_3 are assumed to be negligible, Equation (11.21) reduces to Equation (11.17). This condition holds for practically all the better organophosphate and carbamate inhibitors having k_i values greater than 10^4 $M^{-1}min^{-1}$ at 25°C.

In many experiments in which the steady-state condition is used, conditions are chosen such that $[I] \ll K_d$ and $k_2(1 + K_d/[I])$ then reduces to $k_i[I]$. Substituting k_i for k_2/K_d, Equation (11.21) becomes

$$y = \ln \frac{v - v_{ss}}{v_0 - v_{ss}} = -t([I]k_i + k_3). \qquad (11.22)$$

Values of y were obtained for a range of [I] values using equation (11.22). Equation (11.22) was then rearranged to use the y values so obtained:

$$\frac{y}{t} = -[I]k_i + k_3. \qquad (11.23)$$

The plot of y/t against [I] is straight with a slope of $-k_i$ and an intercept of k_3. This treatment then gives k_i and k_3.

More frequently, k_3 is determined by diluting out the inhibitor (or otherwise removing it) and measuring the recovery rate. The scheme is

$$EC \xrightarrow{k_3} E + \dot{C}. \tag{11.X}$$

From Scheme (11.X) the rate of regeneration is $-d[EC]/dt = k_3[EC]$, which leads to

$$\ln \frac{v_0 - v}{v_0 - v'} = -k_3 t \tag{11.24}$$

where v_0 is the velocity before inhibition, v' the velocity at the beginning of regeneration, and v the velocity at regeneration time t. The plot of $\ln [(v_0 - v)/(v_0 - v')]$ against t is linear, and the slope gives $-k_3$.

The steady-state condition where $d[EC]/dt = 0$ and $k_2[ECX] = k_3[EC]$ leads to

$$\frac{v_{ss}}{v_0 - v_{ss}} = \left(\frac{K_d}{[I]} \times \frac{k_3}{k_2} \right) + \frac{k_3}{k_2}. \tag{11.25}$$

A plot of $v_{ss}/(v_0 - v_{ss})$ against $1/[I]$ is straight. The intercept on the $1/[I]$ axis then gives $-1/k_d$. To use Equation (11.25) experimentally some values of $[I]$ must approach K_d, and the ratio k_3/k_2 must not be too small, a condition that very few good inhibitors will satisfy.

11.5.6. Inhibition in the Presence of Substrates and Reversible Inhibitors

Thus far, only the case of the irreversible inhibitor and enzyme acting alone has been considered. However, the reaction has been studied in the presence of reversible inhibitors and substrates. Inhibition in the presence of substrate can be considered in terms of the following reaction schemes:

$$E + PX \rightleftharpoons EPX \xrightarrow[X]{} EP$$
$$E + AB \rightleftharpoons EAB \xrightarrow[B]{} EA \longrightarrow E + A. \tag{11.XI}$$

Equation (11.17) is then modified to include the substrate term

$$\frac{\ln (v_0/v)}{t} = \rho = \frac{k_2}{1 + (K_d/[I])[1 + ([S]/K_m)]}. \tag{11.26}$$

Equation (11.26) is analogous to that describing purely competitive inhibition in steady-state reactions. To obtain ρ, curving substrate progress curves are used:

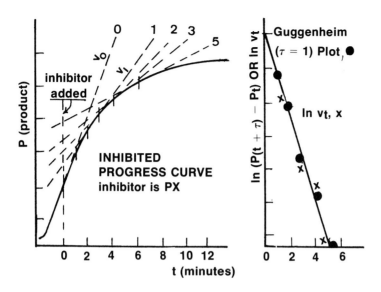

The broken lines are tangents to the slope of the inhibited progress curve. They give the velocities $v_1, v_2, \cdots$ at the corresponding times $t_1, t_2, \cdots$ after inhibition has started. Curving is from progressive inhibition of E by PX during hydrolysis of substrate. Alternatively, the curve can be interpreted by using a Guggenheim plot and

$$\ln \left([P]_{(t+\tau)} - [P]_t\right) = \frac{-k_2[I]K_m t}{([S]K_d + K_d K_m + [I]K_m)} + \ln C \qquad (11.27)$$

where [P] is the concentration of product formed at time t and τ is a selected time constant. The plots of Equations (11.26) and (11.27) are shown on the right-hand side of the sketch above, and, as expected, they give the same slope. To determine k_2 and K_d, K_m must be known.

11.6. Spontaneous Regeneration, Aging, and Reactivators

11.6.1. Spontaneous Regeneration

The inhibitory power and therefore the toxicity of organophosphates and carbamates depends on the stability of the acyl-enzyme intermediates as well as on the rates at which they are formed. Phosphorylated ChE tend to be more stable than carbamylated ChE, but there is nevertheless a wide variation in the stability of phosphorylated ChE. The stability depends on the nature of the groups attached to the phosphate and on the particular ChE. For example, the half-life of dimethylphosphoryl AChE from rat erythrocytes is 2 hr, whereas the comparable half-life of the diethylphosphorylated enzyme is almost 2 days.

With respect to different ChE phosphorylated by the same groups, dimethylphosphoryl AChE from fly head appears to be completely stable after 5 hr, whereas the dimethylphosphoryl AChE from rabbit erythrocytes has a half-life of only 72 min. Similarly, the half-life of diethylphosphoryl ChE from rat serum is 5 hr, whereas the half-life of the diethylphosphoryl BuChE from human serum is 30 days. Substitution of a chlorine atom on the alkyl phosphate group greatly increases the rate of spontaneous regeneration. Dichlorethylphosphoryl BuChE from human serum has, for example, a half-life of about 20 min, whereas the comparable diethylphosphoryl BuChE has a half-life of 30 days, which means it is 2000 times more stable because it contains no chlorine. Table 11.4 lists the half-life values of a number of alkyl substituted phosphoryl ChE. Spontaneous regeneration follows first-order kinetics since one of the reactants, water, is in great excess.

Whereas the half-life values of phosphorylated ChE vary from minutes to weeks, those of the two common carbamylated ChE, the N-methyl and N,N-dimethyl carbamates, appear to be more uniform. For example, the half-life of cow erythrocyte, fly head, and electric eel AChE are 19 min, 24 min, and 38 min, respectively. These values are not strictly comparable since the conditions for

Table 11.4 Rates of Spontaneous Regeneration of Phosphorylated and Carbamylated Cholinesterases

Enzyme	Acyl group	pH	Temp. (°C)	$10^3 k$ (min^{-1})	$t_{1/2}$
	Phosphates				
AChE (rabbit)	$(CH_3O)_2$—P— (O)	7.8	37	8.5	82 min
AChE (human)	$(C_2H_5O)_2$—P— (O)	7.4	37	0.2	58 hr
AChE (eel)	$(C_2H_5O)_2$—P— (O)	7.0	7	0.018	27 days
ChE (human)	$(C_2H_5O)_2$—P— (O)	7.8	37	0.016	30 days
	Carbamates				
AChE (eel)	H_2—N—C— (O)	7.0	25	400	1.7 min
AChE (eel)	HCH_3—N—C— (O)	7.0	25	18	38 min
AChE (bovine)	HCH_3—N—C— (O)	7.4	25	11.3	1 hr
AChE (eel)	$(CH_3)_2$—N—C— (O)	7.0	25	26	27 min
AChE (bovine)	$(CH_3)_2$—N—C— (O)	8.0	25	12	56 min
ChE (human)	$(CH_3)_2$—N—C— (O)	7.4	25	3.3	3–5 hr

each determination varied a little. Carbamylated serum BuChE are somewhat more stable than the carbamylated AChE.

Spontaneous reactivation of both phosphorylated and carbamylated AChE is pH dependent. The curve is bell shaped, indicating ionizing groups of $pK_i = 6.9$ and of $pK_2 = 9.8$ are involved. The pH activity curve for reactivation and the substrate reactions are alike (Figure 11.2).

11.6.2. Aging or Dealkylation

The extent to which phosphorylated ChE can be regenerated, either spontaneously or with reactivators, may depend on the time the inhibited enzyme has been stored. The phosphorylated ChE will undergo one of two possible reactions. The first is regeneration, and the second is the loss of one of the two alkyl groups. The second reaction is aging or dealkylation:

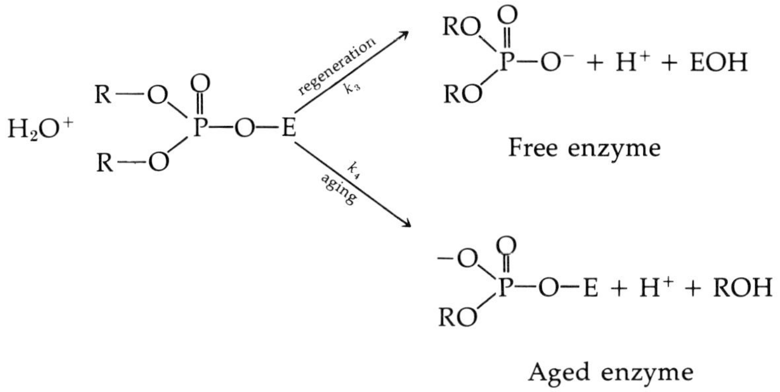

The aged mono-alkyl phosphorylated ChE is much more stable than the dialkyl form; and in the aged form, the ChE cannot be regenerated. The rate of aging depends on the alkyl groups and on the type of ChE.

Both phosphoryl ChE,

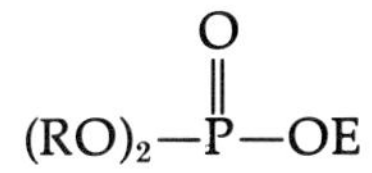

$$(RO)_2-\overset{\overset{\textstyle O}{\|}}{P}-OE$$

and phosphonyl ChE,

$$RO-\overset{\overset{\textstyle O}{\|}}{\underset{\underset{\textstyle |}{\overset{|}{-C-}}}{P}}-OE$$

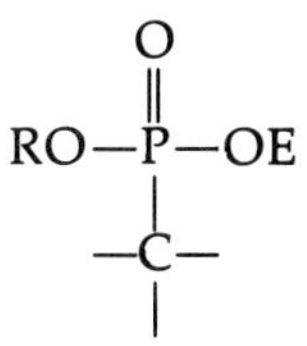

age. The half-life of conversion to the aged form varies from a minute or less to several days. For example, the aging half-life of di*isopropyl*phosphoryl AChE of human erythrocytes is 4.6 hr, whereas the comparable di*ethyl*-phosphoryl AChE aging half-life is 41 hr. The rate of aging increases as the pH decreases, and aging is controlled by an ionizing group with a pK of 6.4. Aging is also temperature dependent. In one example the rate increased about ten times as the temperature increased from 3° to 25°C. Much of the available information has been obtained with phosphonyl ChE, and quite a number of insecticides, such as EPN, are phosphonates:

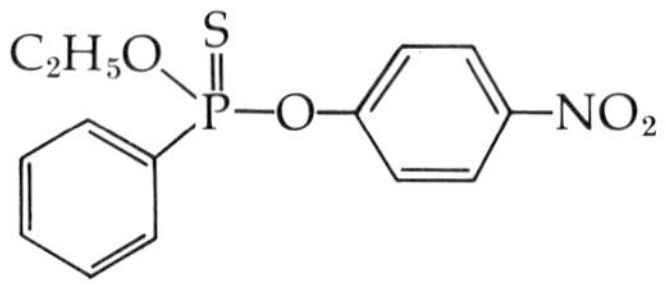

EPN

11.6.3. Reactivators

The origin of reactivators was mentioned in Section 11.3.1 in connection with reactivation by hydroxylamine. These early studies stimulated a search for more powerful reactivators to be used as therapeutic reagents in the treatment of poisoning. Compounds were tested that contained a powerful nucleophile and a quaternary nitrogen–promoting group. Two groups of nucleophilic compounds showed particular promise, the hydroxamic acids and the oximes:

Hydroxamic acid   Oxime

With both oximes and hydroxamic acids, the nucleophile is the oxygen attached to the nitrogen. The hydroxamate anion actually makes the attack, as does the oxime anion:

Hydroxamate anion

$$RHC{=}NOH \;\rightleftharpoons\; RHC{=}NO^- + H^+$$

Oxime anion

Both reactivators can therefore be depicted as RH, where the H is attached to the nucleophilic O. The best reactivators also have a promoting function in the form of a quaternary ammonium group which attaches to the anionic site. Methyl pyridinium is one of the most successful promoting functions; and when combined with an aldoxime, the very potent pyridine aldoxime methiodides (PAM) are formed:

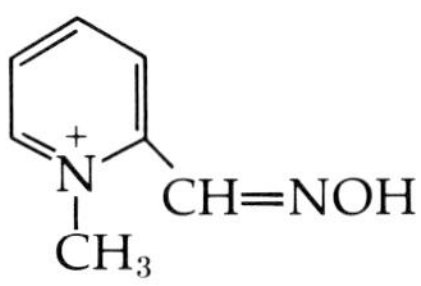

CH=NOH

CH=NOH

CH=NOH

2-PAM 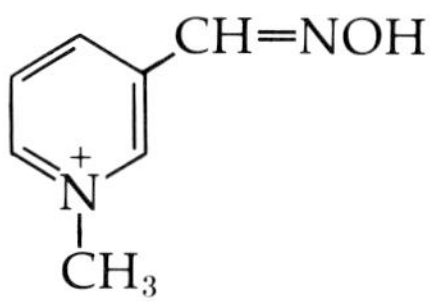   3-PAM 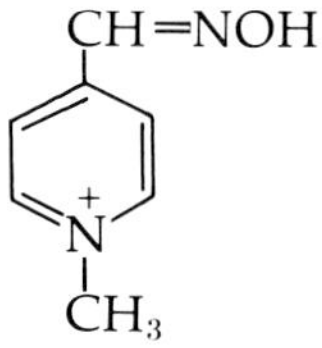   4-PAM

To be fully effective, the reactivator must have not only a charged N function, but the function must be properly oriented. For example, the reactivating potential of the three PAM compounds above varies greatly depending on the position of ring substitution. The 2-PAM compound is almost 30,000 times more effective than 3-PAM and almost 50 times better than 4-PAM. Thus, proper positioning is a crucial factor. These aldoximes exist in syn- and anti-isomeric forms. 2-PAM is believed to exist largely in the syn form.

The effect of the charge on the promoting group on the rate of recovery can be seen by comparing the effectiveness of charged and uncharged pyridine aldoximes. For example, 2-PAM is 50,000 times more effective than the uncharged analog:

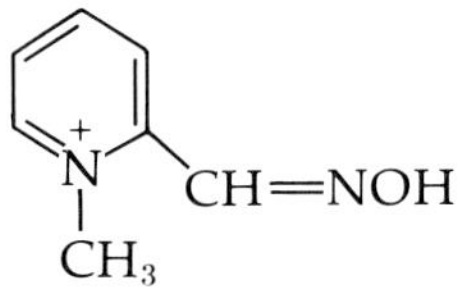

2-PAM 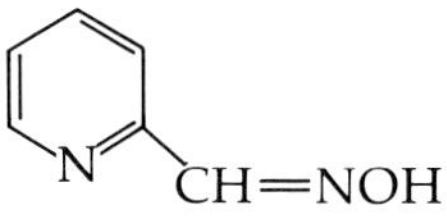   Pyridine-2-aldoxime

Although the effect of introducing the charge is not always so dramatic, the charged compounds are invariably better than the uncharged.

The effectiveness of a reactivator will depend on the nature of the phosphorylated group on the ChE as well as on the ChE itself. For example, diethylphosphoryl AChE is reactivated 30 times faster than the diisopropylphosphoryl AChE (DIPAChE) by nicotine hydroxamic acid methiodide:

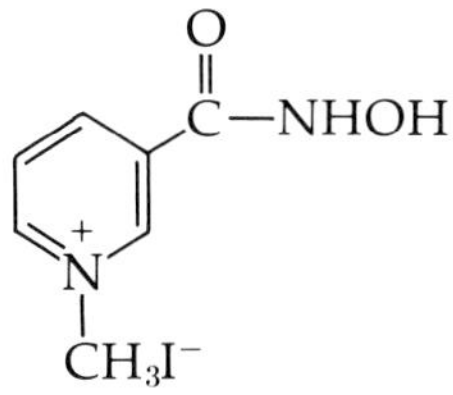

Nicotine hydroxamic
acid methiodide

DIPAChE are in general more difficult to reactivate than n-alkyl homologs. In general, too, the best oxime reactivators are far more effective than the best hydroxamic acid reactivators.

The most powerful reactivators of phosphorylated AChE combine the bisquaternary feature with the 2-PAM structure. They were introduced by Hobbiger and his group in 1958. One of the best, called TMB 4, is shown below.

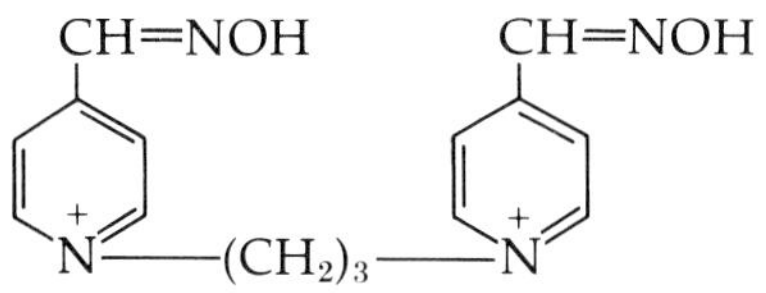

TMB 4

TMB 4 is about 22 times more effective than 2-PAM in reactivating diethylphosphoryl AChE and 52 times more effective with the DIPAChE. TMB 4 has a bridge of 3 methylenes and, while this appears optimal, varying the bridge between 2 and 5 methylenes is not dramatic.

   The effectiveness of the promoting functions suggests that the reactivators act by first forming a reversible binding complex with the phosphorylated ChE, before the free enzyme is regenerated. Reactivation then follows the scheme

$$RH + EP \overset{K_t}{\rightleftharpoons} RHEP \overset{k_2'}{\to} RP + EH \tag{11.XII}$$

where RHEP is the reversible binding complex and the product RP is the phosphorylated oxime. With 2-PAM, RP would be

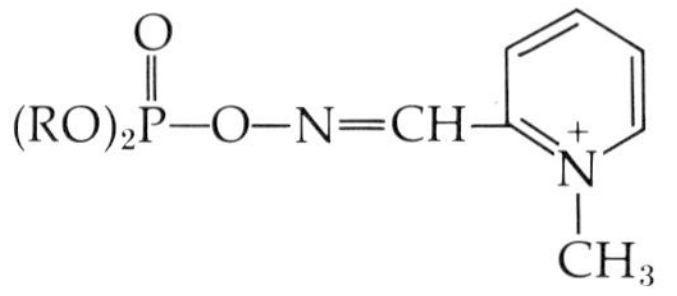

Phosphorylated oximes are potent inhibitors of ChE, but they are often unstable and decompose in water in a few minutes or hours.

   Scheme (11.XII) is essentially the same as Scheme (11.VIII), and thus the kinetics applied to the two schemes are identical. The rate of reactivation is given by $-d[EP]/dt = d[EH]/dt = k_2'[RHEP]$, from which is derived

$$\frac{\ln\left([EP]_0/[EP]\right)}{t} = \frac{k_2'}{1 + K_r/[RH]} \; . \tag{11.28}$$

If $RH \ll K_r$, then

$$\frac{\ln\left([EP]_0/[EP]\right)}{t} = \frac{k_2'[RH]}{K_r} = [RH]k_r \tag{11.29}$$

where k_r is a bimolecular rate constant which holds for poorly binding activators or for conditions where $RH \ll K_r$.

   Various criteria have been used to compare the effectiveness of reactivators. The percent recovery of activity after incubation for arbitrary times in the presence of typically high, but also arbitrary, concentrations of reactivator is often seen. The half-life of recovery at high reactivator concentrations is used since in the presence of excess reactivator the reaction follows first-order kinetics. K_r, k_2, and k_r values are rare, but they are the most informative.

The effects of pH, temperature, and salts have been studied with these compounds, and, as might be expected, reactivation kinetics has much in common with substrate and inhibition kinetics.

11.6.4. Structures of Organophosphate and Carbamate Inhibitors of Cholinesterases

The structures of organophosphate and carbamate insecticides are amazingly diverse, and there are literally thousands of members of each class of compound. The carbamates and organophosphates used as insecticides number well over 100, and each compound is characterized by a unique history and structure.

The structural features are by no means limited to factors promoting inhibitory power. Some features confer selectivity through a variety of mechanisms, while others are involved with penetration, stability, cost, and the kind of insect or pest over which control is sought. In addition to insects, organophosphates and carbamates are used to control parasitic worms, spiders, reptiles, and even mammalian pests such as rats. In spite of this diversity, however, the basic mode of action is the same for all these compounds. They kill by acylating the active sites of ChE, resulting in "irreversible" inhibition. This chapter has been concerned with the details of that basic mode of action. Details of the structures of organophosphate and carbamate insecticides and the mechanisms by which they are detoxicated may be found in chapters 4 and 5 of this book or in the articles and books listed at the end of this chapter.

Suggested Reading

Aldridge, W. N., Reiner, E. Frontiers of Biology, Vol. 26, Enzyme Inhibitors as Substrates. Amsterdam: North-Holland, 1972.

Bulletin of the World Health Organization, 44, No. 1-2-3, 1971, pp. 1–470.

Corbett, J. T. The Biochemical Mode of Action of Pesticides. London: Academic Press, 1974.

Ehrenpreis, S. (Ed.). Cholinergic mechanisms. Ann. N. Y. Acad. Sci. 144 (1967), 383.

Eto, M. Organophosphorus Pesticides: Organic and Biological Chemistry. Cleveland: CRC Press, 1974.

Koelle, G. G. (Ed.). Handbook of Experimental Pharmacology, Vol. 15, Cholinesterases and Anticholinesterase Agents. Berlin: Springer, 1963.

Kuhr R. J., Dorough, H. W. Carbamate Insecticides: Chemistry, Biochemistry and Toxicology. Cleveland: CRC Press, 1976.

Matsumura, F. Toxicology of Insecticides. New York: Plenum Press, 1975.

O'Brien, R. D. Toxic Phosphorus Esters: Chemistry, Metabolism, and Biological Effects. New York: Academic Press, 1960.

O'Brien, R. D. Insecticides: Action and Metabolism. New York: Academic Press, 1967.

Silver, A. Frontiers of Biology, Vol. 36, The Biology of Cholinesterases. Amsterdam: North-Holland, 1974.

Wilkinson, C. F. (Ed.). Insecticide Biochemistry and Physiology. New York: Plenum Press, 1976.

Richard B. Mailman

12

Biochemical Toxicology of the Central Nervous System

12.1. Introduction

The role of the central nervous system (CNS) in cognitive and emotive processes is recognized by both scientists and laymen. However, the essential function of the brain in regulating other critical physiological events (exemplified in the work of Nobel Laureates Roger Guillemin and Andrew Schally) has only more recently been appreciated. These mechanisms involve not only the CNS, but ultimately every tissue in the body through hormonal actions originating in the brain. Despite the importance of the CNS to an organism's welfare, xenobiotic actions on these critical tissues are not yet well understood. The reasons for this are threefold.

First, the complexity of the brain has made many tools that are used to study peripheral functions only marginally useful. This complexity is not only anatomical and morphological, but also biochemical, and has curtailed attempts to understand CNS toxicity. Second, many compounds that may have toxic effects on the CNS also cause lesions of the peripheral nervous system that are ultimately fatal. This result often prevents detailed evaluation of the CNS effects of sublethal doses of the toxicant. Third, CNS toxicity includes events beyond those that cause gross physical signs such as encephalopathy and death. There is sufficient evidence to suspect that subtle lesions, not causing gross physical signs, may still result in important physiological changes for the target organisms. These toxicological changes may only be evident when an environmental challenge (either physical or chemical) is present, but the result is a decreased ability to cope with change. It is of interest to note that childhood minimal brain dysfunction ("hyperkinesis"), which afflicts a significant percentage of children, is felt by many to involve, in part, toxicological changes caused by exposure to lead, various natural and artificial food additives, or other purported etiological agents.

For these reasons, toxicological events in the CNS are of paramount importance, and the study of them will increase as more fundamental knowledge about the CNS is unearthed. However, at present there is a relative paucity of substantive biochemical data about the CNS actions of various xenobiotics. In this chapter, therefore, a general framework of possible biochemical sites of action for toxicants will be presented, along with specific examples when available or relevant. In addition, factors directly relevant to the biochemical toxicology of the CNS will be discussed to provide sufficient information for further study.

12.2. Blood–Brain Barrier

One important reason that xenobiotics that have target sites present in both central and peripheral areas have more demonstrable effects on the latter is the presence of structures that differentially prevent free diffusion of the toxicant. CNS toxicity is dependent upon contact of sufficient concentrations of the chemical with sensitive sites in the brain or spinal cord. Barring breaches in the physical integrity of the head and skull through major trauma, this contact must occur by the passage of chemicals from the blood into the brain through a series of membranous structures. Most tissues have a single membrane (the plasmalemma) separating the intra- from the extracellular compartment. The brain is unique, however, because three membranes divide the intracellular space from the systemic circulation. The blood–brain barrier and the brain-cell membrane are in series, with the choroid plexus parallel to these. The choroid plexus separates the blood from the cerebrospinal fluid, whereas the blood–brain barrier limits the influx of circulating substances into the immediate brain interstitial space. The utilization of histochemical (peroxidase) or electron microscopic techniques have demonstrated that brain capillaries, unlike those in other tissues, are *not* fundamentally porous. For example, a microperoxidase (molecular mass 1800 daltons) that readily transverses capillaries in other tissues will not pass through capillaries in the brain. However, the brain must have a mechanism to obtain needed nutrients, including carbohydrates and amino acids. Since entry of molecules (especially polar ones) into the brain is prevented or retarded, adequate nutrition is dependent on specific blood–brain transport mechanisms. Such systems have been demonstrated for hexoses, carboxylic acids, amino acids (separate ones for neutral, basic, and acidic amino acids), amines, and inorganic ions.

These facts suggest that most toxicants will either be totally excluded from brain tissue, or at least hindered in contacting possibly sensitive sites. It is of teleological interest that the physiological systems essential to survival have these protective features (in the adult the gut membranes, in the developing organism the placental membranes, and in the most sensitive tissue, the brain, the blood–brain barrier). In order to understand the biochemical toxicology of the CNS it is necessary to know whether a toxicant can pass through these protective barriers or can alter or damage them, permitting secondary events to occur. Several generalizations may be made about these events.

First, the passage of large molecules, such as larger peptides or proteins, does not usually occur or is severely retarded. As a consequence, ingestion of a proteinaceous toxin will result in only peripheral toxicity until sufficiently large concentrations "force" the toxin past the blood–brain barrier. It is this fact that often make central effects of the toxicant moot, since the peripheral actions may be lethal.

Second, polar molecules are generally physically excluded from the brain because the blood–brain barrier is a highly lipophilic membrane, as are most biological membranes. However, nonpolar, lipid-soluble molecules penetrate into the brain more easily—a fact that has several important consequences. Alkylated mercury compounds (such as dimethyl mercury) are absorbed from the gastrointestinal tract into the blood and from the blood into the brain several orders of magnitude more readily than are the comparable inorganic ions. Consequently, the environmental conversion of the inorganic mercury to methylated compounds by microbial action, and the subsequent uptake of the latter compounds by fish in the food chain, has resulted in Minamata disease (extreme CNS dysfunction resulting in permanent neurological changes or death). For similar reasons, *rational* drug design utilizes moieties to impart a net charge (at physiological pH) to a molecule, thereby selectively decreasing the action of that drug on central versus peripheral sites.

Third, the specific transport systems cited earlier may facilitate the passage of toxicants into the brain. Though these systems are usually highly specific in nature, potential toxicants with structures analogous to physiological substrates may be transported into the brain, thus bypassing the blood–brain barrier.

A fourth factor to consider is the presence of extra blood–brain barrier structures (known as supraependymal structures) that are bathed in the cerebrospinal fluid and can be exposed to molecules that will not penetrate into deeper brain tissue. A possible role for these structures is to monitor neuroendocrine function, and the presumed function of the fenestrations in the barrier in this region is to permit the access of specific endogenous molecules. However, other chemicals, including putative CNS toxicants, may penetrate through these openings even though they pass through other portions of the blood–brain barrier only with great difficulty. These supraependymal sites may be particularly vulnerable to toxicants.

Finally, many factors can influence blood–brain permeability. The most important of these is the age of the target animal. It is generally accepted that embryonic or fetal forms have higher central accessibility to xenobiotics, and even after birth there appears to be greater passage in the immediate postnatal period than during adulthood. The importance of these differences will be illustrated in later sections.

Alterations in blood–brain barrier function may be caused by many types of toxicant exposure. For example, substances that alter membrane function directly—such as the bile salt sodium desoxycholate or high concentrations of various organic solvents, including alcohols—disrupt the blood–brain barrier. Increases in blood–brain barrier permeability are also seen after exposure to cobra venom, presumably because the phospholipases in these venom hydrolyze membrane lipids. Heavy metals such as lead are also believed to alter blood–brain barrier function, though the specific biochemical site of action is not known. It should be noted that changes caused by these and other agents may be reversible or irreversible and may also profoundly influence the CNS toxicity of subsequent exposure to other materials.

12.3. Toxicant Metabolism in the Central Nervous System

Chapters 2 through 9 of this book have dealt in great detail with the possible fates of xenobiotics. The diversity of mechanisms that can chemically alter foreign molecules, thereby changing both the reactivity of the molecules and their relative affinities for physiological sites of action, has been emphasized. A major difference between the CNS and peripheral tissues is that these detoxification mechanisms are generally considered to be absent from the brain, with the blood–brain barrier providing the major protective mechanisms. However, the synthesis, transport, and degradation of many endogenous molecules is dependent on specific enzymatic systems, and it is possible that these systems may also use possible toxicants as "pseudosubstrates." For example, the compound 2,4,5-trihydroxyphenylalanine is decarboxylated by the same enzymes that decarboxylate 3,4-dihydroxyphenylalanine. Whereas the product of the latter substrate is the neurotransmitter dopamine, the former compound is metabolized to 6-hydroxydopamine, a neurocytotoxin that will be discussed in detail in later sections of this chapter. Since the aromatic amino acid transport mechanisms will also transport 2,4,5-trihydroxyphenylalanine into brain, the importance of considering the structural similarities between endogenous substrates and putative CNS toxicants should be evident.

Finally, both the circulation and cerebrospinal fluid may passively eliminate certain toxicants. However, toxicokinetics after xenobiotic exposure usually reflect primarily peripheral events, as well as factors influencing the passage of the toxicants into the brain, and are only slightly influenced by metabolic alterations of the toxin in the brain. Although cytochrome P-450 has recently been reported to be present in small quantities in brain tissue, whether this mixed-function oxidase serves a biosynthetic (as in the adrenals) or a detoxicative (as in the liver) role has yet to be elucidated. It does seem certain that its activity as a protective mechanism is limited.

12.4. Biochemical Sites of Action of Toxicants

The brain consists of many cell types, but the class that is generally considered most important is the nerve cell, or neuron. The diversity of this class of cells is extensive, but for illustrative purposes a description of a "typical" neuron will be given to exemplify some sites where CNS toxicants may act.

12.4.1. Nerve Cell and Synaptic Transmission

Information passage and integration in the brain is the result of many electrochemical events. These events occur because of the specialized physiology of the nerve cell, an example of which is shown in Figure 12.1. The cell body, or perikaryon, is essential for survival of the processes, which themselves also contain mitochondria. Impulses generally travel unidirectionally from the dendrites to the axon, and the axons terminate in a series of specialized structures called synapses. Whereas electrical stimulation experiments have demonstrated

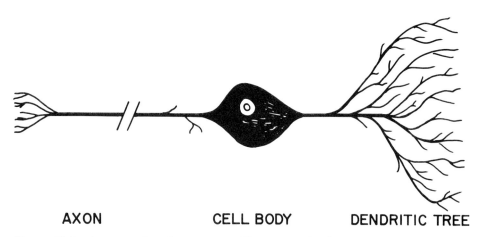

AXON   **CELL BODY**   **DENDRITIC TREE**

Figure 12.1 An example of a neuron. The many dendritic and axonal processes exemplify the numerous intercellular contacts that occur.

that information, in the form of action potentials, may travel bidirectionally in axons, the synapse acts as a rectifier to ensure undirectional flow.

Similar to other cells, the interior of the nerve cell is generally 50 or more millivolts more negative in potential than the exterior. In neurons, however, a reduction in potential (as by electrical stimulation) to approximately −10 mV results in an explosive, self-limiting overshoot such that the interior of the cell actually becomes positive to the exterior. This event, the action potential, is propagated along the course of the nerve.

It has been demonstrated that at the synapse chemical events mediate the transmission of information between neurons. As shown in Figure 12.2, the arriving impulse may cause the release of molecules of a specific type from storage areas on the presynaptic side of impulse propagation. The molecules that are released into the synapse, or cleft, between the axon originally carrying the signal (the presynaptic side) and the cellular projection on the receiving side (the postsynaptic side) are called neurotransmitters. When released into the synaptic cleft, these neurotransmitters interact with highly specific sites, called receptors, to convey chemical information that may be reconverted into electrical signals or modulate other chemical events. Receptors are found not only in the postsynaptic, but also in the presynaptic areas, where they presumably play regulatory roles.

When the neurotransmitter binds to the receptor, it causes perturbations resulting in direct, or allosteric, interactions that ultimately alter the enzyme activity that generates or inhibits further electrical impulses. One of the most important of these interactions is presently believed to involve cyclic nucleotides. Certain receptors have been demonstrated to be associated with the enzyme adenylate cyclase. The interaction between the neurotransmitter and its receptor causes adenylate cyclase to become more active, increasing the synthesis of cAMP from ATP. This results in alterations in intracellular cAMP levels that change the activity of certain enzymes—enzymes that ultimately mediate many of the changes caused by the neurotransmitter. For example, there are protein

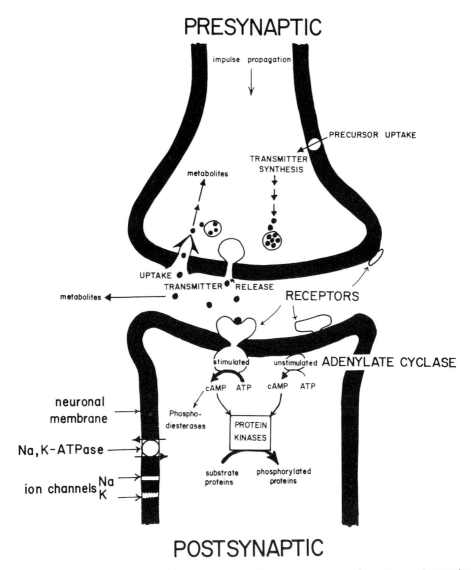

Figure 12.2 Schematic model of a synapse. The presynaptic and postsynaptic terminals are indicated as are some possible biochemical sites of toxicant action.

kinases in the brain whose activity is dependent upon these cyclic nucleotides; the presence or absence of cAMP alters the rate at which these kinases phosphorylate other proteins (using ATP as substrate). The phosphorylated products of these protein kinases are enzymes whose activity to effect certain reactions is thereby altered. One example of a reaction that is altered is the transport of cations (e.g., Na^+, K^+) by the enzyme adenosinetriphosphatase (ATPase). These processes (summarized in Figure 12.2) are all possible loci for biochemical attack by toxicants—events that can markedly alter neural transmission and result in toxicity in the CNS.

12.4.2. Specific Biochemical Sites of Action

12.4.2a. Changes in Transmitter (Modulator) Levels

If the concentration of the neurotransmitter itself is markedly altered, then biochemical and physiological processes that are dependent on it may also be affected. The concentrations of the neurotransmitters in situ are primarily a function of the net of synthesis and degradation, and an agent that either decreases synthesis or increases degradation will have the same net effect—an apparent depletion in neurotransmitter concentrations. Many plant alkaloids known to folklore both as poisons and medicines work through mechanisms that alter neurotransmitter concentrations. For example, the *Rauwolfia* alkaloids cause acute depletions of both central and peripheral stores of the catecholamines norepinephrine and dopamine and the indolamine serotonin. One of these alkaloids, reserpine, appears to cause depletions by releasing the catecholamines from storage vesicles, a result that is not completely reversible. The molecular mechanism for this biochemical effect is not known, but the result is an impairment in processes dependent on the neurotransmitters involved.

The same effect can be induced by drugs that block the synthesis of catecholamines by inhibiting the enzyme that catalyzes the initial reaction in their biosynthesis, tyrosine hydroxylase. One such drug, α-methyl-*p*-tyrosine, is a competitive inhibitor of the enzyme and (unlike reserpine, which depletes stores of the catecholamines) prevents new neurotransmitter synthesis. This results in an eventual depletion of the catecholamines since normal degradative processes are still active. These toxicants have been used frequently in basic research to help assess the role of catecholamines in many physiological responses and have also been used clinically when reduced catecholamine function is desired. These toxicant-induced changes in neurotransmitter levels are demonstrable as acute effects, but long-term secondary changes may also occur. These processes, which are of tremendous importance in evaluating the toxic events in the CNS, are discussed in detail later in this chapter.

12.4.2b. Receptor Interactions

The characterization of many neurotransmitter receptors has provided an invaluable tool for studying the mechanisms by which toxicants or drugs may affect this site of action in the CNS. Major breakthroughs in this area resulted from attempts to characterize a hypothetical "opiate receptor" that would account for the central actions of opiate alkaloids or their derivatives such as morphine and heroin. The analgesic or euphoric actions of these compounds, as well as their acute toxicity (e.g., respiratory depression), were hypothesized to be a result of their binding with specific CNS receptors (opiate receptors). These receptors were thought to be physiological effectors for a previously unknown neurotransmitter that presumably was involved in the normal physiological process that the opiate drugs affect, such as nociception. It has recently been demonstrated that radiolabeled opiates or opiate antagonists bind to certain brain subfractions in a highly specific manner and that this binding correlates well with the actions of these drugs in vivo. For example, the physiologically active opiate levallorphan displaces ^{3}H-diprenorphine from rat brain, whereas dextrallorphan (the inactive enantiomer) has no effect.

The presumed endogenous substrates for these receptors were also isolated and found to be a series of peptides called enkephalins and endorphins. These peptides bound with high affinity to the opiate receptors and would also cause narcoticlike actions when administered in vivo. Increased understanding of the receptors and transmitters involved in the action of opiates has permitted the evolution of a molecular biochemical concept of the physiological sequelae of acute and chronic administration of these xenobiotics. More pertinently, the types of studies illustrated above have resulted in new methodology which provides a powerful tool for future studies on the effects of putative CNS toxicants on central neurotransmitters and receptors.

Molecules that pass the blood–brain barrier may interact with receptors in several ways. First, the interaction may mimic the in situ neurotransmitter and cause agonistlike actions. Second, the molecule may bind to the receptor without causing resultant activation, thereby blocking access of the endogenous ligand (antagonist actions). In either case, if the binding between toxicant and receptor is sufficiently strong, or of sufficient duration, the result may be a substantial alteration in homeostatic, compensatory mechanisms that ultimately may result in a variety of secondary changes.

12.4.2c. Cyclic Nucleotide Biochemistry

The sequence of neural events summarized in Figure 12.2 results in the binding of a neurotransmitter to a receptor with subsequent activation of adenylate cyclase. Increased quantities of cAMP, made from ATP, can then act as a secondary messenger on other receptors, such as protein kinases. Many unanswered questions still exist regarding the definitive roles of cAMP and cyclic guanosine monophosphate (cGMP) in neuronal functioning, but it is assumed that cyclic nucleotide systems probably play a major role in direct impulse transmission as well as in feedback control in the CNS. The evidence for this includes the following observations: alterations in nucleotide levels correlate temporally with physiological events; enzymatic machinery is present in sufficient concentration for rapid synthesis and degradation of the nucleotides; and there are enzymes present whose activities in ion transport, protein phosphorylation, or related processes are markedly altered by cyclic nucleotides.

It is obvious that toxicants that interfere with the levels of cyclic nucleotides via either synthetic or degradive enzymes can markedly alter CNS function. Several alkaloids known to have these actions include the methylxanthines, caffeine and theophylline, which are found in coffee and tea. They affect cyclic nucleotide systems by inhibiting the phosphodiesterase enzymes that degrade cAMP to 5'-AMP and cGMP to 5'-GMP. Chronic administration of high concentrations of caffeine to rats during development is known to cause a condition similar to the Lesch-Nyhan syndrome seen in humans. The mechanisms for this action are unknown but may involve actions on both cyclic nucleotide systems and adenosine receptors in the brain.

12.4.2d. Ion Balance and Flow

The generation and integration of electrical signals in the CNS are ultimately dependent upon the differential distribution of various ionic species at membrane interfaces. This distribution is influenced by many biochemical events, but the two most important are active transport of ions ("pumping") and selective membrane permeabilities. These biochemical foci, and the related processes, are therefore extremely important sites of toxicant action.

The development of electrogenic potentials is dependent upon the active transport of ions, principally sodium and potassium, across nerve cell membranes. This is accomplished by an Na^+, K^+-ATPase, which brings about a coupled transfer of sodium and potassium—sodium to the outside and potassium to the inside. Loss of this activity results in a loss of function of the nerve cell, and it may be effected in two ways. The enzyme is naturally dependent on a continuing supply of ATP, and agents that inhibit oxidative phosphorylation or other steps of energy metabolism indirectly inhibit the ion pumps. Ion transport can also be inhibited by specific agents that affect the enzyme, such as the glycoside ouabain or the lead ion. Many other factors can also influence ATPase activity. For example, studies in vitro have indicated that ATPase activity can be regulated by calcium levels, as well as by the association of calcium with regulator proteins, which can then act as activators of the enzyme. It is also interesting to note that these calcium-binding regulatory proteins are also involved in the control of cyclic nucleotide phosphodiesterases and adenylate cyclases.

The passage of ions through nerve cell membranes after establishment of an electrogenic potential occurs through specific channels in the membrane for both potassium and sodium. Tetrodotoxin, a compound isolated from the ovary and liver of the puffer fish, blocks the increase in conductance in the sodium channel necessary for generation of an action potential. Conversely, a group of plant alkaloids, the grayanotoxins, have been demonstrated to cause increases in the resting sodium permeability.

The regulation of ion flux is essential to the CNS because it allows the integration and modulation of electrical signals between afferent and efferent sites. Changes in ion balance do not always result in direct impulse transmission, but may also regulate membrane events that are reflected in hypo- or hyperpolarizability of the membrane. The latter changes can modulate subsequent neurotransmission.

12.4.2e. Intermediary Metabolism and Miscellaneous Sites of Action

The previous descriptions are indicative of the energy-intensive nature of nerve cell functioning. These requirements for large and constant quantities of ATP make the CNS very sensitive to factors that disrupt intermediary metabolism. Agents that disrupt oxidative phosphorylation or other metabolic systems can damage or kill nerve cells, with subsequent effects on other cells that communicate with the damaged neuron. Similar actions result from agents with specific sites of action, such as the fluoride ion, and more nonspecific chemicals, such as heavy metals.

Another important factor in the functioning of nerve cells is the integrity of membranes and related structures. The axons of many nerve cells have surrounding myelin sheaths consisting of concentric layers of the surface membrane of specialized cells called oligodendrocytes. Myelin sheaths, as well as neuron cell surface membranes, are subject to attack by toxicants. The damage that chemicals such as polychlorinated insecticides (DDT, mirex, etc.) and organic solvents (hexane) cause to the peripheral and central nervous system are presumed to be due to effects on cell membranes.

Finally, many of the specific agents that will be discussed in the following sections that have demonstrable actions in the brain also attack the peripheral nervous system. In many instances, they will damage the sympathetic or parasympathetic nerves sufficiently to terminate respiration or cardiovascular function, indirectly causing brain death. However, because the central actions of these compounds may be important after exposure at lower doses, or because they provide the best examples of a particular point, their mechanisms will be discussed.

12.5. Specific Mechanisms and Examples

12.5.1. Primary and Secondary Actions

12.5.1a. Depletion of Neurotransmitters

Primary actions. CNS toxicants that cause depletion of specific neurotransmitters have been a valuable tool in investigating the response of the brain to challenge. The compound that has been investigated most thoroughly is the catecholamine analog 6-hydroxydopamine. Its use in pharmacological, physiological, and behavioral studies has resulted in a detailed understanding of the complexities of acute toxic effects in the CNS and the mechanisms by which these toxic effects may be overcome. As illustrated in Figure 12.2, 6-hydroxydopamine may interact at those sites where norepinephrine or dopamine are normally present:

6-Hydroxydopamine   Dopamine   Norepinephrine

The mechanism critical to the action of this compound is the synaptic uptake system, which is normally the major way that the action of endogenous catecholamines is terminated. Once taken into the presynaptic process, 6-hydroxydopamine causes the destruction of the nerve terminal, apparently through an oxidative mechanism involving free radical and/or superoxide anion intermediates. Administration to rat brain of quantities of 6-hydroxydopamine as small as 100 μg may cause the *permanent* loss of more than 90% of the brain norepinephrine and dopamine content. Biochemical (loss of enzyme activities) and histological (loss of terminals) methods both indicate that the depletion is due to destruction of the nerve terminals and possibly the nerve cell. It is important to note that the effects of 6-hydroxydopamine may be altered by many factors. Drugs that inhibit the neuronal uptake of norepinephrine, but not dopamine, will spare norepinephrine-containing nerve endings, whereas a drug that inhibits the oxidative breakdown of catecholamines can markedly enhance the toxicity of 6-hydroxydopamine. These factors are indicative of the possibilities that must be considered in evaluating a putative CNS toxicant.

Secondary actions. The physiological results of 6-hydroxydopamine treatment are marked, with treated animals exhibiting severe ataxia, aphagia, and adipsia immediately after treatment. This acute phase of 6-hydroxydopamine toxicity will be lethal to many animals if measures to guarantee adequate nutrition are not instituted. However, if forced feeding is done for several days after treatment, the animals make a remarkable recovery within several weeks after administration of the toxicant. The obvious conclusion is that catecholamine neurons have recovered, with a resultant disappearance of symptoms. However, as stated earlier, autopsy of these "recovered" animals demonstrates that there is still massive depletion of central dopamine and/or norepinephrine. The recovery of physiological functions that are dependent on the catecholamines must therefore involve factors other than the absolute levels of the neurotransmitters.

However, if a xenobiotic that stimulates catecholamine receptors (such as the dopamine agonist apomorphrine) is administered to these recovered animals, the behavioral response observed is much greater than in control animals. This phenomenon is known as supersensitivity and reflects mechanisms designed to recover function after toxicant insult. It is interesting to note that the opposite result, subsensitivity, has also been documented after different types of treatments. In either case, one result of these compensatory changes is a diminished response of the target organism to challenges of either an environmental or chemical nature. It should also be observed that these compensatory changes, after a recovery period, will tend to obscure long-term neural deficits. Assessment of the effects of putative CNS toxins should include paradigms utilizing pharmacological or other challenges to attempt to discover latent alterations.

There are many mechanisms that may be involved in recovery from neural injury; many of which cause evident morphological changes. Biochemical changes also occur; the most interesting that have been demonstrated are alterations in neurotransmitter receptors in response to xenobiotic injury. It has been demonstrated that 6-hydroxydopamine treatment causes an increase in the density of the affected catecholamine receptors. Presumably, when decreased amounts of dopamine or norepinephrine become available (due to destruction of the presynaptic nerve terminal), unknown mechanisms (which may involve cAMP) are initiated that cause a proliferation of the affected receptor and, possibly, increased affinity of the receptor for the neurotransmitter. This is believed to be the reason, in large part, for the recovery of normal function. Furthermore, it is this increased receptor activity that causes the supersensitive response after administration of apomorphine, a dopaminergic agonist, to recovered dopamine-depleted animals.

Scope and variety of neurotransmitters. The previous sections, as well as certain material which follows, emphasize brain catecholamine systems primarily because there is a paucity of information about other neurotransmitters. For example, many agents are known to cause similar effects on brain levels of the neurotransmitter 5-hydroxytryptamine (serotonin).

Decreased catecholamine systhesis and content are observed after inhibition of the enzyme tyrosine hydroxylase by α-methyl-p-tyrosine. Similarly, p-chlorophenylalanine decreases central stores of serotonin by inhibiting a necessary enzyme in serotonin biosynthesis, tryptophan decarboxylase. In addition, serotonin levels in the CNS can also be permanently depleted by administration of the serotonin analogs 5,6- or 5,7-dihydroxytryptamine:

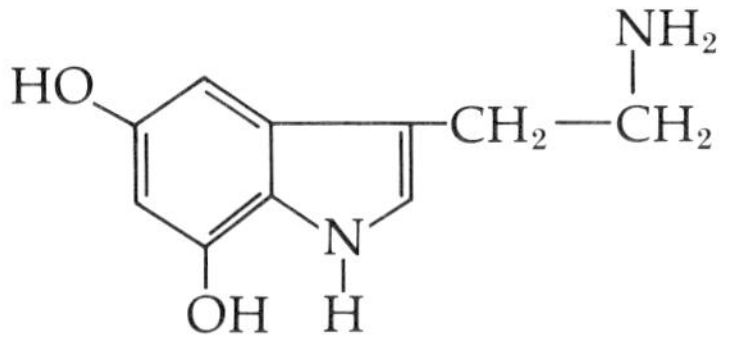

$$\text{5,7-Dihydroxytryptamine} \qquad \text{Serotonin}$$

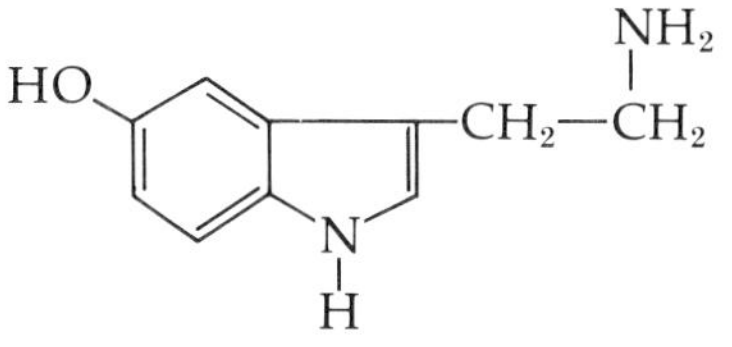

These toxicants are taken up into the presynaptic serotonin neuron (Figure 12.2), where by unknown mechanisms they cause the destruction of the nerve terminal and sometimes the remainder of the presynaptic cell. However, as with 6-hydroxydopamine toxicity, the serotonin postsynaptic receptors are not damaged since they do not have the uptake mechanisms. Thus, the amount of releasable serotonin is dramatically reduced, causing alterations in behaviors dependent upon serotonin pathways in the brain. Another result of this treatment is supersensitivity toward drugs, such as certain ergot alkaloids that have actions on serotonergic receptors.

Depletion of neurotransmitters may result through other mechanisms. Peripheral administration of large doses of monosodium glutamate (a normal cellular constituent) to young rats causes disruption of normal endocrine function, resulting in an extremely obese animal. This obesity results from loss of food intake regulation caused by specific lesions of one area of the hypothalamus, the arcuate nucleus. It appears that these cells are killed because the young animal has an immature blood–brain barrier that permits high concentrations of the amino acid to penetrate to cells that utilize glutamate as a neurotransmitter. The molecular mechanisms by which these cells are then destroyed is not known.

A major difficulty in assessing the action of possible CNS toxicants is the plethora of putative and purported neurotransmitters. As displayed in Table 12.1, these materials cover a wide range of chemical structures and are indicative of the complexities that are encountered in studying the brain. A major concern of toxicologists in the future will be the application of new methods to study xenobiotic effects on these many systems.

12.5.2. Natural Toxins

The majority of drugs that are or have been used clinically are products derived from living organisms. The traditional use of plant, animal, and microbial products in folk medicine is a reflection of the toxicopharmacological actions of these materials. Some examination of the diversity of actions of materials of natural origin will illustrate the scope of the possible toxicological problems that are present.

12.5.2a. Plant Products

The use of herbal extracts for millenia has recently been rationalized by the development and application of modern chemical techniques that allow elucidation of the active principles of these potions. The particular extract that has affected the greatest number of people and has also been an important biomedical tool is morphine, an alkaloid of the opium poppy. The observation of both

Table 12.1 Molecules with Demonstrated or Purported Roles as Neurotransmitters or Neuromodulators in the Central Nervous System

Amines	Peptides and proteins
Catecholamines	*"Opiate-like"*
Dopamine[a]	β-Endorphin[b]
Norepinephrine[a]	Enkephalin(s)[b]
Epinephrine[a]	
Miscellaneous	*Miscellaneous*
Serotonin[a]	Substance P[b]
Acetylcholine[a]	Vasopressin
Histamine[b]	Angiotensin II
Octopamine[b]	Thyrotropin-releasing hormone (TRH)
Tyramine	Neurotensin
β-Phenylethylamine	Somatostatin
Carnosine	Luteinizing hormone–releasing hormone (LHRH)
	Corticotropin (ACTH)
Amino acids	Cholecystokinin
γ-Aminobutyric acid (GABA)[a]	Vasoactive intestinal polypeptide (VIP)
Glycine[a]	Gastrin
Taurine[b]	Prolactin
Glutamic acid[b]	Insulin
Aspartic acid[b]	Glucagon
Proline	Follicle-stimulating hormone (FSH)
Cysteic acid	Oxytocin
Homocysteic acid	
β-Alanine	

Note: Many molecules found in the brain are believed to have roles as neuroregulatory substances. However, to be considered a neurotransmitter, these molecules must fulfill the following criteria: (a) be localized in neurons; (b) have excitatory or inhibitory effects on neurons; (c) be released from neurons; and (d) have the same effect at the synapse as does electrical stimulation of the pathway.

[a] Fulfill all criteria listed below.

[b] Fulfill most criteria (or all criteria in lower species) listed below. The remaining materials have either been found to have profound CNS activity or have been localized in the brain, but have not met most of the listed criteria.

the acute analgesic–euphoric action of opiate derivatives and the dependence syndrome has led to an understanding of important brain mechanisms, as well as the design and use of drug analogs for a variety of purposes. These studies led to the identification of a brain "opiate receptor," a series of receptors that bind morphine with high affinity (see Section 12.4.2b). The presence of receptors in the brain indicates that an endogenous physiological substrate exists, and several such substances have been isolated. These compounds have been isolated from animal brains and are peptides called endorphins and enkephalins (Table 12.1). These opiatelike materials appear to originate from a prohormone which, when cleaved, yields both the endorphin precursor and the peptide known as ACTH. It has been demonstrated that smaller peptide fragments of ACTH also have powerful effects on the CNS when administered directly into the brain, as do the endorphins and enkephalins. These endogenous neurotransmitter–modulators naturally provide a site for toxicant action. Interestingly, alkaloid effectors of other peptide receptors have not yet been documented, but this area may be important in future toxicological investigations. Table 12.1 lists some of the peptides that have been proposed to have transmitter–modulator functions in the CNS.

There have been many other plant derivatives documented to have dramatic physiological actions, but a great many of the common ones (such as the anticholinergic belladonna alkaloids) possess CNS as well as important peripheral actions. Because the latter effects can lead to death through alterations of respiration or circulation, the central actions of many of these drugs are rendered superfluous by the blood–brain barrier. Similarly, the alkaloid colchicine has been used clinically for the treatment of gout and is used experimentally as a mitotic poison. Colchicine is a CNS toxin because it prevents tubulin formation, on which axonal transport mechanisms are dependent. However, the inherent peripheral toxicity of the compound and the ability of the blood–brain barrier to prevent central influx of the alkaloid minimizes its central effects.

The grayanotoxins, discussed in Section 12.4.2d, are found in leaves of plants of the Ericaceae family. Veratridine is a steroidal alkaloid (found in *Veratrum* and *Zygadenus* species) that also depolarizes nerve membranes. Saxitoxin, which blocks sodium channels in nerve membranes as tetrodotoxin does, is found in dinoflaggelate phytoplankton. These are just a few of many well-documented plant-derived neurotoxins, many of which do not have a documented mechanism of action. Consultation of any pharmacology text for a history of drug development will indicate the importance of botanical species to both toxicology and pharmacology.

12.5.2b. Microbial and Fungal Toxins

Accidental intoxications by microbial products have been numerous, presenting both public health challenges and research possibilities. This group of toxins includes those of bacterial and fungal origin. An important group of bacterial toxins are proteins produced by numerous species of the genus *Clostridium*. Though gas gangrene is a result of the growth of *Cl. perfringens* on necrotic tissue, more is known of the mechanisms of *Cl. tetani.* This bacterium produces a protein of 70,000 daltons called tetanospasmin, which is believed to be moved through nerve cells via retrograde axonal transport until it binds, or is fixed, to gangliosides in the brain stem or cord. There it blocks inhibitory synaptic input on spinal motor neurons, resulting in spastic paralysis.

The proteinaceous products of *Cl. botulinum* are probably the most toxic materials known. These are a series of neurotoxins produced by several *Cl. botulinum* strains that bind to presynaptic nerve terminals of cholinergic neurons. At these sites, the proteins inhibit the release of the acetylcholine, with resulting loss of function. The action of these toxins on the peripheral nervous system is critical since, as with the belladonna alkaloids, loss of cholinergic control of circulatory and respiratory functions causes death. However, the toxins are also thought to affect the CNS, and in cases in which sufficient antitoxin (immunoglobulin G) is given therapeutically to arrest the peripheral actions, there may still be residual brain damage, presumably resulting from the action of botulinum toxins that penetrated the blood–brain barrier. The botulinum toxins are sufficiently potent that submicrogram doses are lethal to adult humans.

There are many neurotoxins that are constituents of various fungal species—

toxins that make the art of mushroom picking a nonroutine hobby. These include derivatives of the peyote cactus, one of which, mescaline, is a drug that is believed to cause central actions via interactions with catecholamine- or serotonin-containing neurons. The same systems are believed to be affected by ergot fungus alkaloids that include lysergic acid diethylamide (LSD). Poisonings resulting from ingestion of ergot-contaminated grain have been hypothesized to be responsible for certain tales of medieval European cities becoming possessed by the devil and even for the Salem (Massachusetts) witch trials. LSD has been shown to interact with both dopamine and serotonin receptors, explaining at least part of its biological actions. The *Amanita* species mushrooms also produce a series of cyclic octapeptides, the amanitines, that have a delayed cerebrotoxicity. The mechanism of action of these compounds may be related to their actions to specifically inhibit nuclear RNA polymerase, thus killing the cell.

12.5.2c. Animal Products

The animal products most often associated with human health are snake venoms and venoms from other reptiles such as Gila monsters. These materials are covered in detail in Chapter 20, but it is important to reiterate that the deadliest venoms almost always have a neurotoxin constituent. Another interesting, though less alarming, source of potent neurotoxins is the globe or puffer fish, which can engorge air and "blow" itself up to ferocious dimensions. The principle factor is tetrodotoxin (found in the livers and ovaries of these fish), which inhibits the sodium channel in nerve cell membranes. Another interesting and potent neurotoxin is one of the toxic principles contained in the secretions from the skin of the Colombian arrow poison frog, *Phyllobates aurotaenia*. It is a potent steroid-based molecule with actions similar to those of grayanotoxins.

12.5.3. Pharmaceutical Agents

12.5.3a. Major Tranquilizers

The development of chlorpromazine during the 1950s for use in the treatment of schizophrenia was the first effective use of a synthetic compound in treating mental illness. The clinical use of the major tranquilizers (neuroleptics), which include chlorpromazine and related phenothiazines and the butyrophenones, has spurred research into their possible mechanisms of action. This research, in turn, has led to many hypotheses about the etiology of mental illnesses. It has been proven that these drugs, when given acutely, bind to the receptors in the CNS that are normally responsive to dopamine. Many of the acute actions of drugs that mimic dopamine (including the dopamine precursor L-dihydroxyphenylalanine or L-dopa) are antagonized by these drugs, suggesting that this effect is somehow related to their mechanism of clinical action. Chronic administration of these drugs results in a supersensitivity to dopaminergic agonists for several days after cessation of the neuroleptic. Furthermore, long-term administration sometimes results in a condition called "tardive dyskinesia," which presumably results from compensatory changes initiated by the receptor blockade. Despite the tremendous clinical importance of these findings, the mechanisms responsible have not yet been elucidated.

12.5.3b. Ethanol

Alcohol has been studied for decades because of the problems its abuse has presented to many societies. To date, there is no defined, specific action of alcohol on the CNS that explains its many actions. The inability to find specific biochemical modes of action (as has been done with the major tranquilizers) has led many investigators to suggest that alcohol may act nonspecifically on many neuronal tracts, presumably by actions on membranes. It also appears that varied actions of alcohol may result from its interactions with genetic, environmental, and other xenobiotic factors. For example, it has been shown that ethanol, by altering the oxidation–reduction environment, or by means of its primary metabolite, acetaldehyde, can lead to the formation of compounds that may undergo further reaction under physiological conditions. These compounds, salsolinol or 3,4-dihydroxyphenylacetaldehyde, may condense with dopamine to yield the compound tetrahydropapaveroline and related molecules:

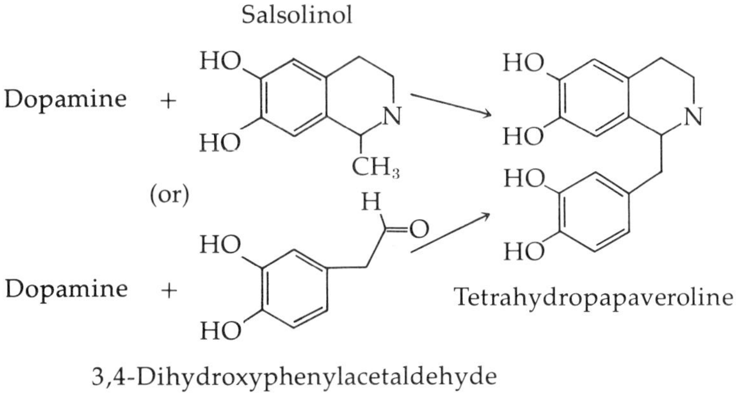

Recent work has demonstrated that tetrahydropapaveroline (after infusion at low doses into rat or monkey brain) causes the development of a marked preference for alcohol solutions over water, which is not a generally demonstrable phenomenon in animals. It is believed by some that this may provide a toxicological basis for the development of alcoholism in certain susceptible humans.

12.5.3c. Anesthetics

The use of anesthetic agents has provided a tool that has allowed modern surgery to convert life-threatening conditions into routine medical practice. Despite their tremendous utility, the mechanism of action of many classes of anesthetic agents has not been well defined. Empirical studies have lead to refined usage, but there is still a dearth of understanding about how agents with diverse effects cause anesthesia. It is generally assumed that these materials, like ethanol, may act nonspecifically. Many of these agents, including ether, halothane, nitrous oxide, etc., are very lipid soluble; they tend to penetrate the blood–brain barrier and may penetrate other lipophilic membranes, such as those in nerve cells. Slight changes in these membranes can have profound physiological effects, and one may surmise that the general CNS depression one finds in anesthesia may be the result of alterations in neural function in many systems. Local anesthetics, however, are believed to act by blocking sodium conductance, which prevents depolarization. The available empirical evidence, which correlates time and depth of anesthesia with different central agents, may be an expression of differential sensitivity or accessibility of neural membranes. The high incidence of complications from anesthesia is evidence that more detailed pharmacological/toxicological information is needed about these agents in the CNS.

12.5.4. Heavy Metals

Trace elements are ubiquitous as cofactors in biological systems. Because calcium is known to have numerous regulatory roles in the CNS, it is unremarkable that other elements that are polyvalent cations and are able to form coordination compounds may interfere with normal physiological functioning when present at sufficient levels to compete or interact with the endogenous metals. Heavy metals, so named because they are of greater atomic weight than the physiologically necessary elements, have been documented to have many CNS actions.

Mercury, because of its ability to bind to organic molecules, has been used both experimentally and clinically as a gastrointestinal helminthicide and as a topical skin agent. Its safe use is a result of low penetration of inorganic mercury through the gut and blood–brain barriers. However, human consumption of fish that had been exposed to dimethyl and methyl mercury (formed by biomethylation of inorganic mercury in sediments of the waters near Minamata, Japan), resulted in an epidemic of mercury poisoning. Because methyl mercuries penetrate biological membranes nearly two orders of magnitude more effectively than inorganic forms of mercury, this resulted in more than 100 cases of illness and dozens of deaths. The symptoms of what is now called Minamata disease are a compendium of CNS disturbances: loss of cognitive functioning, palsied movements, and often permanent mental retardation. The young and the unborn were markedly more sensitive to the effects of the mercurials (see Section 12.5.5b). It may be that toxic effects on the brain are due to inorganic mercury after in situ demethylation of the absorbed compounds. The molecular site of action is unknown, but it is suspected that flavoproteins involved in energy metabolism may be particularly sensitive.

The evaluation of subacute lead toxicity has also recently become an important question. Exposure to high levels of lead is known to cause permanent alterations of the central and peripheral nervous systems in both humans and laboratory animals. It is less certain how lead affects the CNS when lower levels of exposure (detected in humans via measurement of blood lead and alterations in protoporphyrin biosynthesis) occur. Pediatric studies suggested that lead burdens lower than those causing clinical symptoms were correlated with both behavioral and cognitive deficits. Despite valid methodological criticism of these studies, they spurred the search for animal models of low-level developmental lead exposure. Recent research has found that exposure of rodents to lead during postnatal developmental periods will cause a series of subtle, but consistent alterations in behavioral and pharmacological responses mediated through the CNS. The specific biochemical mechanisms by which these changes occur is not yet known, though it is probable that they result from the interaction of lead with numerous loci. Some data also suggest that rats exposed to lead after critical development periods do not show that same neural changes seen in younger animals that have been exposed. The high incidence of lead exposure of infants and juveniles in urban areas, certain industrial populations, and, until recently, populations in areas located near major automotive thoroughfares, makes the potential effect of these lead-induced CNS alterations very important.

12.5.5. Considerations in Long-Term or Chronic Toxicant Exposure

The previous discussions on selected toxins of the CNS have dealt with both acute (e.g., grayanotoxins) and chronic (e.g., lead) exposures. These examples have indicated important compensatory changes that may occur after toxicant exposure—responses that may be more profound than the acute actions. An understanding of these compensatory mechanisms is essential to the proper evaluation of biochemical toxicology in the CNS.

12.5.5a. Types of Changes Occurring After Toxicant Exposure

The changes that occur after exposure to a toxicant may fall into certain discrete categories. First, there is the acute exposure in which the biochemical effects of the xenobiotic are dependent on the continued presence of the toxin at appropriate sites. The actions of many drugs, such as the opiates or neuroleptics discussed earlier in this chapter, are examples of this. Second, the acute effects of the toxin may cause an immediate lesion that will remain even after the disappearance of the agent. The mode of action of 6-hydroxydopamine or the organophosphate cholinesterase inhibitors may be considered to be examples of this. Finally, there are situations in which exposure to the toxin occurs over long periods of time, whether deliberately (as in clinical situations) or inadvertently (as in environmental exposures).

In evaluating the effects of xenobiotics on the CNS it is essential to consider all these changes and the effects of not only the primary biochemical changes, but also the secondary, compensatory changes that may occur. A few examples of the latter changes have been given, but many others are known. As illustrated in Figure 12.1, one nerve cell makes contact with many other cells, and the latter cells may utilize other neurotransmitters for their communication. For example, a cell that releases dopamine as its neurotransmitter may have a synaptic contact with a cell that releases γ-aminobutyric acid (GABA) at its synapses. The cell that is receptive to GABA may be a cholinergic neuron. From the number of known and suspected neuroregulatory materials (Table 12.1), it becomes obvious that full assessment of possible compensatory mechanisms is a difficult task, yet one with important consequences. This aspect of toxicological assessment will be dependent on fundamental advances that are being or will be made in neurobiology.

12.5.5b. Developmental Factors in Nervous System Toxicology

During the ontogenesis of the CNS, a series of morphological and biochemical changes occur that may be altered by xenobiotic exposure. The observed cellular changes may be summarized as follows:

1. Proliferation of cells, followed by migration, aggregation, and cytodifferentiation.
2. Axonal outgrowth and synaptogenesis.
3. Functional validation accomplished by the withdrawal of processes and dying back of certain cells.

In general, though these gross anatomical changes are well documented, little information is available about the molecular and biochemical systems that control these events. Certain predictions about the consequences of toxicant exposure may, nonetheless, be made.

There is generally assumed to be a "critical period" during which the death of a single or several cells may have extreme consequences for the differentiating nervous system. Because some of this development may occur postnatally, it is evident that toxicant exposure that may cause little effect in the adult may have permanent and severe results in the developing animal. The critical period may also be reflected in changes that occur during axonal outgrowth and other "sprouting" phenomena, during which toxicant exposure may prevent normal synaptogenesis from occurring and, as a consequence, cause the occurrence of compensatory changes. It is interesting to note, however, that developing animals do exhibit greater "plasticity" (ability to recover from damage) than do adults. For example, after surgical sectioning of a nerve, the young animal shows more sprouting and, in turn, greater recovery than the adult. Thus, the extent and consequences of toxicant exposure in the developing animal are dependent on when exposure occurs during ontogenesis and whether the biochemical site of action is specifically on either nerve cell body or processes. Age-dependent changes in the blood–brain barrier also influence these phenomena.

In humans, it is estimated that as many as 5–10% of all children suffer from the syndrome called minimal brain dysfunction, evidenced by both behavioral and cognitive difficulties. Several correlations have been made between the occurrence of minimal brain dysfunction and exposure to certain toxicants.

Several research groups observed an apparent correlation in some children of increased blood lead levels with the occurrence of learning and behavioral disabilities. These reports spurred studies on animal models, and some investigators found that exposure of rats or mice to lead during developmental periods caused behavioral alterations that appeared similar to minimal brain dysfunction. These animals also appeared to have specific alterations in catecholamine and acetylcholine neuronal systems in the brain, though mechanisms for these changes were not found. It has also been found that levels of developmental lead exposure that cause no observable pathological changes cause permanent alterations in certain pharmacological responses known to be dependent on dopamine neurons in the brain. If further studies can associate these animal studies with human exposure, it may indicate that presently tolerated levels of lead exposure will have to be reevaluated. It is interesting to note that adult animals similarly exposed to equivalent lead levels do not exhibit similar changes.

More recently, it was reported that minimal brain dysfunction in certain children was linked to the ingestion of specific food additives and natural constituents. The "Feingold hypothesis" (named after the California pediatrician who proposed it) suggests that dietary factors, through unknown mechanisms, significantly alter brain function, resulting in clinically observable symptoms. Proponents of this hypothesis suggest that elimination of the offensive agents through dietary manipulation can markedly improve many children. Evidence does not yet support these claims, but it suggests both the difficulty and importance of toxicological assessments.

12.6. Conclusions

The purpose of this chapter was not to provide an overview of CNS toxicology, a task that would have required several volumes. Rather, the intent has been to highlight specific aspects of brain function and to indicate the complex and fascinating way that changes may occur after toxic insult. If the reader has concluded that the study of toxic events in the CNS has been a neglected area, then the chapter has succeeded in its first purpose. If the reader has been instilled with an interest in how particular toxicants alter the functioning of the CNS, and therefore that of the whole organism, then all of the author's goals have been achieved. The references cited below must be considered a reflection of personal prejudices and interests and should be regarded only as a starting point for further study. It is explicit that successful investigation of the biochemical toxicology of the CNS is dependent on first understanding fundamental aspects of neurobiology.

Suggested Reading

Breese, G. R. Chemical and immunochemical lesions by specific neurotoxic substances and antisera. In Iversen, L. L., Iversen, S. D., Snyder, S. H. (Eds.). Handbook of Psychopharmacology, Vol. 1. New York: Plenum Press, 1975, pp. 137–189.

Breese, G. R., Cooper, B. R. Chemical lesioning: Catecholamine pathways. Myers, R. D. (Ed.). Methods in Psychobiology, Vol. 3. New York: Academic Press, 1977, pp. 27–46.

Cooper, J. R., Bloom, F. E., Roth, R. H. The Biochemical Basis of Neuropharmacology, third edition. New York: Oxford University Press, 1977.

Cuatrecasas, P. Membrane receptors. Ann. Rev. Biochem. 43 (1974), 169.

Cuatrecasas, P. (Ed.). The Specificity and Action of Animal, Bacterial, and Plant Toxins: Receptors and Recognition, Series B, Vol. 1. New York: Halsted Press, 1977.

Mailman, R. B., Krigman, M. R., Mueller, R. A., Mushak, P., Breese, G. R. Lead exposure during infancy permanently increases lithium-induced polydipsia. Science 201 (1978), 637.

Myers, R. D., Melchoir, C. L. Alcohol drinking: abnormal intake caused by tetrahydropapaveroline in brain. Science 196 (1977), 554.

Narahashi, T. Neurotoxins: Pharmacological dissection of ionic channels of nerve membranes. In Brady, R. O. (Ed.). The Nervous System, Vol. 1, The Basic Neurosciences. New York: Raven Press, 1975, pp. 101–110.

Pardridge, W. M., Connor, J. D., Crawford, I. L. Permeability changes in the blood–brain barrier: Causes and consequences. CRC Crit. Rev. Toxicol. 3 (1975), 159.

Phillis, J. W. The role of cyclic nucleotides in the CNS. Can. Sci. Neurol. 4 (1977), 151.

Roisin, L., Shiraki, H., Grcevic, N. (Eds.). Neurotoxicology. New York: Raven Press, 1977.

Shankland, D. L., Hollingworth, R. M., Smyth, T., Jr. (Eds.). Pesticide and Venom Neurotoxicity. New York: Plenum Press, 1978.

Silbergeld, E. K., Goldberg, A. M. Lead-induced behavioral dysfunction: An animal model of hyperactivity. Exp. Neurol. 42 (1974), 146.

Donald E. Moreland

13

Effects of Toxicants on Oxidative and Photophosphorylation

13.1. Oxidative Phosphorylation and Respiration

Energy obtained from the oxidation of foods is converted to and stored as bond energy by mitochondria in a compound called adenosine triphosphate (ATP). The energy so stored is utilized by all plant and animal cells to drive or power all of the mechanical, transport, and biosynthetic work done by the cell. Hence, ATP is a pivotal metabolic compound and interference with its production or utilization by xenobiotics could have a lethal effect.

13.1.1. Introduction

Mitochondrial oxidative phosphorylation is the primary process by which aerobic cells produce ATP by esterification of adenosine diphosphate (ADP) with inorganic phosphate. Tremendous effort by a large number of researchers has been devoted to understanding the pathways and mechanisms through which ATP is generated. However, many details and aspects are still highly speculative and controversial. Consequently, firm knowledge about oxidative phosphorylation is frustratingly meager.

Mitochondria are found in all aerobic eukaryotic cells. The general structure and function of plant, mammalian, and insect mitochondria appear to be alike. The number of mitochondria per cell range from 20 up to many thousands, depending on the organism concerned. The more metabolically active cells possess the greater number. The number also varies with the type of tissue or organ and the maturation state of the tissue. For example, liver cells average 1000–2500 mitochondria per cell, paramecia about 1000, and *Euglena* 15–20. Mitochondria are typically about 3 μm long and 1 μm in diameter and are spear shaped, but size may vary and transient changes in shape are exhibited. The organelle consists of a sophisticated membrane system within which are incorporated the enzymes that mediate cellular respiration. Located in the mitochondria are all of

the Krebs cycle enzymes, the enzymes associated with electron transport and
oxidative phosphorylation, enzymes for phospholipid synthesis, enzymes for
fatty acid oxidation, and the enzymes for elongation of fatty acids by addition of
acetyl-CoA. Mitochondria also possess DNA that differs from nuclear DNA,
RNA, and a capacity for protein synthesis.

Electron micrographic studies have been helpful in elucidating mitochondrial
structure. A diagrammatic representation of the membrane systems and spaces
of mitochondria is shown in Figure 13.1A. The two membrane systems are the
outer membrane and the inner membrane. The inner membrane is made up of
two sectors—the inner boundary membrane, which parallels the outer membrane, and the cristal membranes, which are invaginations of the inner membrane. The space within the cristae and between the two membrane systems is
called the intracristal space; the space in the interior of the mitochondrion is
called the matrix space. The membranes are 5–7 nm thick. The outer membrane
is smooth and freely permeable to many substances. Only the inner membrane
is considered to be semipermeable. There may be considerable variation in the
number, size, and shape of cristae among mitochondria of different cell types. A
large number of cristae per mitochondrion is associated with the capacity for
high metabolic activity. When mitochondria are negatively stained, dense
granules are revealed that line the inner surface of the cristal or peripheral inner
membrane (Figure 13.1B). These particles appear to be attached to the mem-

Figure 13.1 Diagrammatic representation of (**A**) cross-section of a mitochondrion, (**B**)
detail view of cristael morphology, and (**C**) tripartite repeating unit.

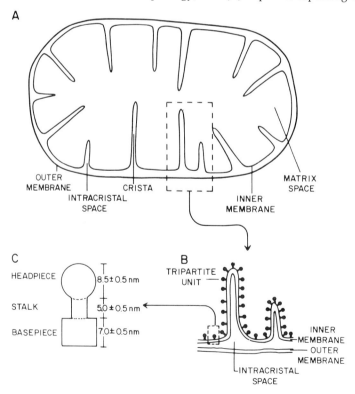

brane by means of a short neck, and they protrude into the matrix. These granules and their stalks are called inner membrane subunits, and they constitute a portion of the tripartite unit. This tripartite structure consists of three bonded sectors: basepiece, stalk, and headpiece (Figure 13.1C). The stalk and headpiece can be detached without compromising the intactness of the membrane.

Phospholipids account for approximately 30% of the weight of the basepiece and the remaining 70% is protein. Approximately 50% of the protein is catalytic and 50% is noncatalytic. Noncatalytic protein plays a role in membrane biogenesis and the organizational pattern of the sectors of the repeating unit.

The enzymes responsible for electron transport appear to be contained in the basepiece of the tripartite repeating unit. The coupled synthesis of ATP by the union of ADP and inorganic phosphate (Pi) is catalyzed by enzymes located in the headpiece–stalk sector.

13.1.2. Electron Transport and Phosphorylation

The inner membrane basepiece sectors have been fractionated into four complexes, each of which contains several of the components of the electron transport chain. The components of the respective complexes and their oxidation–reduction sequences are shown in Figure 13.2. Each complex is the smallest unit in which a sector of the electron transfer chain can be isolated without a loss of native characteristics, such as the ability to react with natural electron acceptors, to show susceptibility to selective inhibitors, and to maintain the appropriate redox values of the component proteins.

Complex I consists of NADH dehydrogenase (Fp · D) and four or five nonheme iron proteins with differing redox potentials. FMN is the flavin component and it is not covalently bound to the dehydrogenase. Complex I is reduced by NADH and oxidized by coenzyme Q (NADH–CoQ reductase). Complex II is composed of succinic dehydrogenase (Fp · S), a b-type cytochrome, and three nonheme iron proteins. It is reduced by succinate and oxidized by CoQ (succinate–CoQ reductase). The flavin component, FAD, is covalently linked through a histidine residue to the peptide chain of the dehydrogenase. Complex III consists of at least one type of cytochrome b, 1 mole cytochrome c_1, and 1 mole nonheme iron protein. It is reduced by CoQ and is oxidized by cytochrome c (CoQ–cytochrome c reductase). Complex IV contains cytochromes a and a_3 in addition to two copper centers, but no nonheme iron protein. It is reduced by reduced cytochrome c and is oxidized by molecular oxygen (cytochrome c oxidase).

Each complex has a molecular mass of approximately 300,000 daltons. If isolated in pure form and added back together in the presence of phospholipids, the system can be reconstituted.

Phospholipid is required for the complexes to form membranes, for electron transfer activity to occur, and for the interaction between the complexes and mobile components. CoQ and cytochrome c, which link the complexes, are associated with the phospholipid. The components are considered to move freely from one complex to the other within the membrane continuum.

There appears to be no fixed stoichiometry between the complexes. Instead, the stoichiometry may be of genetic determination.

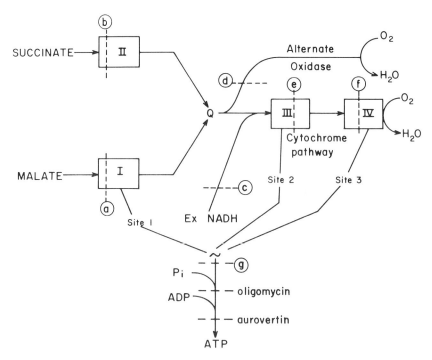

Figure 13.2 Schematic presentation of electron transport and phosphorylation in mitochondria showing postulated sites of action of inhibitors. Abbreviations used: I, II, III, and IV: complexes I, II, III, and IV, respectively; site 1, 2, and 3: phosphorylation sites 1, 2, and 3; alt. oxid.: terminal components of the alternate (cyanide-resistant) pathway; ExNADH: exogenous NADH; Q: ubiquinone; a, b, c, d, e, f, and g: postulated sites of action of inhibitors. See text for details.

The number of ATP molecules synthesized during the oxidation of substrates via the respiratory chain by molecular oxygen is defined as the P/O or ADP/O ratio. The theoretical ratio for the oxidation of NAD-linked substrates such as malate is 3 and for succinate it is 2.

13.1.3. Mechanism of Electron Transfer

The classical concept of electron transport considered that there was a continuous flow of electrons from one redox component to the next as presented diagramatically in Figure 13.2. However, newer evidence suggests that a discontinuous flow of electrons may be involved, i.e., the redox components may not be in electronic communication at all times. When electrons are delivered to a complex, a conformational rearrangement is thought to occur. Only then is electronic communication established between the complexes. The conformational changes result from the shift of a component from its oxidized to its reduced state, or vice versa. Shifts in conformation then lead to the making and breaking of electronic interactions. The mobile carriers such as CoQ and cytochrome c transfer electrons between the complexes. Electron transfer generates electrostatic energy, and this electrostatic energy is transduced into conformational energy.

13.1.4. ATP Generation

The machinery for coupled synthesis of ATP by the union of ADP and Pi is located on the matrix side of the inner membrane. Coupling involves the interdigitation of the electron transport chain and the ATP generating system. In an uncoupled system, substrate is oxidized, electron transport occurs, oxygen is utilized, but no ATP is generated.

The exact mechanism through which ATP is synthesized is not known. Most hypotheses of the mechanism of oxidative phosphorylation differ mainly in what is assumed to be the nature of the primary intermediate, the energy of which is derived from redox energy and subsequently used for ATP synthesis. Three hypotheses have been advanced to explain the coupling of oxidation and phosphorylation. All of the hypotheses have experimental support, but no one hypothesis has been accepted universally.

13.1.4a. Chemiosmotic Hypothesis

The most widely accepted hypothesis is the chemiosmotic, which is based on the principles that the mitochondrial inner membrane has selective permeability to cations and that electron transfer reactions across it are vectorial. The primary energy-conserving reaction that is coupled to electron transport involves the translocation of protons from the inside to the outside of the inner membrane. Because the inner membrane is relatively impermeable to protons and many other ions, an electrochemical gradient results. Energy is considered to be stored as a combination of a pH gradient and membrane potential in varying ratios. ATP is synthesized from ADP and Pi with the energy derived from the movement of protons down the electrochemical gradient by a reversible, proton-translocating ATPase. Some experimental observations conflict with the chemiosmotic hypothesis. Most relate to measurements that have been made on the membrane potential and pH gradient that are inconsistent with the requirements of the hypothesis. In addition, the hypothesis does not account for observed energy-related changes in mitochondrial configuration.

13.1.4b. Chemical Hypothesis

The chemical hypothesis envisions the coupling process as involving the transformation of redox energy into chemical energy that is stored in a few reactive bonds of a chemical intermediate. The hypothesis assumes that the transfer of electrons through the respiratory chain results in the formation of high-energy intermediates that are responsible for the synthesis of ATP. To date, none of the chemical intermediates has been isolated. These are needed to validate the hypothesis. The hypothesis does not consider the relationship between energy state and structural configuration.

13.1.4c. Conformational Coupling Hypothesis

The conformational coupling hypothesis assumes that as a result of the coupling event, potential energy is stored in the conformational state of a protein and, therefore, distributed over many bonds that are distorted with respect to their ground state. The hypothesis relies on the inner membrane being composed of elementary particles. Oxidative phosphorylation is thought to result from the transduction of electrical energy, provided by electron transport, to mechanical energy in the form of configurational changes in the mitochondrial membrane. The mechanical energy can be used for the formation of ATP. The inner membrane supposedly exists in three forms. In the nonenergized form, the headpiece and stalk are compressed into the basepiece (Figure 13.1C). During electron transfer, the headpiece and stalk extend from the basepiece to result in the energized conformation. Addition of Pi results in a further extension of the headpiece and stalk to form the energized twisted configuration. The nonenergized conformation is thermodynamically stable and occurs under anaerobic conditions. The energized and energized twisted structures are metastable and revert to the nonenergized form during anaerobiosis. This hypothesis is attractive, but the existence of the elementary particles is questioned by some investigators.

13.1.5. Methods of Study

Warburg manometry was once the favorite method for studying oxygen utilization by isolated mitochondria. In recent years, however, oxygen uptake has been measured polarographically with the platinum (Clark) electrode and changes in potential are monitored with a strip-chart recorder.

Examples of oxygen utilization by plant mitochondria as measured with a Clark electrode are shown in Figure 13.3. for responses obtained with a hypothetical inhibitor "X." In the first trace (trace A) the pattern of succinate oxidation by mitochondria is shown; it reflects the stimulation of oxygen uptake (state 3 respiration) by the addition of a small amount of ADP, followed by the decrease in respiration upon the exhaustion of the added ADP (state 4 respiration). This sequence can be repeated by further addition of ADP until anaerobiosis occurs, thus demonstrating respiratory control that is required for the evaluation of the action of inhibitors on the energy transfer sequence. This control manifested by ADP will only be evident when the mitochondria are tightly coupled. The relative efficiency of energy transduction of a mitochondrial preparation is indicated by the respiratory control ratio (RC). The RC ratio is obtained by dividing the fast state 3 rate by the slow state 4 rate. RC values for both animal and plant mitochondria range between 3 and 8. ADP/O ratios can be calculated directly from the traces because the amount of ADP added is known and the moles of oxygen consumed are measured.

Trace B shows the stimulation of state 4 or ADP-limited respiration by the compound X when added at a concentration of 1 μM. This reflects uncoupling action and is obtained in the absence of ADP. All control exerted by ADP is lost. Electron transport continues at an accelerated rate along with oxygen utilization, but no ATP is synthesized.

Trace C reflects the circumvention of oligomycin-inhibited respiration by compound X at an uncoupling concentration of 1 μM. In this trace, inhibition of state 3 respiration with ADP present in nonlimiting concentrations is shown by oligomycin. An uncoupler then relieves or circumvents the inhibition imposed by oligomycin. Oligomycin is considered to inhibit respiration by blocking the formation of a high-energy intermediate required for ATP production. Circum-

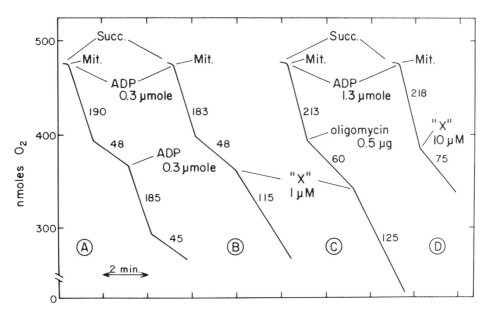

Figure 13.3 Representative polarographic traces depicting oxygen utilization obtained with plant mitochondria for succinate oxidation. Trace A, respiratory control obtained in the absence of an inhibitor. Trace B, stimulation of state 4 respiration by a hypothetical inhibitor "X" (1 μM). Trace C, circumvention of oligomycin-inhibited respiration by "X" (1 μM). Trace D, inhibition of state 3 respiration by "X" (10 μM). Rates of oxygen utilization (nmoles O_2/min/mg protein) are indicated above the traces. Mitochondria (Mit) containing 0.4 mg protein, succinate (8.5 μmoles), ADP, oligomycin, and "X" were added at the points indicated. Concentrations of components are shown as μmoles (succinate and ADP), or μg (oligomycin) supplied to, or as the final molarity ("X") in, the 2-ml reaction medium.

vention of oligomycin-inhibited respiration has prompted investigators to place the site of action of uncouplers, such as 2,4-dinitrophenol (DNP) and the compound X used here, prior to that of oligomycin on the energy-transfer pathway.

Trace D shows the inhibition of state 3 respiration obtained in the presence of nonlimiting concentrations of ADP by an uncoupler such as compound X when added at concentrations greater than those required to express uncoupling action. In this case, compound X was added at a concentration of 10 μM. This response is characteristic of that obtained with electron transport inhibitors.

13.1.6. Differences Between Plant and Animal Mitochondria

Mammalian mitochondria, especially from rat liver, have been used in many studies because of their ease of preparation. The mitochondria can be isolated by homogenization in a sucrose medium followed by differential centrifugation. They stay coupled for many hours, even overnight. On the other hand, isolation of intact, time-stable mitochondria from plant cells is considerably more difficult. Plant tissues have tough cell walls that have to be broken to release the cytoplasmic contents. Rough and/or prolonged homogenization and isolation procedures damage the mitochondria. In addition, plant cells have vacuoles that contain acidic constituents. Hence, when plant cells are homogenized, vacuolar contents are released and the pH of the homogenization medium is lowered. Consequently, the pH of the extracting medium must be maintained at about 7.1–7.4. If the pH should drop much below 7.0, irreversible changes occur and the mitochondria are unsuitable for use in critical studies.

The composition of the electron transport and phosphorylation pathways in plant and animal mitochondria is similar in some respects, but different in others. Intact plant mitochondria readily oxidize exogenous NADH and malate, but isolated animal mitochondria do not. A cyanide- and antimycin A–insensitive pathway (Figure 13.2) is present in many plant mitochondria, but absent from animal mitochondria. Plant, animal, and insect mitochondria are affected similarly by inhibitors and uncouplers; however, their relative sensitivities to the compounds may differ. For example, plant mitochondria are less sensitive to rotenone and antimycin A but more sensitive to oligomycin than are animal mitochondria.

13.1.7. Classification of Inhibitors

Many compounds of widely different chemical structure are known to affect oxidative phosphorylation in different ways. They have played important roles in the formulation of current theories of oxidative phosphorylation and in the elucidation of components of the electron transport and ATP generation pathways. Classically, inhibitors have been placed in one of three categories, depending upon how they affect the various reactions mediated by mitochondria.

13.1.7a. Electron Transport Inhibitors

Experimentally, electron transport inhibitors are characterized by their ability to interrupt electron flow at some point in the respiratory chain by acting on one of the complexes. When electron flow is interrupted, the coupled phosphorylating reactions are also inhibited. The chemicals are thought to combine with one of the electron carriers in some manner so as to prevent the formation of a redox couple. Amytal, rotenone, and piericidin A are complex I inhibitors (Figure 13.2, site a). They prevent the oxidation of malate and other NADH-linked substrates. Malonate is a competitive inhibitor of succinate and interferes with the oxidation of succinate. Antimycin A and 2-heptyl-4-hydroxyquinoline-N-oxide (HOQNO) interfere with complex III (Figure 13.2, site e). Cyanide, azide, and carbon monoxide interfere at complex IV (Figure 13.2, site f). Cyclic hydroxamates, such as salicylhydroxamic acid (SHAM), inhibit the cyanide-insensitive pathway in plant mitochondria (Figure 13.2, site d).

13.1.7b. Uncouplers

At appropriate concentrations, uncouplers prevent the phosphorylation of ADP without interfering with electron transport (Figure 13.2, site g). In general, any compound that promotes the dissipation of energy generated by electron transport, other than for production of ATP, may be regarded as an uncoupler. Uncouplers, when added in vitro to tightly coupled mitochondria, stimulate oxygen uptake by eliminating the regulatory influence normally exerted by Pi and ADP. To be classified as an uncoupler, a compound should do the following:

1. Stimulate state 4 respiration in media deficient in either ADP or Pi.
2. Induce ATPase activity (intact mitochondria contain an inducible ATPase; the induction process is inhibited by oligomycin).
3. Circumvent inhibition of state 3 respiration imposed by oligomycin.
4. Inhibit various exchange reactions catalyzed by mitochondria in the absence of substrate —these exchange reactions involve ADP, Pi, ATP, and water.

Pentachlorophenol (PCP) and DNP are classical examples of uncouplers that have been used as pesticides for many years. Most halogenated and nitrophenols possess uncoupling activity. Their activities vary, depending upon the substituents present on the benzene ring, in that some are insecticides, acaricides, ovicides, fungicides, or herbicides. Substituted 2-trifluoromethyl-benzimidazoles are also uncouplers with a wide range of biological activity. Some are insecticides, acaricides, molluscicides, or herbicides. Others possess antiviral and antibacterial activities. Additional compounds identified as being uncouplers of oxidative phosphorylation include dicoumarin (an anticoagulant), carbonyl cyanide phenylhydrazones, salicylanilides, atebrin (the antimalarial drug), and various anesthetic gases such as halothane.

Classically, uncouplers have been considered to have a pKa in the range of 4–6 and to be quite lipophilic. One concept relative to their action was that uncouplers penetrated the mitochondrial membrane in an un-ionized form. Inside the mitochondrion they were considered to dissociate or ionize and adsorb to catalytic proteins in the ionized form. However, many of the newer pesticides are neutral molecules and do not dissociate under physiological pH.

Many pesticides are detoxified by hydroxylation of their phenyl rings. This occurs in the microsomal system of animals, plants, and soil microorganisms. Whereas the unaltered parent molecule may not be an uncoupler, the hydroxylated degradation forms are potential uncouplers if they are not rapidly complexed as glucosides or glycosides in the plant or as glucuronides in the animal.

13.1.7c. Energy Transfer Inhibitors

Compounds in this group inhibit phosphorylating electron transport when the energy-conserving apparatus of the mitochondria is intact. They are considered to combine with an intermediate in the energy-coupling chain and hence block the phosphorylation sequence that leads to the production of ATP. Oligomycin is the prototype. Aurovertin also affects ATP generation by acting at a locus closer to ATP formation than that affected by oligomycin. Other compounds in this group include the organotins, some of which are pesticides.

13.1.7d. Multiple Types of Inhibition

The action of a given inhibitor is frequently complex. Overlaps in action occur that are sometimes related to the concentration of the inhibitor. Many herbicides (N-phenylcarbamates, 2,6-dinitroanilines, and phenylamides) and some insecticides (cyclodienes) act as uncouplers at low molar concentrations and inhibitors of electron transport at high molar concentrations. This action is shown in Figure 13.3 for the hypothetical compound X. From the various interferences measured with various electron mediators, evidence can he obtained for the following sites of action:

1. ATP generating pathway by stimulation of state 4 respiration, circumvention of oligomycin-imposed state 3 respiration, and induction of ATPase activity.
2. Complex I.
3. Complex II.
4. Exogenous NADH pathway prior to complex III (plant mitochondria).
5. Cyanide-insensitive pathway after the branch point (plant mitochondria).

No evidence has been obtained for interference by herbicides with a site associated with either complex III or IV.

Most investigators who have studied the action of xenobiotics on mitochondria have mainly measured effects on state 3 and state 4 respiration, and related the interferences to the action expressed by classical reference compounds. However, most of the inhibitory insecticides, herbicides, pharmaceuticals, and anesthetics do not structurally resemble the classical inhibitors and uncouplers of oxidative phosphorylation. Conceivably, the action of these many compounds may be different from that of the classical chemicals. All are lipophilic and hence can partition into the nonpolar regions of the inner membrane. Partitioning could produce alterations in the fluidity and permeability properties of the membrane that result in perturbational and conformational shifts to the constituent redox components. These alterations then could be responsible for the observed effects on state 3 and possibly state 4 respiration.

The production of alterations in the fluidity and permeability properties of the mitochondrial inner membrane by cyclodiene insecticides and some herbicides is evidenced by the induction of swelling of rat liver mitochondria and plant mitochondria in a sucrose and mannitol medium, respectively, and in isotonic potassium chloride. Inhibitory herbicides have also been shown to inhibit the rate of valinomycin-induced swelling. Valinomycin is a mobile carrier of potassium, and a restriction in its movement across the membrane may indicate that the fluidity of the membrane has been decreased.

Additional evidence for a change in the permeability of the inner membrane is provided by the action of the cyclodiene insecticides on rat liver mitochondria relative to the oxidation of exogenous NADH. The oxidation of endogenous NADH is catalyzed by a dehydrogenase located on the inside (matrix side) of the inner membrane. Under normal conditions, tightly coupled animal mitochondria do not oxidize substrate levels of NADH because the NADH does not penetrate the inner membrane. Animal mitochondria do not have an externally located NAD-linked dehydrogenase enzyme, whereas plant mitochondria do. The oxidation of exogenous NADH by rat liver mitochondria, however, is promoted by low concentrations of cyclodiene insecticides. This observation suggests that the cyclodienes increase the permeability of the inner membrane to NADH.

13.2. Photophosphorylation and Photosynthesis

13.2.1. Introduction

Chlorophyllous higher plants and microorganisms are able to convert solar energy to chemical energy. This conversion occurs in organelles called chloroplasts. Chloroplasts, like mitochondria, contain their own DNA and RNA and synthesize specific proteins.

Leaf mesophyll cells contain a variable number of chloroplasts, typically 40–50. Chloroplasts of higher plants are lens shaped, bounded by a double membrane, 4–10 μm in diameter, and 1–3 μm thick. Chlorophyll, the light-absorbing pigment, is concentrated in substructures within the chloroplasts called grana, which are about 0.4 μm in diameter. Under the electron microscope (Figure 13.4), the grana appear as highly organized, precisely stacked, membranous sacs that are called thylakoids. Surrounding the thylakoids is the stroma matrix. The light and associated electron transport reactions take place in the thylakoids, whereas the enzymes involved in the fixation of carbon dioxide are located in the stroma.

13.2.2. Photoinduced Electron Transport

Photoinduced electron transport and the coupled phosphorylation reactions as they are postulated to occur in chloroplasts are presented schematically in Figure 13.5. Not all investigators agree on the details of the scheme; some even ques-

Figure 13.4 Electron micrograph of an ultrathin section through a chloroplast showing the double membrane envelop (E), grana (G) consisting of stacks of thylakoids, starch (St), and the stromal matrix (S).
SOURCE: *Courtesy of K. E. Muse.*

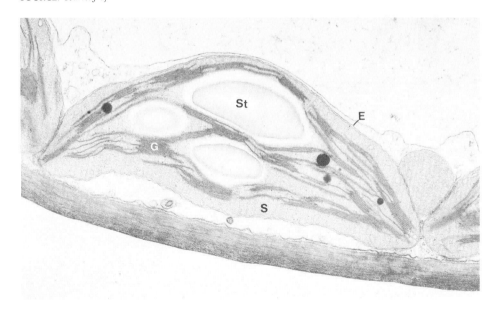

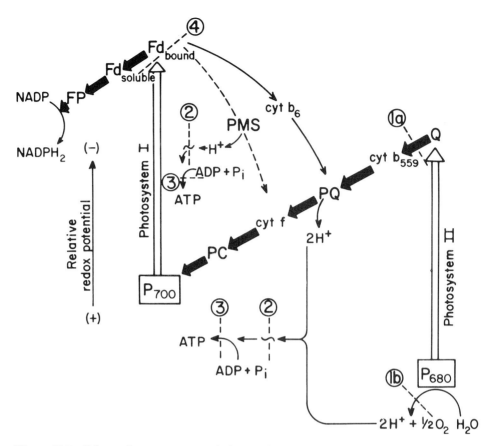

Figure 13.5 Schematic presentation of photoinduced electron transport and phosphory-lation reactions considered to occur in chloroplast lamellae. Open arrows indicate light reactions, solid arrows indicate dark reactions, and the narrow lines represent the cyclic pathway. Abbreviations used: PS I, photosystem I; PS II, photosystem II; P_{680}, reaction center chlorophyll of photosystem II; Q, primary electron acceptor for photosystem II; PQ, plastoquinones; cyt b_{-559} and cyt b_6, b-type cytochromes; cyt f, cytochrome f; PC, plastocyanin; P_{700}, reaction center chlorophyll of photosystem I; Fd, ferredoxin; PMS, phenazine methosulfate; FP, ferredoxin-NADP oxidoreductase. The numbers 1a, 1b, 2, 3, and 4 indicate postulated sites of action by herbicides. See text for details.

tion the sequence of the intermediates. The numbers and locations of the phos-phorylation sites also remain to be identified precisely. However, the scheme is a reasonable approximation based on available information. Reactions that occur in the light are represented by open arrows, and the solid arrows repre-sent electron transfers connecting the two photosystems that are not strictly light dependent.

Through a series of oxidation–reduction reactions driven by two light reac-tions operating in series and involving several hundred chlorophyll molecules, electrons flow from water to NADP (Figure 13.5). A chlorophyll a molecule with an absorption maximum at 680 nm (P_{680}) is postulated to serve as the reaction center of photosystem II, with Q (possibly a bound quinone) as the primary electron acceptor and water as the ultimate source of electrons. Involved sequentially on the electron transport chain that connects the two photosystems are cytochrome b_{559}, plastoquinone (PQ), cytochrome f, and plastocyanin (PC): P_{700} (a specialized chlorophyll a molecule), with an absorption maximum at 700 nm, serves as the reaction center of photosystem I, and a bound form of ferredoxin (Fd_{bound}) is thought to be the electron acceptor. In noncyclic electron flow, electrons then flow through a soluble ferredoxin ($Fd_{soluble}$) and a flavoprotein (FP) to NADP.

Ferredoxin can also transfer electrons to cytochrome b_6, which in turn reduces plastoquinone (Figure 13.5). This type of electron transport, which involves only photosystem I, is termed cyclic electron flow. An artificial cyclic pathway not involving soluble ferredoxin or plastoquinone can be induced with the cofactor phenazine methosulfate (PMS) (Figure 13.5, broken line).

Most investigators agree that a proton gradient across the thylakoid membrane is either the driving force or a precursor of the driving force for phosphorylation. During the transport of two electrons from water to NADP (noncyclic electron transport), four protons are deposited within the thylakoid space. Two arise from the oxidation of water and two are transported during the oxidation of reduced plastoquinone (Figure 13.5). An efflux of protons from the thylakoid space drives the synthesis of ATP. The reaction is catalyzed by the chloroplast coupling factor, and it is thought that movement of three protons is required to form one molecule of ATP.

The ATP and NADPH are used by enzymes in the stroma to fix carbon dioxide.

Artificial electron acceptors, such as ferricyanide, can be substituted for NADP. These give rise to oxygen evolution but do not involve the entire electron transport chain. This partial reaction is known as the Hill reaction, and compounds that disrupt it are known as Hill inhibitors.

13.2.3. Classification of Inhibitors

Herbicides that inhibit the photochemical reactions of isolated chloroplasts have been referred to routinely as inhibitors of the Hill reaction. This has been done primarily for convenience and because, for many years, their action was evaluated under nonphosphorylating conditions, frequently with ferricyanide as the electron acceptor. In recent years, more sophisticated studies have been conducted with herbicides, and more is known about their differential actions. Consequently, herbicidal inhibitors of the photochemically induced reactions can now be separated into the following classes: (a) electron transport inhibitors, (b) uncouplers, (c) energy transfer inhibitors, (d) inhibitory uncouplers, and (e) electron acceptors.

A full comprehension of the specific sites involved in the inhibitory action of herbicides and the mechanisms through which inhibition is produced will be achieved only when the uncertainties surrounding the sequence and interrelation of components in the electron transport pathway, numbers and locations of phosphorylation sites, and mechanism of phosphorylation have been resolved.

13.2.3a. Electron Transport Inhibitors

Electron transport is inhibited when one or more of the intermediate electron transport carriers are removed or inactivated. The site of action of most herbicidal electron transport inhibitors is considered to be associated closely with photosystem II. Consequently, reactions coupled to photosystem II are inhibited, such as basal electron transport, methylamine-uncoupled electron transport, and noncyclic electron transport with water as electron donor and ferricyanide or NADP as electron acceptor. The coupled phosphorylation is inhibited by the action on the reductive reaction. Partial reactions not dependent on photosystem II, such as cyclic phosphorylation or the photoreduction of NADP with an electron donor that circumvents photosystem II [ascorbate plus 2,6-dichlorophenolindophenol (DPIP)], are either not inhibited or are inhibited only weakly. These herbicides also do not inhibit mitochondrial oxidative phosphorylation.

The action of diuron has been studied more intensively and extensively than that of any other herbicide. However, the site at which inhibition is expressed has not been resolved to the satisfaction of all investigators. Some investigators have shown that diuron acts on the reducing side of photosystem II between Q and plastoquinone (Figure 13.5, site la). However, other investigators have suggested that diuron may act on the oxidizing side of photosystem II (Figure 13.5, site 1b) or directly on P_{680}. The action of many other diversely structured compounds is compared frequently to that of diuron; however, their site(s) of action has not been resolved beyond the general area around photosystem II. The mechanism through which inhibition is imposed, even by diuron, is unknown.

Herbicides that seem to have a single site of action on the photochemical pathway that is associated closely with photosystem II are the chlorinated phenylureas, biscarbamates such as phenmedipham, chlorinated s-triazines, substituted uracils, pyridazinones, diphenyl ethers, 1,2,4-triazinones, azido-s-triazines, cyclopropane-carboxamides, p-alkylanilides, p-alkylthioanilides, aminotriazinones, and urea carbamates.

13.2.3b. Uncouplers

Uncouplers dissociate electron transport from photophosphorylation. Both noncyclic and cyclic phosphorylation are inhibited, but electron transport reactions are either unaffected or stimulated. Because uncouplers relieve the inhibition of electron transport imposed by energy transfer inhibitors, they are considered to act at a site closer to the electron transport chain than the site of phosphate uptake. In Figure 13.5, they are shown (site 2) as dissipating some form of conserved energy represented as $\sim$ on the noncyclic and cyclic ATP generating pathways. Perfluidone is the only herbicide identified to date that functions as a pure uncoupler at pH 8.0. Compounds that uncouple photophosphorylation also uncouple mitochondrial oxidative phosphorylation.

13.2.3c. Energy Transfer Inhibitors

Energy transfer inhibitors act directly on phosphorylation. Like electron transport inhibitors, they inhibit both electron transport and phosphorylation in coupled systems. However, the inhibition of electron flow (but not of ATP formation) is released by the addition of an appropriate uncoupler. No herbicide has been shown to act as an energy transfer inhibitor in photophosphorylation. Nonherbicides that behave in this way include the antibiotic Dio-9 and phlorizin. Energy transfer inhibitors are depicted as affecting site 3 on the noncyclic and cyclic ATP generating pathways in Figure 13.5.

13.2.3d. Inhibitory Uncouplers

Inhibitory uncouplers inhibit the responses affected by both electron transport inhibitors and uncouplers. Hence, they inhibit basal, methylamine-uncoupled, and coupled electron transport with ferricyanide as electron acceptor and water as the electron donor, much as electron transport inhibitors do. Coupled noncyclic photophosphorylation is inhibited and the phosphorylation reaction is slightly more sensitive than the reduction of ferricyanide. Cyclic photophosphorylation is also inhibited. NADP reduction, when photosystem II is circumvented with ascorbate plus DPIP, is not inhibited; however, the associated phosphorylation is inhibited. Hence, inhibitory uncouplers act at both sites 1 and 2 (Figure 13.5).

Herbicides that act as inhibitory uncouplers include the dinitrophenols, N-phenylcarbamates, acylanilides, halogenated benzonitriles, substituted imidazoles, substituted benzimidazoles, bromofenoxim, substituted 2,6-dinitroanilines, pyridinols, and substituted 1,2,4-thiadiazoles.

13.2.3e. Electron Acceptors

Compounds classified as electron acceptors can compete with some component of the electron transport pathway and subsequently be reduced. Ferricyanide, PMS, and FMN, which are used to study partial reactions of the photochemical pathway, operate in this manner. However, they are not phytotoxic.

Bipyridyliums with redox potentials in the range of -300 to -500 mV, such as diquat and paraquat, can accept electrons in competition with the acceptor of photosystem I (Figure 13.5, site 4) and have herbicidal activity. Interception of electron flow from photosystem I essentially shunts the electron transport chain. The bipyridyliums support both noncyclic and cyclic photophosphorylation, are photoreduced by illuminated chloroplasts under anaerobic conditions, and inhibit the photoreduction of NADP. This inhibition is not circumvented by the addition of reduced DPIP.

13.2.4. Studies with Intact Plants

Insofar as they have been studied, all herbicides classified as electron transport inhibitors also inhibit photosynthesis of intact plants and photosynthetic microorganisms. Phytotoxicity is produced only in the light, and severity of the response is proportional to light intensity. Studies with light quality have indicated that the chlorophylls are the principal absorbing pigments involved in the production of phytotoxicity.

The development of toxic symptoms in plants treated with pure electron transport inhibitors, such as simazine, diuron, and the uracils, can be prevented if the plants are supplied exogenously with a respirable carbohydrate. This observation suggests that the glycolytic or the mitochondrial system can provide sufficient energy to prevent the appearance of phytotoxic symptoms if respirable substrates are provided. In contrast, carbohydrate protection cannot be obtained with herbicides classified as inhibitory uncouplers or uncouplers because these also interfere with oxidative phosphorylation.

Suggested Reading

Arnon, D. I. The light reactions of photosynthesis. Proc. Natl. Acad. Sci. U.S.A. 68 (1971), 2823.

Corbett, J. R. The Biochemical Mode of Action of Pesticides. London: Academic Press, 1974.

Good, N. E., Izawa, S. Inhibition of photosynthesis. In Hochster, R. M., Kates, M., Quastel J. H. (Eds.). Metabolic Inhibitors, Vol. 4. New York: Academic Press, 1973, pp. 179–214.

Govindjee, Govindjee, R. The primary events of photosynthesis. Sci. Am. 231 (1974), 68.

Govindjee. Bioenergetics of Photosynthesis. New York: Academic Press, 1975.

Green, D. E., Baum, H. Energy and the Mitochondrion. New York: Academic Press, 1970.

Ikuma, H. Electron transport in plant respiration. Ann. Rev. Plant Physiol. 23 (1972), 419.

Izawa, S. Good, N. E. Inhibition of photosynthetic electron transport and photophosphorylation. In San Pietro, A. (Ed.). Methods in Enzymology, Vol. 24. New York: Academic Press, 1972, pp. 355–377.

Kirkland, R. C. Action on respiration and intermediary metabolism. In Audus, L. J. (Ed.). Herbicides: Physiology, Biochemistry, Ecology, Vol. 1. London: Academic Press, 1976, pp. 444–492.

Lehninger, A. L. The Mitochondrion: Molecular Basis of Structure and Function. New York: Benjamin, 1964.

Lehninger, A. L. Bioenergetics. Menlo Park, N. J.: Benjamin, 1971.

Moreland, D. E., Hilton, J. L. Actions on photosynthetic systems. In Audus, L. J. (Ed.). Herbicides: Physiology, Biochemistry, Ecology, Vol. 1. London: Academic Press, 1976, pp. 493–524.

Palmer, J. M. The organization and regulation of electron transport in plant mitochondria. Ann. Rev. Plant Physiol. 27 (1976), 133.

Slater, E. C. Uncouplers and inhibitors of oxidative phosphorylation. In Hochster, R. M., Quastel J. H. (Eds.). Metabolic Inhibitors, Vol. 2. New York: Academic Press, 1963, pp. 503–516.

Slater, E. C. Application of inhibitors and uncouplers for a study of oxidative phosphorylation. In Estabrook, R. W., Pullman, M. E. (Eds.). Methods in Enzymology, Vol. 10. New York: Academic Press, 1970, pp. 48–57.

David J. Holbrook, Jr.

14

Effects of Toxicants on Nucleic Acid and Protein Metabolism

14.1. Introduction

Toxicants may exert primary or secondary effects on various aspects of nucleic acid or protein metabolism. It is obviously of interest to identify the direct and indirect effects of the toxicants and the specific biochemical processes involved. The topics to be presented include some of the basic principles of the metabolism of nucleic acids and proteins, the methodology that may be used to examine the effects of toxicants, and examples of the application of this information to specific toxicants. Many of the studies to be described are conducted in the liver. This tissue is commonly selected because the properties of nucleic acid and protein metabolism in the liver are well established, the liver is able to convert most nonreactive toxicants to reactive metabolites, and regenerating liver following partial hepatectomy provides a convenient model system for controlled active synthesis of the macromolecules. Some of the toxicants selected as examples in this chapter are carcinogens since their effects on nucleic acid and protein metabolism have been extensively studied. The carcinogens are also discussed in Chapter 16 in relation to DNA damage and repair.

14.1.1. Precursor Incorporation into Macromolecules

In whole-cell experiments, the incorporation of radioactive precursors into macromolecules is commonly used as an indicator of the synthesis of the appropriate macromolecule. Thymidine is generally used as the precursor for incorporation into DNA; either orotate, uridine, or orthophosphate is used as the precursor for incorporation into RNA; and an amino acid is used as the precursor for incorporation into protein.

A toxicant-induced alteration in precursor incorporation into a macromolecule may reflect direct effects on the process under study. For example, a decrease in thymidine incorporation into DNA or orotic acid or uridine incorporation into RNA after treatment with a toxicant may be due to a direct inhibition of the appropriate polymerase (or the accessory proteins necessary for replication or transcription) or damage to the DNA, which is manifested by interference with its normal utilization as template by the appropriate polymerases. Likewise, inhibition of amino acid incorporation into cellular proteins may reflect the interference by the toxicant with one of the components involved in protein synthesis. However, it should be recognized that actions of a toxicant on various processes, such as energy production or transport across membranes, may markedly affect the incorporation of a precursor into a macromolecule in an indirect manner. Thus, the inhibition of precursor *incorporation* into a macromolecule, although indicative, does not demonstrate inhibition of the *synthesis* of that macromolecule by the toxicant.

The synthesis of DNA, RNA, and protein are energy-requiring processes; likewise, the entrance of a precursor into a cell may be an energy-requiring process. It is obvious that a toxicant that interferes with mitochondrial structure, oxidative phosphorylation, or other energy-yielding reactions is *indirectly* an inhibitor of the syntheses of DNA, RNA, and protein. It is likely that a specific toxicant is acting in such a manner if it is found that the toxicant inhibits the synthesis of all three macromolecules by comparable levels in dose–response experiments or in similar temporal relationships in treatment duration–response experiments.

Toxicants often do not exhibit highly selective action against the synthesis of, or precursor incorporation into, a single type of macromolecule. In some instances, the toxicant may initiate a direct effect on energy production or cellular nucleotide concentration, and the toxicant effects on macromolecular synthesis may represent indirect actions that are a consequence of the cellular energy deficiency. The acute effects of carbon tetrachloride on hepatic RNA and protein metabolism are discussed in Section 14.7. However, the *hepatic* ATP levels are decreased by one-third to three-fourths 1–36 hr after the oral administration of carbon tetrachloride. At this time it is not known to what extent the effects of carbon tetrachloride on RNA and protein synthesis and on ATP levels are related, or whether one effect initiates the others during the acute phase after toxicant administration. The depression in ATP levels also is observed during the manifestation of other toxicants. The hepatic ATP level is decreased by more than one-half following the 6-day administration of ethionine. As in other instances, the decreased energy availability—as ATP—is only one of a number of toxic manifestations of ethionine (see Section 14.3.3). Galactosamine is a hepatotoxicant, and the hexosamine is converted to phosphorylated and uridine nucleotide-containing metabolites. The resultant decrease in hepatic cellular UTP (and UMP and UDP) appears to exert a number of secondary biochemical effects, including inhibition of precursor incorporation into RNA (due to a decrease in one of the requisite ribonucleoside triphosphates) and into DNA (due to a decrease in the metabolic intermediates leading to the deoxyribonucleoside triphosphates). There is also a decrease in cellular UDP glucose and UDP galactose with an accompanying inhibition of the glycosylation of protein and lipid and of the conjugation reactions to yield glucuronides.

14.1.2. Correlation of Precursor Incorporation and Rate of Macromolecular Synthesis

The rate of precursor incorporation into a macromolecule may not reflect the rate of synthesis of that macromolecule. When a tracer dose of radioactive precursor of a nucleic acid is used, the metabolites (nucleosides and nucleoside phosphates) of the labeled precursor are diluted by the endogenous pools of each of the intermediates. Thus, a toxicant that alters the size of each of the intermediate pools markedly changes the dilution of the radioactive precursor by endogenous metabolites and consequently alters the specific radioactivity (e.g., $dpm/\mu mole$) of the immediate precursors of the nucleic acids (i.e., the appropriate nucleoside triphosphates). Treatment with a toxicant that elicits cell death and necrosis is accompanied by a period of release of bases and nucleosides and of amino acids from the degraded macromolecules of autolyzed cells. In addition, cells that are stimulated to undergo nucleic acid synthesis exhibit increased activities of the enzymes involved in the anabolism of precursors (conversion to nucleoside triphosphates) and decreased activities of the enzymes involved in the catabolism of the precursors or their metabolites.

Under ideal conditions, the precursor incorporation into a macromolecule in control and toxicant-treated animals is experimentally adjusted for the specific radioactivity of the penultimate metabolic intermediate (e.g., thymidine triphosphate (dTTP) when radioactive thymidine is used or UTP and cytidine triphosphate (CTP) when labeled orotate or uridine is used) in the cold perchloric acid–soluble or cold trichloroacetic acid–soluble fraction. Upon occasion the specific radioactivity is measured for the entire pool of nucleoside phosphates (the mixture of the mono-, di-, and triphosphates of a single nucleoside) since the pool sizes are often small, the specific radioactivities change during the incorporation interval, and there is generally a moderately rapid interconversion among the nucleoside phosphates of a single nucleoside. There is evidence for and against the existence of several discrete nucleotide pools within mammalian cells. It is possible that only one of these pools serves as the nucleotide source during DNA or RNA synthesis. In spite of these difficulties, the measurement of the specific radioactivity in nucleoside triphosphates or other nucleotide pools and its use in the calculation of the quantity (e.g., $\mu moles$) of precursor incorporated into a macromolecule are desirable steps if the aim is to correlate the effects of a toxicant on the rate of macromolecular *synthesis*. It is now recognized that the rate of precursor *incorporation* into a macromolecule should not be equated to or referred to as *synthesis* of the macromolecule.

It is apparent from the following description of the effects of toxicants on the metabolism of nucleic acids and proteins that many of the studies have been limited to precursor incorporation into macromolecules. In the future it is anticipated that studies in biochemical toxicology will be extended in order to establish more precisely the individual steps that are being affected by the toxicant. For example, studies on precursor incorporation into macromolecules may appropriately include pool sizes and rates of synthesis, separation and measurement of incorporation into individual RNAs (mRNA or poly(A)-containing mRNA, rRNA, etc.), or the effects on individual polymerases or individual steps in protein synthesis.

14.1.3. Cellular Heterogeneity Within Tissues

The cell population in any tissue is heterogeneous. The liver is composed of the parenchymal cells (or hepatocytes), bile duct cells, Kupffer cells, and cells lining the blood vessels. As anticipated, the various cell types differ in characteristics of macromolecular synthesis, susceptibility to certain toxicants (which in part may be due to the ability of the cell to convert a nonreactive toxicant to a reactive metabolite), and other characteristics. For example, the enzymatic complement of certain lysosomal enzymes differs appreciably between parenchymal and nonparenchymal cells in rat liver. Toxicant-initiated cell death in different cell types results in the release of lysosomal enzymes with various patterns of degradative properties.

The measurement of macromolecular metabolism in the liver and in almost any other tissue reflects contributions of the different cell populations. In normal rat liver, the parenchymal cells constitute approximately 75% of the cell number and approximately 90% of the tissue mass (because of the larger size of the parenchymal cells). In addition to the differing metabolic characteristics between cell types, the biochemical characteristics differ among parenchymal cells within the liver depending on the proximity to afferent blood vessels. In adult rats and mice, tetraploid parenchymal cells are usually found, rather-than the diploid cells normally seen in young animals. Approximately 90% of the parenchymal cells are tetraploid in the liver of adult rats. The increased ploidy of the parenchymal cells makes the comparison of the macromolecular metabolism in the predominantly tetraploid parenchymal nuclei with the predominantly nonparenchymal diploid nuclei amenable because separation of the classes of hepatic nuclei can be attained by centrifugation through a discontinuous sucrose gradient. The more dense tetraploid parenchymal nuclei are collected as a pellet after centrifugation through 2.3 M sucrose. The diploid nonparenchymal nuclei are then isolated from the less dense sucrose layers. The parenchymal and nonparenchymal nuclei sometimes differ in their properties related to nucleic acid synthesis, such as the incorporation of precursors into nucleic acids in normal and in toxicant-treated animals. Furthermore, the parenchymal tetraploid and nonparenchymal diploid nuclei isolated from rodent liver differ in relation to the activities of the DNA polymerase and RNA polymerase retained in the nuclei.

14.1.4. Interrelationships in the Synthesis of Macromolecules

Consideration must be given to the temporal relationships of toxicant effects on DNA, RNA, and protein synthesis because these processes are interdependent to a large extent. The enzymes of nucleoside anabolism and the polymerases have limited half-lives that can vary depending on the anabolic state of the cell. For example, in normal rat liver, the half-lives of thymidine kinase, thymidylate kinase, and total RNA polymerase are 2.6, 18, and 12 hr, respectively. Treatment with a toxicant that has a primary effect on the synthesis of messenger RNA will be followed shortly by the conversion of cytoplasmic polyribosomes to monoribosomes and ribosomal subunits. The dissociation of polyribosomes is accompanied by a cessation of protein synthesis. In view of the rapid turnover of certain enzymes or their mRNAs, a toxicant with a primary effect on mRNA or protein synthesis may have a subsequent but often rapid effect on the synthesis of and/or the precursor incorporation into any of the macromolecules.

14.2. DNA Synthesis

14.2.1. Cell Cycle and DNA Synthetic Phase

The cell cycle of mitotically active mammalian cells can be divided into four distinct stages. The M phase is the mitotic stage and its duration is approximately 1 hr. The G_1 phase is an active stage of RNA and protein synthesis but no DNA synthesis occurs; its duration is approximately 8–10 hr. The S phase is the period of active DNA replication and generally has a duration of 6–8 hr. The levels of RNA and protein synthesis generally are less during the S phase than in the G_1 or G_2 phase. The S phase is followed by the G_2 phase of 6–8 hr. During the G_2 phase there is active synthesis of RNA and protein but no synthesis of DNA. Cells that are not mitotically active, such as circulating lymphocytes, are often referred to as being in a G_0 phase (or an extended G_1 phase).

14.2.2. DNA Replication

The replicon is the replicating unit of DNA. DNA replication is initiated at a fixed site (the origin) on the chromosome and proceeds bidirectionally along the chromosome away from the origin. In *Escherichia coli,* there is only one replicon for the single circular DNA molecule. In contrast, each mammalian chromosome is many-fold larger than a bacterial chromosome and contains multiple and shorter (nucleotide-length) replicons. None of the mammalian DNA polymerases is capable of initiating a DNA chain; DNA polymerases are capable only of extending a preexisting polynucleotide (either DNA-like or RNA-like) chain. A polynucleotide chain is initiated by the action of an RNA polymerase, which produces a short (30–100 nucleotides) polynucleotide primer. One of the DNA polymerases then extends the polynucleotide primer by the attachment of deoxyribonucleotides to produce a nascent DNA fragment (or Okazaki fragment). There are many such nascent fragments at each replicating fork. The RNA-like primer is removed by a nuclease, and a DNA polymerase (using the adjacent nascent fragment as primer) polymerizes nucleotides to fill the gap left after removal of the primer. DNA ligase, which requires ATP in mammalian cells, then seals the nicks to join the adjacent nascent fragments.

14.2.3. DNA Polymerases

The mammalian DNA polymerases exist in distinct multiple forms and are named, by Greek letters, in their sequence of discovery: DNA polymerases α, β, and γ. The original nomenclature scheme included polymerase mt (mitochondrial); however, since most of the properties of polymerase γ are similar to those of polymerase mt, these polymerase activities may be identical. A fourth non-mitochondrial polymerase activity (polymerase δ) has been reported. The mammalian polymerases differ in their biophysical properties (molecular weight, sedimentation coefficient, and isoelectric point) and their enzymatic characteristics (notably, the ability to use various polynucleotide templates and susceptibility to inhibition by sulfhydryl-reactive reagents). The activity of DNA polymerase α, the first discovered, usually is measured in the cytosol when cellular fractionation is carried out in aqueous media of moderate ionic strength. Although not accepted by all groups, appreciable evidence indicates that polymerase α is a nuclear enzyme but is easily and extensively extracted into the cytosol when the nuclei are subjected to certain aqueous solutions.

When quiescent cells are stimulated to undergo DNA synthesis and subsequent mitotic activity (e.g., regenerating rat liver), there is a marked increase in DNA polymerase α activity but very little increase in polymerase β activity. Consequently, it generally is concluded that polymerase α is responsible for most of the nucleotide polymerization during DNA replication. However, such a conclusion does not exclude the participation of the other polymerases at various stages during replication. The proposal has been made that polymerase β may function during DNA repair, but such a proposal is in need of further study. Polymerase γ represents only a minor portion of the total cellular DNA polymerase activity.

The studies of the effects of toxicants on individual DNA polymerases generally have not progressed to the detail seen in comparable studies on RNA polymerases (Section 14.5.2). Most studies on DNA polymerases have examined the total polymerase activity rather than the activity of the individual DNA polymerases. However, since polymerase α is the predominant activity in highly proliferative cells, the observed effects of toxicants probably reflect effects on that polymerase when such cells are used experimentally.

Under favorable conditions, prokaryotic and eukaryotic DNA polymerases utilize polydeoxyribonucleotide templates with a high degree of fidelity in nucleotide pairing. Many of the prokaryotic polymerases possess a 3'-to-5' exonuclease and a polymerase activity within the same protein. It is proposed that the nuclease functions as a "proofreading" mechanism by removing mispaired nucleotides from the nascent DNA chain and thereby partially contributes to the high degree of fidelity exhibited by the prokaryotic polymerases. Eukaryotic DNA polymerases normally exhibit a high degree of fidelity, but most of the highly purified mammalian polymerases lack an associated exonuclease that is part of the same protein molecule. DNA polymerase δ may represent an exception. This polymerase appears to possess an associated 3'-to-5' exonuclease, and it is proposed that this polymerase may perform a proofreading function during DNA replication. Alternatively, other cellular exonucleases may function to remove mispaired nucleotides incorporated into nascent DNA chains. A defect in the normal high fidelity of replication by polymerases may be of importance in error-prone DNA repair, somatic mutation, and carcinogenesis (Chapter 16).

Numerous examples exist of agents inhibiting DNA or RNA polymerases by interaction either with the template DNA or with the polymerase. One technique that is indicative of the mechanism of inhibition is an examination of the percentage inhibition when the concentration of the template is varied (at constant polymerase and inhibitor concentrations) and when the concentration of the polymerase is varied (at constant template and inhibitor concentrations). If the percentage inhibition is decreased when the template concentration is increased, it is probable that inhibition is due to interaction of the inhibitor with the template. Conversely, if the percentage inhibition is decreased when the polymerase concentration is increased, the mechanism of inhibition probably involves the interaction of the inhibitor with the polymerase.

14.2.4. Precursors Incorporated into DNA

Radioactive thymidine is the most commonly used precursor for incorporation into DNA, but orotate, orthophosphate, and other compounds have also been used as precursors. At times, the attempt has been made in experiments with radioactive thymidine to equate the incorporation into DNA with the total radioactivity measured in the tissue macromolecules (i.e., the sediment obtained by precipitation with cold perchloric acid or cold trichloroacetic acid). Such an abbreviated experimental procedure should be viewed with skepticism. In certain tissues, the radioactive thymidine undergoes catabolic reactions, and the radioactive degradative products can be incorporated into or nonspecifically bind to macromolecules such as protein and glycogen. Consequently, the DNA should be separated from other tissue macromolecules in such labeling experiments before the measurement of thymidine incorporation into the DNA.

14.2.5. Liver Regeneration and Partial Hepatectomy
as a Model System

The loss of viable liver tissue in rodents is followed by the production of new cells (hyperplasia) to replace the missing mass of liver. The initial loss of viable liver may be experimentally induced by surgical removal (partial hepatectomy) of one-third to two-thirds of the liver or by treatment with a hepatotoxicant such as carbon tetrachloride, which results in the death of an appreciable fraction of the liver cells. The processes involved in nucleotide and nucleic acid metabolism following partial hepatectomy have been extensively studied. In many cases, comparable changes in metabolism appear to occur in the liver after treatment with a hepatotoxicant resulting in hepatic necrosis. Based on the properties of regenerating liver as a model system, there are a number of characteristics that should be considered in the study of the effects of toxicants on the synthesis of nucleic acids and proteins. Pool sizes, cell types, and the cellular location within the hepatic lobule alter the synthetic properties and, in some cases, the capabilities of a hepatic cell to convert a nonreactive toxicant to a damaging reactive metabolite.

The changes related to RNA synthesis appear to occur early (prior to 6 hr) during liver regeneration. In contrast, many of the changes directly related to DNA synthesis are not apparent at 12 hr after partial hepatectomy. Beginning at 15–18 hr, there are increases in the anabolic enzymatic activities associated with DNA synthesis: thymidine kinase, deoxycytidylate deaminase, thymidylate synthetase, thymidylate kinase and total DNA polymerase. The first peak in thymidine incorporation into DNA occurs at approximately 24–26 hr, and the first peak in mitosis occurs at 30–32 hr after two-thirds hepatectomy. The pool size (pmoles/μg DNA) of each of the deoxyribonucleoside triphosphates increases 4–10-fold approximately 26 hr after partial hepatectomy. The activities of the anabolic enzymes and of thymidine incorporation return to near normal levels by 96 hr after partial hepatectomy.

After partial hepatectomy, all of the remaining cells do not participate in thymidine incorporation during the first peak in DNA synthesis. The cellular location within the hepatic lobule markedly affects the extent of thymidine incorporation into DNA. At 18 hr after partial hepatectomy, autoradiographic studies with radioactive thymidine show that 80% of the labeled hepatocytes are in the periportal (portal vein and hepatic artery) zone, 15% in the midzonal area or intermediate zone, and 5% in the perivenous (hepatic vein) zone. Usually a second peak in DNA synthesis is observed 42–48 hr after partial hepatectomy. This appears to correlate with an increased percentage of labeled hepatocytes in areas other than the periportal zone.

The DNA synthesis and accompanying thymidine incorporation into DNA of the liver of normal *adult* rodents is relatively low. In order to increase the experimental sensitivity in studies of the *inhibitory* effects of a toxicant on DNA synthesis, it is a common practice to utilize animals that are undergoing a greater level of hepatic DNA synthesis. For example, the effect of a toxicant may be measured in partially hepatectomized rats (or very young rats), which have a rapid rate of hepatic cell formation.

14.3. Modification of DNA Metabolism by Toxicants

14.3.1. Toxicants and Thymidine Incorporation into DNA

The administration of a toxicant often results in an acute or short-term inhibition of the incorporation of thymidine or other precursors into DNA. However, in many cases, such inhibitory effects are observed only during the first 12 hr after treatment with the toxicant. For example, the administration of 7,12-dimethylbenzanthracene to young rats inhibits the incorporation of thymidine into hepatic DNA. The inhibition is apparent at 2 hr, and the maximal inhibition (greater than 75%) is observed 6 hr after injection of the toxicant. Thymidine incorporation returns nearly to the normal level at 24 hr. An equal dose of dimethylbenzanthracene does not appreciably alter orotate incorporation into hepatic nuclear RNA during the first 24 hr. However, most toxicants do not show such highly specific effects on precursor incorporation into DNA without some concurrent effect on precursor incorporation into RNA.

In contrast, the administration of a single dose of a hepatotoxicant in a sufficiently high amount to cause hepatic necrosis is followed within several days by a regenerating process similar to that observed during the first 1–3 days after two-thirds hepatectomy, although the toxicant-induced effects on macromolecular synthesis and mitotic activity are usually delayed by approximately 0.5 day. The increased thymidine incorporation observed 12 hr or longer after the administration of hepatocarcinogens or other hepatotoxicants may be attributable to DNA replication preparatory to the replacement of cells lost by cell lethality and necrosis and/or deoxynucleotide polymerization during the repair of DNA in the surviving cells. Thymidine incorporation into hepatic DNA is markedly increased 1–3 days after the administration of various toxicants, including carbon tetrachloride, thioacetamide, diethylnitrosamine, and galactosamine. For example, the administration of the hepatocarcinogen diethylnitrosamine causes hepatic necrosis and, after several days, a regenerating process. Thymidine incorporation into hepatic DNA of hamsters is marginally decreased 4–8 hr after injection of diethylnitrosamine. However, on the second through the seventh day after injection of the nitrosamine derivative, the thymidine incorporation into hepatic DNA is appreciably increased and attains a maximum incorporation of five to ten times the control level. The periodic intraperitoneal injection of thioacetamide or carbon tetrachloride for 1–3 weeks increases thymidine incorporation into hepatic DNA by at least tenfold.

In addition to the increased thymidine incorporation observed in the regenerative state after toxicant-induced hepatic necrosis, increased DNA synthesis occurs in other tissues after cellular destruction by certain toxicants. The daily injection of ethionine for 10 days results in the destruction of 90% of the rat pancreatic acinar cells; within several weeks after cessation of ethionine administration, there is a regenerative process that results in a return of the total pancreatic mass and normal ultrastructural and cytochemical patterns. On the third to fifth day after cessation of ethionine administration, the incorporation of thymidine into total pancreatic DNA (biochemical studies) and the percentage of thymidine-incorporating nuclei of acinar, ductal, and interstitial cells (autoradiographic studies) reach peaks that are 10- to 20-fold the control levels. At 3–4 weeks after cessation of ethionine administration, the parameters related to thymidine incorporation return to control levels.

14.3.2. Toxicants and Cellular Heterogeneity in Liver

The different cell types within a single tissue may not respond in a similar manner to the effects of a specific toxicant. The dissimilar responses among cells may arise from differences in the properties of the macromolecular synthesis preceding mitotic activity and repair, or the ability to convert metabolically an inert toxicant to a reactive species (e.g., epoxide, reactive ester, or free radical) that causes the tissue damage.

The dietary administration of the hepatocarcinogen 3'-methyl-4-dimethyl-aminoazobenzene for 2–7 weeks causes a marked increase in thymidine incorporation into the DNA of the tetraploid (predominantly parenchymal) nuclei and the diploid (predominantly nonparenchymal) nuclei in rat liver. Either the replacement of cells following necrosis or the repair of DNA in surviving cells may contribute to the observed increase in labeling, but the total amount of hepatic DNA also increases. The incorporation of thymidine and of orotate into the DNA (dpm unit quantity of DNA) of tetraploid nuclei usually exceeds by twofold or greater the incorporation into the diploid nuclei. A companion autoradiographic study conducted on the material used in the biochemical study confirmed the heterogeneous pattern of thymidine incorporation into the nuclei of various cell types and the importance of the separation of parenchymal and nonparenchymal nuclei of liver during the examination of thymidine incorporation into the parenchymal nuclei. However, during the early stages in hepatic carcinogenesis induced by 3'-methyl-4-dimethyl-aminoazobenzene, the proliferative characteristics differ appreciably among the multiple cell types included in the nonparenchymal diploid nuclei (of bile duct cells, mesenchymal and endothelial cells, and hemopoietic cells). Thus, as one might anticipate, a biochemically heterogeneous population exists even within the diploid nuclei.

Ethionine also exhibits varying effects on thymidine incorporation into the different cell types within the liver and pancreas. In intact young rats, parenchymal, ductal, and other cells of the liver and the pancreas exhibit thymidine incorporation (autoradiographic studies) in control animals. The 2-day administration of ethionine blocks thymidine incorporation in the parenchymal cells of both the liver and pancreas but does not block incorporation in the ductal and other cells within these tissues. The differential inhibition in various cell types apparently is not due to differences in ethionine uptake into the cells. The affected and unaffected cell types may differ in the ability to convert ethionine to a toxic derivative (for example, S-adenosylethionine) and/or in the effects of the toxicant on RNA synthesis, which is possibly a prerequisite to DNA synthesis. The cell types in which ethionine inhibits thymidine incorporation into DNA also show an apparent inhibition of RNA synthesis. In contrast, in the cell types that do not exhibit an inhibition of thymidine incorporation by ethionine, RNA synthesis is apparently unaffected by ethionine.

14.4. RNA Synthesis

14.4.1. Synthesis of Multiple Forms of RNA

Each of the major multiple forms of cellular RNA (mRNA, rRNA, and tRNA) is synthesized by a different RNA polymerase and, in some cases, at a different nuclear site. In addition, each form of the RNAs is synthesized initially as a high molecular weight product during transcription, and the primary transcript undergoes subsequent processing or maturation to yield the functional RNA molecule.

14.4.1a. Ribosomal RNA

The high molecular weight units of rRNA are synthesized in the nucleolus by RNA polymerase I. The initial product or primary transcript is a precursor rRNA which has a sedimentation constant of 45S or somewhat greater and which rapidly associates with proteins previously synthesized on the cytoplasmic ribosomes. Regions of the 45S RNA undergo enzymatic methylation, predominantly on the 2'-hydroxyl groups of the ribose moieties. A succession of nuclease reactions produces a series of intermediates. One of the nuclear products, a 60S RNA–protein complex is transposed into the cytoplasm. The cytoplasmic 60S particle contains three rRNAs: 28S, 5.8S (formerly referred to as 7S), and 5S. Only the first two RNAs are derived from scissions of the nucleolar 45S precursor rRNA; the 5S rRNA is synthesized by RNA polymerase III in the nucleoplasm. A second nuclear product is a 40S RNA–protein complex which contains a 20S RNA derived from scission of the 45S precursor rRNA. The 40S complex is transposed to the cytoplasm, where both the final methylation of the RNA and the conversion of 20S RNA to 18S rRNA occur. In normal resting cells such as lymphocytes, a major portion of the 45S precursor rRNA is degraded rather than being converted to cytoplasmic rRNAs. If such cells are stimulated to synthesize proteins, the "wastage" of the precursor rRNA is decreased and a greater fraction of the precursor rRNA is converted to cytoplasmic rRNA—compatible with the increased need for functional ribosomes for cytoplasmic protein synthesis.

14.4.1b. Messenger RNA

Heterogeneous nuclear RNA (HnRNA) is synthesized in the nucleoplasm by RNA polymerase II. Most (approximately 90%) of the HnRNA is degraded within the nucleus. A portion of the remainder is the precursor of cytoplasmic mRNA. The maturation to yield mRNA may involve four processes: limited methylation, hydrolytic cleavage, polyadenylation, and "capping." After the transcription coded by the template DNA is complete, a polyriboadenylate "tail" of approximately 150–200 riboadenylate units is attached to the 3'-hydroxyl end of the transcript by a nuclear polyriboadenylate polymerase. However, usually only 70% of the RNA that undergoes conversion to cytoplasmic mRNA contains an attached poly(A) fragment, and the poly(A) fragment is shortened in the cytoplasm. Approximately 30% of the cytoplasmic mRNA, including the mRNA for the histones, lacks the poly(A) fragment.

The rapidly labeled RNA that enters the cytoplasm can exist as aggregates sedimenting at 100S–300S, i.e., associated with polyribosomes, or as a protein–RNA complex sedimenting at 40S and greater. The latter complex is sometimes referred to as an informasome, or its RNA component is sometimes referred to as messengerlike RNA (mlRNA).

The presence of the poly(A) fragment on some mRNAs is often used in the experimental separation of this class of mRNA from other labeled RNA. The poly(A) fragment results in the adsorption of the poly(A)-containing mRNA to nitrocellulose filters (e.g., Millipore) or to complementary oligonucleotide fragments coupled to polysaccharide supports (e.g., oligo(dT)-cellulose or poly(U)-Sepharose).

14.4.1c. Transfer RNA

Transfer RNA, like mRNA and the large rRNAs, is synthesized as a primary transcript that must undergo maturation to yield the functional RNA. The primary transcript is synthesized by RNA polymerase III in the nucleoplasm. A 4.5S precursor tRNA is produced and subsequently converted to 4S tRNA. The maturation includes some methylation of the tRNA by cytoplasmic methylases that use S-adenosylmethionine as the methyl donor.

14.4.2. Mammalian RNA Polymerases

Three major classes of mammalian nuclear RNA polymerases generally are distinguished. Although various criteria are used in the classifications and nomenclature schemes, the most common scheme designates the classes of DNA-directed RNA polymerases in the order of elution from DEAE-Sephadex. Each of the major classes is capable of being resolved into subclasses: polymerase I can be resolved into IA and IB, polymerase II into IIA and IIB, and polymerase III into IIIA and IIIB. On occasion, another class or other subclasses are distinguished. In an alternative, commonly used nomenclature system, the class I polymerases are designated as class A, and the class II polymerases are designated as class B. The three major classes of RNA polymerases differ markedly in sensitivity to inhibition by α-amanitin, a toxin from the poisonous mushroom *Amanita phalloides.*

RNA polymerase I, a nucleolar enzyme, is responsible for the synthesis of precursor rRNA. Polymerase I is resistant to inhibition by α-amanitin. RNA polymerase II, a nucleoplasmic enzyme, is responsible for the synthesis of HnRNA and, therefore, mRNA. Polymerase II is very sensitive to inhibition by α-amanitin and is completely inhibited at relative low concentrations of the inhibitor. RNA polymerase III is a nucleoplasmic enzyme. RNA polymerase III is responsible for the transcription yielding precursor tRNA and 5S rRNA. RNA polymerase III is inhibited by α-amanitin at intermediate concentrations but not at low concentrations.

α-Amanitin is a useful reagent in the identification of isolated polymerases and in the measurement of a specific polymerase in a mixture of the polymerases, e.g., in an extract of nuclei. The inhibition by α-amanitin is due to an interaction of the toxin with the polymerase, whereas most substances inhibit polymerases by interaction with the template DNA. Although the requisite concentrations of α-amanitin vary somewhat depending on the mammalian source of the polymerases, a comparison of the relative sensitivities of the polymerases I, II, and III can be made from data obtained with polymerases from HeLa cells. Polymerase I is not inhibited by the toxin at very high concentrations (>400 μg/ml), polymerase II is inhibited by 50% at an α-amanitin concentration of 0.003 μg/ml, and polymerase III (or polymerase IIIA or IIIB) is inhibited by approximately 50% at a toxin concentration of 15 μg/ml. α-Amanitin is also a selective inhibitor of part of the RNA polymerase activity measured in vitro in isolated nuclei. For example, the syntheses of 4.5S precursor tRNA and 5S rRNA (i.e., RNA polymerase III) in isolated nuclei of HeLa cells are inhibited 50% by 15 μg/ml α-amanitin and are almost totally abolished by a toxin concentration of approximately 130 μg/ml. The sensitivities of mammalian (or vertebrate) RNA polymerases to inhibition by α-amanitin exhibit a number of qualitative and quantitative differences when compared to the RNA polymerases of yeast. These differences include a reversal of the relative sensitivities to α-amanitin of polymerases I and III.

Each of the RNA polymerase classes exists in two functional states within isolated nuclei. For each polymerase, there is a bound (chromatin-associated or "engaged") state, which is extracted with difficulty from the nuclei and actively engaged in transcribing endogenous template. In addition, each polymerase also exists in a free state, which is easily extractable from nuclei (e.g., with 0.34 M sucrose or 0.15 M ammonium sulfate) and is not engaged in transcription within the nuclei.

In addition to the three classes of nuclear RNA polymerases, a distinct RNA polymerase also occurs within mitochondria. The mitochondrial RNA polymerase isolated from rat liver is not affected by α-amanitin but is inhibited by rifampicin, an established inhibitor of prokaryotic RNA polymerases.

The antibiotic actinomycin D is a potent inhibitor of the DNA-directed RNA polymerases, and the inhibition is due to the interaction of the antibiotic with the deoxyguanosine moieties of the template DNA. However, since actinomycin D does not bind to synthetic DNA-like polymers such as poly(dA-dT) or poly (dI) · poly(dC) which lack deoxyguanosine, the RNA polymerase is not inhibited by the antibiotic when the latter polynucleotides are used as templates for the polymerase. Thus, in a mixture containing RNA polymerase, actinomycin D, natural DNA, and DNA-like polynucleotides *lacking deoxyguanosine,* the free RNA polymerase can utilize the DNA-like polynucleotides as template even though the use of the deoxyguanosine-containing natural DNA by the chromatin-bound RNA polymerase is suppressed by the antibiotic.

14.4.3. Precursor Incorporation into RNA

The most commonly used radioactive precursors for labeling RNA are orotate, uridine, and orthophosphate. In addition, methyl-labeled methionine serves as a precursor for the enzymatically methylated RNAs in whole-cell experiments in which the methionine can be converted to the active methyl donor, S-adenosylmethionine. As in the case of studies of thymidine incorporation into DNA, studies of a toxicant effect on precursor incorporation into RNA should consider the possible effects of the toxicant on the relative activities of the anabolic and catabolic pyrimidine-metabolizing enzymes, the size of the nucleotide pools, and the cellular energy-yielding processes. Uridine is an efficient precursor in the labeling of RNA in mice. In rats, however, the activities of uridine-degradative enzymes are high, and relatively little uridine is incorporated into RNA. Consequently, orotate is generally the radioactive precursor of choice for studies in rats except in certain short-term labeling experiments.

The importance of adjusting precursor incorporation into RNA for the specific radioactivity of the nucleoside triphosphate is demonstrated in a comparison of fed and fasted rats. In *fed* rats, there is an increased *incorporation* of orotate into RNA (dpm/g tissue or dpm/mg DNA) after partial hepatectomy. An increased *synthesis* of RNA is also observed when the specific radioactivity of the RNA is adjusted for the specific radioactivity of the uridine nucleotides. In fasted rats, the pool size of UTP (μmoles/mg DNA) is markedly increased 3–12 hr after partial hepatectomy, and thus the radioactivity of the entering precursor is diluted in the larger pool. In 12-hr fasted, 12-hr partially hepatectomized rats, orotate *incorporation* into RNA (dpm/mg DNA) does *not* differ from that in the newly hepatectomized control. However, in the latter experiment, if the orotate incorporation into RNA is adjusted for the decreased specific radioactivity (dpm/μmole) in the UTP pool (due to the increased pool size), the RNA *synthesis* observed in fasted rats is comparable to the *synthesis* observed in fed rats 12 hr after partial hepatectomy.

Useful but limited information can be obtained from measurements of precursor incorporation into total cellular RNA. However, the rates of precursor incorporation into the various types of RNA sometimes differ markedly even in normal cells, and toxicants may initiate selective effects on the metabolism of a single type of RNA. Consequently, the more informative studies on toxicants include methodology that distinguishes the actions on the basis of types and/or cellular sites of the affected RNAs.

Four basic techniques are used to measure precursor incorporation into cytoplasmic mRNA. One technique, the most commonly used, involves the separation of the poly(A)-containing mRNA of the cytoplasmic polyribosomes or the cytoplasm by a method dependent on the presence of the poly(A) fragment. A major disadvantage, however, is that the poly(A)-containing mRNA constitutes only approximately 70% of the cytoplasmic mRNA, and thus the remaining 30% of the cytoplasmic mRNA is ignored in such studies. A second technique is to measure the precursor incorporation into cytoplasmic polyribosomes at relatively short intervals after administration of the radioactive precursor. In rat liver, the synthesis of rRNA and its transport to the cytoplasm requires approximately 45 min. Consequently, the radioactivity in the high molecular weight RNA of the cytoplasmic polyribosomes in rat liver is present exclusively in the mRNA when polyribosomes are isolated after a 15–30 min labeling interval. A third technique to distinguish between the precursor incorporation into mRNA and that into rRNA is dependent on the greater sensitivity of mRNA to ribonuclease. In this technique, the cytoplasmic polyribosomes or the total ribosomes are isolated after the administration of the radioactive precursor and then subjected to a mild treatment with exogenous ribonuclease. The ribonuclease-solubilized RNA reflects predominantly mRNA and can be separated from the rRNA, which is relatively ribonuclease resistant when complexed with ribosomal proteins. A fourth technique to differentiate precursor incorporation into mRNA and rRNA is dependent upon the greater sensitivity of rRNA synthesis to actinomycin D. Although high doses of actinomycin D inhibit the synthesis of both mRNA and rRNA, low doses inhibit only the rRNA synthesis. Thus, precursor incorporation into the RNA of cytoplasmic polyribosomes reflects only, or at least predominantly, the incorporation into mRNA after the administration of low doses of the inhibitor.

Cellular heterogeneity within a tissue is reflected in the synthesis of, or precursor incorporation into, various types of RNA. In both sham-operated and partially hepatectomized rats, the orotate incorporation (expressed as the specific radioactivity of the RNA) into HnRNA and nuclear rRNA of parenchymal nuclei exceeds by several-fold the incorporation into the respective RNA species of nonparenchymal nuclei. The percentage increase in orotate incorporation due to partial hepatectomy is greater in the nonparenchymal nuclei and may imply a greater proliferative response in these nuclei during the early intervals (i.e., 2–20 hr) after partial hepatectomy. Furthermore, it has been demonstrated that the parenchymal tetraploid and nonparenchymal diploid nuclei differ in the activities of RNA polymerase in rat and mouse liver.

14.5. Modification of RNA Metabolism by Toxicants

14.5.1. Effects of Toxicants on Precursor Incorporation into Total Cellular, Nuclear, and Cytoplasmic RNAs

There are many examples of toxicants that exert short-term inhibition of precursor incorporation into RNA. For example, the hepatocarcinogens 3'-methyl-4-dimethylaminoazobenzene, dimethylnitrosamine, and tannic acid initiate ultrastructural abnormalities of the nucleoli in rat liver. The formation and reversibility of the ultrastructural changes are accompanied by a reversible inhibition of uridine incorporation into nuclear RNA. A maximum inhibition of uridine incorporation exceeding 50% is seen for each toxicant 6–48 hr after its administration, and at least partial recovery is observed at 72 hr. In addition, there is generally at least a 50% decrease in the RNA polymerase measured in vitro in the isolated nucleoli of the toxicant-treated rats. The enzymatic activity measured in the nucleoli presumably reflects RNA polymerase I, which is responsible for the synthesis of 45S precursor rRNA.

There are many instances in incorporation experiments in which the fractionation of the cellular RNA is essential in order to study effectively the molecular alterations induced by a toxicant or drug. Phenobarbital, an inducer of hepatic microsomal mixed-function oxidases, increases the nuclear content of RNA and of 45S precursor rRNA. The *incorporation* of orotate into cytoplasmic 28S and 18S rRNA is increased 4–16 hr after a single injection of phenobarbital. However, such a finding does not necessarily imply an increased *synthesis* of precursor rRNA. For example, neither the incorporation in vivo of radioactive orotate or adenine into nuclear 45S precursor rRNA nor the incorporation in vitro of labeled nucleotides into RNA of isolated nucleoli is enhanced by phenobarbital.

These observations and additional data are consistent with the proposal that phenobarbital increases the labeling of cytoplasmic rRNAs by an increase in the posttranscriptional stability of nuclear 45S precursor rRNA, and a greater proportion of the precursor rRNA is processed to yield cytoplasmic rRNA.

The administration of carbon tetrachloride brings about a disaggregation of polyribosomes to monosomes and/or ribosomal subunits and a concomitant decrease in the synthesis of some but not all proteins. The effects of carbon tetrachloride on various parameters of RNA synthesis have been studied extensively. Precursor incorporation into *total cellular* RNA of rat liver is not altered at early intervals by carbon tetrachloride. It is apparent, however, that the effects of carbon tetrachloride vary with different fractions of RNA. After carbon tetrachloride administration in vivo there is a marked increase in the total orotate incorporation into the RNA of the polyribosomal region (after centrifugation of the postmitochondrial supernatant on a sucrose gradient), although there is appreciably less RNA in that region due to the disaggregation of the polyribosomes. The nature of the increased precursor incorporation into the RNA of the polyribosomal fraction of carbon tetrachloride–treated rats is still to be resolved but it may reflect newly synthesized mRNA for a few selected proteins.

The possible importance of toxicant-induced differences in macromolecular synthesis in the various cell types of a tissue has been emphasized. However, there are instances in which cellular heterogeneity does not appear to alter the *relative* responses to a toxicant. For example, the effects of the hepatocarcinogen N-hydroxy-2-acetylaminofluorene on the incorporation of orotate into HnRNA and rRNA are the same in the parenchymal as in the nonparenchymal nuclei of rat liver. In sham-operated animals, the hepatocarcinogen inhibits by approximately 50% the orotate incorporation into HnRNA and rRNA of parenchymal nuclei and HnRNA and rRNA of nonparenchymal nuclei. In regenerating liver, which normally shows a greater incorporation into hepatic RNA than normal liver, the orotate incorporation into each type of RNA in each class of nuclei is inhibited by approximately 75%. Therefore, N-hydroxy-2-acetylaminofluorene is essentially equally toxic to both parenchymal and nonparenchymal cells, as reflected by this parameter of toxicity.

14.5.2. Effects of Toxicants on RNA Polymerases

Treatment with a toxicant may result in a decrease or an increase in the levels of specific RNA polymerases. A toxicant-induced decrease in the activity of an RNA polymerase may occur due to (a) toxicant damage to the template DNA, (b) damage to the polymerase molecule (or to one of the accessory regulatory proteins involved in transcription), or (c) inhibition of the synthesis of sufficient new polymerase to compensate for the loss of polymerase during normal turnover and therefore to maintain the basal level. The inhibition of enzyme synthesis can be due to a direct effect on the process of protein synthesis or to a secondary effect, e.g., inhibition of mRNA synthesis. Various toxicants appear to exert their effects by mechanism (a) or (b), but the role of mechanism (c) is difficult to exclude in many cases.

Measurements of polymerase activities may be conducted on isolated hepatic nuclei. The distinction between the specific classes of polymerases is accomplished by incubation at low ionic strength with low levels of α-amanitin. Since the toxin inhibits polymerase II but does not affect polymerases I and III in the incubated nuclei, the residual activity reflects the latter polymerases. Alternatively, the isolated nuclei are incubated at high ionic strength (0.25 M ammonium sulfate) without α-amanitin, and the measured polymerase activity reflects polymerase II. For example, the treatment of rats with allylisopropylacetamide results in porphyria and is accompanied by an increase in hepatic nuclear RNA synthesis. When isolated hepatic nuclei were assayed for RNA polymerase activities under conditions of low salt concentration and in the presence of α-amanitin (to measure the sum of the activities of polymerases I and III), or at high ionic strength in the absence of α-amanitin (to measure polymerase II), it was found that treatment with allylisopropylacetamide results in an increase in the combined activities of polymerases I and III 4–12 hr after treatment but no change in RNA polymerase II.

A number of studies on toxicants have included an examination of the chromatographically separated polymerases. The intraperitoneal administration of the hepatocarcinogen aflatoxin B_1 to rats inhibits the subsequent in vitro incorporation of UTP into RNA of hepatic nuclei isolated 2–9 hr after treatment with the aflatoxin. Separation of polymerases I and II by chromatography on DEAE-Sephadex and assay of the polymerases with *exogenous* DNA indicate that treatment with aflatoxin B_1 in vivo has no effect on the nucleolar polymerase I but decreases markedly the activity of the nucleoplasmic RNA polymerase II.

In a more detailed study of the effect of aflatoxin B_1 on RNA synthesis, rat liver nuclei were isolated 2 hr after a single intraperitoneal injection of aflatoxin B_1. The RNA polymerase activity in isolated nuclei (i.e., dependent on *endogenous* template) was markedly reduced. When the RNA polymerase activity in the nuclei was measured in the presence of α-amanitin (i.e., to abolish the activity of RNA polymerase II), the percentage inhibition was somewhat greater. These observations imply that the activities of polymerase I and/or polymerase III were inhibited to a greater extent than the activity of polymerase II. However, when the total nuclear RNA polymerases, specifically the free forms, were measured in the presence of an exogenous template (namely poly(dI-dC) in the presence of actinomycin D to prevent utilization of endogenous template by the chromatin-bound polymerases), inhibition was observed only in the α-amanitin–sensitive polymerase II. These and subsequent experiments on the chromatographically separated polymerases—both the free enzymes easily extractable from nuclei and the transcriptionally active bound enzymes—indicate that the inhibition of the activities of polymerases I and/or III was due to the damage by aflatoxin of the appropriate DNA template, whereas the inhibition of the polymerase II activity was due to a decrease in the active polymerase II molecules. The decrease in active polymerase II may potentially be attributed to direct inactivation of this polymerase by an aflatoxin metabolite. However, polymerase II normally appears to have a rapid turnover; consequently, aflatoxin may decrease the synthesis of polymerase II (or its mRNA) and cause insufficient replacement to maintain the basal level of this enzyme. The decreased activity of chromatographically separated RNA polymerase II was reflected in both the free and in the bound fractions when each was assayed in the presence of exogenous template.

Thioacetamide administration results, within 1 or 2 days, in the enlargement of the nucleolus and enhanced synthesis of ribosomal RNA. In more detailed studies, the free forms of the polymerases were separated from the bound, chromatin-associated forms, and polymerase I and II were chromatographically separated from each form. At 24 hr after thioacetamide administration, the amount of the transcriptionally active, bound polymerase I, which synthesizes precursor rRNA, was increased to three times the level found in control nuclei (per unit quantity of nuclear DNA). Each of the other three forms (free polymerase I, free and bound polymerase II) exhibited only 30–50% increases. Subsequent experiments were consistent with the intrepretation that the increased activity of bound RNA polymerase I was due to an increased number of polymerase molecules rather than an increased turnover of the polymerase or the presence of a nuclear stimulatory factor in the liver of thioacetamide-treated rats.

As discussed in Section 14.5.1, the hepatocarcinogen N-hydroxy-2-acetylaminofluorene inhibited in vivo the orotate incorporation into both HnRNA and rRNA of rat liver. In subsequent studies, nuclei were isolated from partially hepatectomized rats 2 hr after the intraperitoneal injection of the hepatocarcinogen. When the isolated nuclei were assayed for RNA polymerases using endogenous nuclear template and conditions favorable for the nucleolar RNA polymerase I (low ionic strength and Mg^{2+}) or the nucleoplasmic RNA polymerase II (high ionic strength and Mn^{2+}), each polymerase activity was decreased by 50–70%. When the enzymatic activities were separated by chromatography on DEAE-Sephadex, there was an increase (50–100%) in the activity (nucleotide incorporated/mg protein) of the nucleolar polymerase I and a decrease (60–70%) in the activity of the nucleoplasmic polymerase II. The apparent decrease in the number of enzymatically active molecules of RNA polymerase II in hepatic nuclei of rats treated with N-hydroxy-2-acetylaminofluorene was consistent with a direct inhibitory action on polymerase II but did not exclude an interference with the synthetic replacement of an enzyme that may have a rapid turnover.

In this study of RNA polymerase I, as in other studies of the effects of certain carcinogens on RNA synthesis and RNA polymerases, the observations are consistent with, but do not prove, the proposal that the toxicant damaged and prevented the full template activity of nuclear DNA. In these situations, nuclear RNA polymerase activity was increased as measured with *exogenous* template, and the activity was unchanged or decreased as measured with *endogenous* template. However, the decreased synthesis of precursor rRNA in nuclei of the carcinogen-treated rats was not explained fully. Treatment of rats in vivo with the carcinogen apparently did not significantly decrease the ability of the purified hepatic DNA to serve in vitro as template for polymerase I or polymerase II. Since no overt inhibitory effects were observed on either the template function of the purified DNA or the RNA polymerase I molecules, the speculation was made that the effects on precursor rRNA synthesis by N-hydroxy-2-acetylaminofluorene may have been due to the effects of the carcinogen on a polymerase I regulatory protein or another chromosomal protein. Such an action may cause the displacement of the polymerase from its normal template.

14.6. Protein Synthesis

14.6.1. Sequential Steps in Protein Synthesis

The synthesis of protein involves the participation of various processes: energy production, RNA synthesis, and the sequential steps in protein synthesis. The amino acid undergoes an activation requiring ATP and resulting in an enzyme-bound aminoacyl adenylate. The activated amino acid is then transferred to the 2′-OH and/or 3′-OH of the terminal adenylate moiety of a cognate tRNA. Both reactions are catalyzed by the same amino acid–specific enzyme, aminoacyl-tRNA synthetase (also called aminoacyl-tRNA ligase or amino acid–activating enzyme). There is a distinct aminoacyl-tRNA synthetase for each of the "major" amino acids (each of the 20 amino acids including glutamine and asparagine but excluding hydroxyproline and hydroxylysine). An aminoacyl-tRNA synthetase recognizes only the cognate amino acid and a cognate tRNA. There are typically several cognate tRNAs, referred to as isoaccepting tRNAs, for each amino acid, and the isoaccepting tRNAs for a single amino acid differ in primary structure (i.e., nucleotide sequence).

Peptide synthesis is initiated by the interactions of methionyl-tRNA, mRNA, a 40S ribosomal subunit, a 60S ribosomal subunit, initiation factors, and guanosine triphosphate (GTP) to yield an 80S initiation complex. Polypeptide chain elongation consists of the following steps: (a) the binding of an aminoacyl-tRNA as dictated by the antiparallel hydrogen bonding of the anticodon region of the tRNA with the complementary region of the mRNA and the binding of the aminoacyl-tRNA to the A site (aminoacyl-tRNA site or acceptor site) of the 80S ribosome; (b) the formation of the peptide bond, the peptidyltransferase reaction, by the transfer of the peptidyl group (or the initiating methionyl group if it is the first peptide bond formed) from the peptidyl-tRNA in the ribosomal P site (peptidyl-tRNA site or donor site) to the amino acid moiety of the aminoacyl-tRNA in the A site; (c) the translocation, which involves the release of the uncharged or "empty" tRNA from the P site, the movement of the peptidyl-tRNA from the A to the P site, and the movement of the mRNA relative to the monoribosome, resulting in the next codon on the mRNA being aligned with the A site of the ribosome; and (d) the participation of elongation factors and the hydrolysis of GTP during several of the enumerated steps. Three nucleotide triplets of mRNA (namely, UAA, UAG, and UGA) serve as termination signals for peptide synthesis but do not code for an amino acid. Peptide chain termination at a termination codon involves the hydrolysis of the bond between the carboxy-terminal amino acid and the tRNA of the peptidyl-tRNA, with the release of the polypeptide, the tRNA, and the monoribosome or the ribosomal subunits. Release factors participate in the chain termination.

Polypeptide chain elongation proceeds from the 5′ terminus to the 3′ terminus of the mRNA and from the amino-terminal amino acid (namely, methionine) to the carboxy-terminal amino acid of the polypeptide. Each 80S mammalian monoribosome extends only over a region of approximately 80 nucleotides on the mRNA. Consequently, multiple copies of the same polypeptide in various stages of completion may exist on a polyribosome, but the extent of completion of each polypeptide depends on the relative position of its attached monoribosomal moiety on the mRNA.

Some agents are highly specific inhibitors of protein synthesis and do not directly affect the synthesis of other macromolecules. Cycloheximide inhibits the peptidyltransferase activity of the 60S ribosomal subunit. The result is that the movement of monoribosomal units along the mRNA is halted, and the polyribosomes remain intact—even when animals are treated concurrently with toxicants, such as carbon tetrachloride, which result normally in polyribosomal disaggregation. Puromycin, a second highly specific inhibitor of protein synthesis, is structurally similar to the aminoacyladenosine moiety of aminoacyl-tRNA. When puromycin is bound to the A site of the ribosome, an amide bond is formed enzymatically between the peptidyl moiety of peptidyl-tRNA and puromycin. The peptidyl puromycin blocks further elongation of the peptide, dissociates from the ribosome, and in effect causes premature peptide chain termination. Both cycloheximide and puromycin are commonly used as experimental tools, and processes that are blocked by these agents are assumed to require protein synthesis. Unfortunately, sometimes the fact that cycloheximide tends to stabilize mRNA is ignored. Treatment with a toxicant that inhibits the synthesis of mRNA is expected to cause disaggregation of polyribosomes because of the lack of replacement of mRNA. However, the mRNA that maintains the polyribosomal structure generally appears to be susceptible to degradation only when the polyribosome is actively engaged in protein synthesis. Concurrent treatment with an inhibitor of mRNA synthesis (toxicant) and cycloheximide results in the maintenance of the polyribosomal structure because its constituent mRNA is not susceptible to enzymatic degradation. This phenomenon is discussed below with regard to the toxic effects of carbon tetrachloride. Diphtheria toxin also is a highly specific inhibitor of protein synthesis. The toxin catalyzes the transfer and covalent reaction of an ADP-ribose moiety from NAD to elongation factor 2 (EF-2 or translocase) and thereby inactivates the factor.

Mammalian mitochondria possess a protein synthetic system that is distinct from the system in the cytosol-cytoplasmic ribosomes. The mitochondrial system is characterized by distinct tRNAs and mitochondrial ribosomes that are smaller than the mammalian 80S ribosomes. Chloramphenicol, a noted inhibitor of prokaryotic protein synthesis, also inhibits protein synthesis in mitochondria but does not interfere with protein synthesis in the nonmitochondrial cytoplasmic system.

14.6.2. Synthesis of Proteins on Free and Membrane-Bound Polyribosomes

The nonmitochondrial ribosomes may exist either free within the cytoplasm or membrane bound, that is, bound to the outer surface of the endoplasmic reticulum and the outer nuclear membrane. In rodent liver and pancreas approximately 70–75% of the ribosomes in the postmitochondrial supernatant are membrane bound. A further experimental and functional distinction sometimes is made between loosely membrane-bound and tightly membrane-bound ribosomes. There is a consensus that many (but not all) of the proteins that remain within the cell are synthesized predominantly on the free ribosomes and that many (but not all) of the secreted proteins are synthesized predominantly on the membrane-bound ribosomes. An observation that is consistent with the separation of function is that membrane-bound ribosomes are abundant in hepatic cells, which synthesize and secrete the bulk of the plasma proteins, and in pancreatic exocrine cells, which synthesize and secrete digestive proenzymes.

Albumin, the major protein in plasma, is synthesized within the liver in precursor forms (preproalbumin and proalbumin), processed, and eventually exported to the blood. Albumin is synthesized almost exculsively (more than 95%) on the membrane-bound ribosomes. The distribution of the mRNA coding for albumin exhibits a very similar distribution. Ferritin is an intracellular iron-binding protein, and increased synthesis in the liver is induced by the administration of iron salts. In the liver of normal rats, only approximately one-half of the immunoprecipitable ribosome-bound ferritin is associated with the free ribosomes. Because the free ribosomes represent only one-fourth of the total ribosomes, the ribosome-associated ferritin level is approximately three times greater in the free than in the membrane-bound ribosomes if expressed per quantity of ribosomal poly(A)-containing mRNA (or per quantity of ribosomes). If ferritin synthesis is induced by iron administration, the ferritin level per quantity of poly(A)-containing mRNA is approximately eightfold greater in the free ribosomes. There are a few examples, however, of retained cellular proteins that may not be synthesized predominantly on the free ribosomes.

14.7. Modification of Protein Metabolism by Toxicants

Although numerous toxicants bring about a cessation of protein synthesis, in many cases the effects on protein synthesis are secondary and subsequent to actions of the toxicant on another process (e.g., energy production or synthesis of mRNA). In some cases, it is difficult to establish whether the alteration of protein synthesis by a toxicant is a primary or secondary effect.

The hepatotoxin carbon tetrachloride initiates cellular necrosis, and the sequence of events and the possible role of altered protein synthesis in cellular necrosis is still debated. In the liver of carbon tetrachloride–treated rats, the polyribosomes undergo disaggregation to monoribosomes and/or ribosomal subunits. The disaggregation of polyribosomes occurs in both the free and membrane-bound polyribosomes, and the fraction of polyribosomes that undergo disaggregation is essentially equal in both types. In addition, although membrane-bound polyribosomes undergo disaggregation to membrane-bound monoribosomes, the disaggregation is not accompanied by a release of the monoribosomes from the endoplasmic reticulum. The disaggregation of both free and membrane-bound polyribosomes implies that carbon tetrachloride causes the polyribosomal dissociation by alteration of a structural component (mRNA, rRNA, or ribosome-associated protein) of the polyribosome rather than by damage to the membraneous components of the endoplasmic reticulum and a resultant release of ribosomes. As in other instances of toxicant-induced disaggregation of polyribosomes, there are decreases in amino acid incorporation into hepatic total cellular protein and in the synthesis of most proteins. As discussed above (Section 14.5.1), the orotate incorporation is increased in the RNA of the larger hepatic polyribosomes after carbon tetrachloride administration, and it has been proposed that the increased orotate incorporation reflects the preferential association of a limited amount of newly synthesized mRNA with the small amount of surviving larger polyribosomes. However, others have found that when RNA is prelabeled with orotate shortly before the administration of carbon tetrachloride, the toxicant appears to depress the amount of poly(A)-containing mRNA entering the cytoplasmic polyribosomes.

Carbon tetrachloride may exert markedly divergent effects on the synthesis of specific mRNAs and specific proteins. The treatment of rats with hydrocortisone induces the synthesis of tryptophan oxygenase (accompanied by the concomitant increase in immunologically reactive enzyme protein), and the synthesis appears to be dependent on the coordinate synthesis of RNA (presumably including the synthesis of the mRNA for tryptophan oxygenase). Administration of carbon tetrachloride suppresses the induction of tryptophan oxygenase by hydrocortisone, as would be expected from the polyribosomal disaggregation and inhibition of protein synthesis by the toxicant. Tyrosine aminotransferase is a second hepatic enzyme that is inducible by hydrocortisone. In contrast to the inhibitory effects seen on tryptophan oxygenase, carbon tetrachloride both increases the activity of tyrosine aminotransferase when given alone and enhances the induction of tyrosine aminotransferase when given with hydrocortisone. The increase in aminotransferase by carbon tetrachloride is prevented by high doses of actinomycin D. Thus, carbon tetrachloride may enhance the synthesis of certain hepatic enzymes by an increase in the synthesis of the respective mRNA (i.e., consistent with the increased orotate incorporation into the RNA of the heavier polyribosomes), although the synthesis of total cellular protein, including tryptophan oxygenase, is markedly depressed.

Agreement has not been reached as to the primary defect in hepatic protein synthesis in carbon tetrachloride–treated animals. Evidence has been presented for defects at various sites, including the following: a modification of mRNA, but not a degradation of mRNA, which decreases the ability of the mRNA to recycle ribosomes during protein synthesis; a decrease in the availability of poly(A)-containing mRNA in the cytoplasm; an alteration in one of the components involved in the recycling of mRNA during protein synthesis; and a selective inhibition of the synthesis of rRNA.

The question has been raised as to whether the effects of carbon tetrachloride on hepatic protein synthesis are of significance in regard to hepatic necrosis or are instead passive responses. The administration of cycloheximide prior to carbon tetrachloride both prevents the disaggregation of polyribosomes and depresses the carbon tetrachloride–induced hepatotoxicity as measured by elevations in serum glutamate–oxaloacetate transaminase or in hepatic triglycerides. The prior administration of cycloheximide does not prevent the carbon tetrachloride–induced destruction of microsomal cytochrome P-450 or the conversion of radioactive carbon tetrachloride to metabolites that react covalently with microsomal protein or lipid. Since the interruption of protein synthesis protects against the *necrotic* manifestations of carbon tetrachloride, perhaps continued but limited protein synthesis is necessary for the development of necrosis. Alternatively, perhaps only the dissociated components of the polyribosomes are susceptible to damage by the toxicant, and the cycloheximide-maintained polyribosomal structure protects a susceptible component against damage. A subsequent release from the cycloheximide-induced inhibition may then permit synthesis of enzymatic and structural proteins to repair the cells before necrosis is manifested. The prior administration of cycloheximide also protects against the hepatotoxicity of other toxicants.

Upon occasion, toxicants can induce the synthesis of a specific protein. There are several metal-binding proteins that are capable of sequestering metallic cations and thereby ameliorating some but not all of the toxic actions. The metal-binding proteins metallothionein (which binds zinc, cadmium, mercury, and other ions) and copper-chelatin (which binds copper ions) are discussed elsewhere (Chapter 19, Section 19.2.2). The amino acid analyses of both proteins show a high molar content of cysteine, and the metallic cations appear to bind to the sulfhydryl groups. The metallothionein normally exists at low levels in the cytosol of hepatic cells and is presumably bound to Zn^{2+}. The administration of high levels of Zn^{2+} or Cd^{2+} is followed within 4–8 hr by the synthesis of high levels of metallothionein. The pattern of results obtained in studies with inhibitors of RNA and protein synthesis are consistent with an induced synthesis of the appropriate mRNA and a subsequent increased synthesis of the protein.

In a representative study, the synthesis of Cd-thionein was measured by the incorporation of radioactive cystine and radioactive Cd^{2+} into a soluble low molecular weight hepatic protein separated by gel chromatography. The injection into rats of a trace amount of radioactive Cd^{2+} at a molar level that does not induce Cd-thionein resulted at 42 hr in negligible cystine incorporation into the Cd-thionein but labeling of the Cd-thionein with radioactive Cd^{2+}, perhaps by displacement of endogenous Zn^{2+} from the protein. In contrast, if a mixture of radioactive and nonradioactive Cd^{2+} was injected at a molar level sufficient to induce the synthesis of Cd-thionein, there was incorporation of cystine into the chromatographic fraction containing the Cd-thionein along with a 16,000-fold increase in the total Cd^{2+} present in the fraction. The administration of cycloheximide or actinomycin D *prior* to the Cd-thionein–inducing dose of Cd^{2+} markedly decreased cystine incorporation and appreciably decreased Cd^{2+} uptake into Cd-thionein. In contrast, when actinomycin D was given 3 hr *after* the Cd-thionein–inducing dose of Cd^{2+} (presumably after an interval which permitted synthesis of the appropriate mRNA during the induction), the incorporation of cystine into the Cd-thionein was not appreciably altered. Thus, the results imply that Cd^{2+} induces the formation of the mRNA of Cd-thionein and the subsequent use of the mRNA in protein synthesis.

The copper-induced synthesis of copper-chelatin has properties similar to those seen in the Cd^{2+}-induced synthesis of metallothionein. Amino acid incorporation into and Cu^{2+} binding to copper-chelatin were observed after the injection of Cu^{2+}. The induced synthesis was inhibited by the prior administration of cycloheximide or actinomycin D but was not inhibited when the actinomycin D was administered after the inducing dose of Cu^{2+}.

14.8. Summary

It is difficult to systematize the effects of toxicants on the metabolism of nucleic acids and proteins, in part due to the difficulty of distinguishing the primary and secondary effects of toxicants. Certain patterns of results are often observed: (a) Some of the acute effects are undoubtedly secondary to the effects of toxicants on energy production and on mitochondrial ultrastructure. (b) Toxicants that cause hepatic necrosis typically initiate DNA synthesis after several days, and such synthesis is preliminary to increased mitotic activity of the tissue regenerative stage. (c) Toxicants that react covalently with DNA, i.e., most organic carcinogens, initiate nucleotide incorporation into DNA during repair processes

(Chapter 16). (d) The toxicity of a number of substances (carbon tetrachloride or toluene) is manifested by the disaggregation of hepatic polyribosomes, which leads to decreased protein synthesis, but the molecular site of damage remains to be established (Section 14.7). (e) The effects on protein synthesis may be highly selective in some cases. While the synthesis of the majority of proteins is inhibited, the synthesis of specific proteins may be induced: e.g., the mixed-function oxidases of the endoplasmic reticulum after treatment with aromatic compounds, and the metal-binding proteins after administration of certain toxic metallic salts. In the latter cases, there is also presumably an induced synthesis of the appropriate mRNA which precedes the synthesis of the protein. (f) Although a number of toxicants are known to affect certain overall processes, the enumeration of specific steps altered must await further study in many cases. Certain carcinogens, such as aflatoxin B_1 and 2-acetylaminofluorene derivatives, have been studied in sufficient detail to establish the identities of the RNA polymerases inhibited and the probable molecular mechanism of inhibition (Section 14.5.2).

Suggested Reading

Importance of the Nucleotide Pool in the Correlation of Precursor Incorporation with the Rate of Synthesis of a Macromolecule

Bucher, N. L. R., Swaffield, M. N. Ribonucleic acid synthesis in relation to precursor pools in regenerating rat liver. Biochim. Biophys. Acta 174 (1969), 491.

Stambrook, P. J., Sisken, J. E. The relationship between rates of (³H) uridine and (³H) adenine incorporation into RNA and the measured rates of RNA synthesis during the cell cycle. Biochim. Biophys. Acta 281 (1972), 45.

Yu, F.-L., Feigelson, P. Effects of cortisone on orotic acid transport and RNA synthesis in rat liver. Arch. Biochem. Biophys. 141 (1970), 662.

Mammalian DNA Polymerases

Bollum, F. J. Mammalian DNA polymerases. Prog. Nucleic Acid Res. Mol. Biol. 15 (1975), 109.

Craig, R. K., Keir, H. M. Nuclear DNA polymerases. In Busch H. (Ed.). The Cell Nucleus, Vol. 3. New York: Academic Press, 1974, pp. 35–66.

Loeb, L. A. Eucaryotic DNA polymerases. In Boyer P. D. (Ed.) The Enzymes, Vol. 10. New York: Academic Press, 1974, pp. 173–209.

Weissbach, A. Eukaryotic DNA polymerases. Ann. Rev. Biochem. 46 (1977), 25.

Mammalian RNA Polymerases

Chambon, P. Eucaryotic RNA polymerases. In Boyer P. D. (Ed.). The Enzymes, Vol. 10. New York: Academic Press, 1974, pp. 261–331.

Jacob, S. T. Mammalian RNA polymerases. Prog. Nucleic Acid Res. Mol. Biol. 13 (1973), 93–126.

Roeder, R. G. Eukaryotic nuclear RNA polymerases. In Losick, R., Chamberlin, M. (Eds.), RNA Polymerase. Cold Spring Harbor, N. Y.: Cold Spring Harbor Laboratory, 1976, pp. 285–329.

Weil, P. A., Blatti, S. P. HeLa cell deoxyribonucleic acid dependent RNA polymerases: Function and properties of the class III enzymes. Biochemistry 15 (1976), 1500.

Effects of Toxicants on DNA and RNA Metabolism

de Bruin, A. Biochemical Toxicology of Environmental Agents. Amsterdam: Elsevier/North-Holland, 1976, pp. 605–654.

Leonard, T. B., Jacob, S. T. Alterations in DNA-dependent RNA polymerases I and II from rat liver by thioacetamide: Preferential increase in the level of chromatin-associated nucleolar RNA polymerase IB. Biochemistry 16 (1977), 4538.

Yu, F.-L. Mechanism of aflatoxin B₁ inhibition of rat hepatic nuclear RNA synthesis. J. Biol. Chem. 252 (1977), 3245.

Mammalian Protein Synthesis

Arnstein, H. R. V. (Ed.). Synthesis of Amino Acids and Proteins. London: Butterworths, and Baltimore: University Park Press, 1975.

Effects of Toxicants on Protein Synthesis

de Bruin, A. Biochemical Toxicology of Environmental Agents. Amsterdam: Elsevier/North-Holland, 1976, pp. 655–685.

Squibb, K. S., Cousins, R. J. Control of cadmium binding protein synthesis in rat liver. Environ. Physiol. Biochem. 4 (1974), 24.

Daniel S. Grosch

15

Genetic Poisons

15.1. Introduction

A genetic poison can be defined as any agent that acts upon the gametogenic cells of the gonad (a) to decrease the number of gametes produced, or (b) to alter deleteriously the genetic information of gametes. The latter category includes the more drastic mutations which cause death of the zygote during an early state of development, as well as less serious alterations of the phenotype. Mutations may also be induced in the cells of somatic tissues, but these are not passed on to future generations. A chief concern is their contribution to carcinogenesis (Chapter 16).

In the gonad the effects of genetic poisons are reflected quantitatively in degrees of fecundity and fertility. Fecundity is synonymous with prolificacy. Because the number of fertilized eggs produced by the female is the limiting factor, fecundity is often expressed as the yield in number of eggs per unit period of time. Fertility is the ability to produce live offspring. In the genetic literature this is often expressed as egg hatchability or seed germination. Infertility may be induced in either sex. By definition it is distinguished from the failure of young plants or animals to survive to maturity. If genetic in origin, premature death is said to be due to a lethal factor (often a single mutant gene).

Gonad tissue can be lost without decreasing health or adult life span. Even if the agent destroys all the gametic cells and germ-line stem cells, no significant decrease in life span should occur, provided somatic tissues are not irrevocably damaged. Indeed, female rodents freed of the stresses of pregnancy and birth by localized radiation castration tend to live longer than controls. Few chemical agents are so selective in mammals, but increased life span can be demonstrated in chemically castrated adult holometabolous insects which lack proliferative somatic tissues.

On the other hand, gamete development and dispensation depend upon the normal functioning of somatic tissues. Therefore, effects on organism physiology must be distinguished from genetic poisons. Sublethal doses of insecticides can decrease reproductive performance by causing poor appetite or poor utilization of food so that yolk deposition or fetal nutrition is inadequate. Furthermore, a variety of toxic agents can disturb hormonal equilibria in birds and mammals. A consequence of neural disorders may be an alteration of mating behavior. Small quantities of pesticides similar in concentration to those of environmental contamination alter male cricket stridulation to a degree causing rejection of males by the females. Detailed discussion of such matters is beyond the scope of this chapter, which concerns agents attacking the germ-line cells of the gonads.

The consequences of directive selection on the heterogeneous gene pools of natural populations must be distinguished from the action of genetic poisons. The appearance of a toxicant-tolerant or pesticide-resistant strain does not result from mass mutation. Instead, the presence of a chemical agent eliminates sensitive individuals, so that over several generations an ever-increasing proportion of the population is made up of individuals that are resistant. In other words, selection acts at the phenotype level to determine the parents of future generations. The consequence is selective pressure on the genetic makeup of the pest population. These situations have occurred in many parts of the world and have given rise to strains resistant to each of the major classes of insecticide.

Even when germinal cells are under direct attack, a distinction must be made between agents that are (a) cytotoxic, (b) cytostatic, or (c) mutagenic. Many cytotoxic agents kill cells by overwhelming nonspecific effects such as anoxia, protein coagulation, increased membrane permeability, etc. When death of the cell occurs promptly from heat shock or cytological fixatives, the cell structure does not undergo alterations visible with the light microscope. Recourse must be made to electron microscopy. Slow death is accompanied by moribund changes. A common nonspecific change in nuclear appearance is pyknosis, in which the diffuse chromatin condenses into a solid structureless mass. A usually reliable criterion of cell death employed by physiologists is the penetration into and homogeneous staining of cytoplasm by dyes that normally remain outside or are accumulated in circumscribed vacuoles. Cytostatic and mutagenic agents are discussed in the following sections.

15.2. Cytostatic Agents

15.2.1. Specific Spindle Poisons

A major exception to the rule that heritable changes are caused by attacks on DNA is the case of agents that attack the spindle of eukaryotic cell division. Changes in ploidy result from doses that only inhibit the spindle temporarily. In turn, compensatory changes in nuclear, cell, tissue, and organ size result from the increase in sets of chromosomes. In addition, with increases in gene dosage, amounts of vitamins, alkaloids, and other products of quantitative genes are elevated in the higher plants in which polyploidy has been a major factor in evolution.

Detection of changes in ploidy involves light microscopic examination of preparations obtained by standard cytological procedures. Microscopy is also used in studying individual cell responses, which are so characteristic that it has become conventional to refer to the metaphase appearance resulting from colchicine treatment as "c-metaphase."

For over 40 years colchicine has been employed extensively to produce polyploid plants. Seeds or growing parts are bathed in 0.1–0.8% solutions, although higher doses are required to inhibit mitosis in the source plant itself which contains amounts within this range. More dilute solutions are used for animal cells. About 0.00005% solutions seem safe for treating newly fertilized eggs and for the initial testing of animal cell cultures (although some strains of cultured tumor cells respond to much lower concentrations). Frogs and fish from cool waters tolerate higher concentrations of colchicine, but this difference from mammals, birds, and incubator-reared insects disappears when the temperature is raised for the aquatic animals.

Few attempts to produce polyploid animals have succeeded. The exceptional individuals obtained in swine, rabbit, and chicken experiments either died young or were sterile. Erythrocytes and sperm were demonstrably larger and a rooster had greatly elongated tail feathers. The hematopoietic and other proliferative cells of the somatic tissues of vertebrates are vulnerable to all types of mitotic inhibitors. Sterility is inevitable in bisexual organisms because polyploidy upsets the sex-chromosome mechanisms associated with heterogamety.

Colchicine (Figure 15.1) is extracted from the Egyptian or autumn flowering crocus *Colchicum autumnale* L. Because it reduces the inflammatory response to urates, it has been used since antiquity to treat gout, on occasion fatally. In the dividing cell, colchicine combines with tubulin, a protein component of the microtubules that associate to form spindle fibers. While the microtubules are in a dynamic state, colchicine prevents successful polymerization, and the result is spindle dissolution. The existence of microtubules in nerve cells accounts in part for the toxicity in animals. At concentrations sufficient to block mitosis colchicine does not inhibit DNA, RNA, or protein synthesis. In the chick brain colchicine binds solely to the microtubule protein at concentrations below 10^{-4} M. At higher colchicine concentrations, considerable nonspecific binding occurs.

Colchicine interferes with the same stage in the cell cycle of all species. Thus there is no selectivity through differences in comparative biochemistry. Small changes in the molecular structure alter its potency. Interchanging the methoxy and oxo groups at positions 14 and 15 in the C ring produces isocolchicine, with effectiveness decreased 100 times. Replacing the acetylamide group of the B ring with methylamine provides colcemid, which is less toxic in animals but somewhat less effective on plant spindles (Table 15.1). In addition, more than a dozen derivatives with small changes in molecular structure have been investigated, all less effective than colchicine by the *Allium* test.

Other botanical drugs such as vinblastine, vincristine, and podophyllotoxin reversibly disrupt the mitotic spindle. The vinalkaloids were isolated from *Vinca rosea* L. Vincristine differs from vinblastine only at one carbon, which carries an N-formyl instead of an N-methyl group. Higher concentrations of the former are required for spindle dissolution. These two *Vinca* compounds do not use the colchicine combining site on tubulin. Furthermore, the spontaneous decay of colchicine–tubulin binding is prevented by *Vinca* alkaloids without interfering with the colchicine attachment.

Toxicologically, the effects of *Vinca* alkaloids on mammalian cells are less

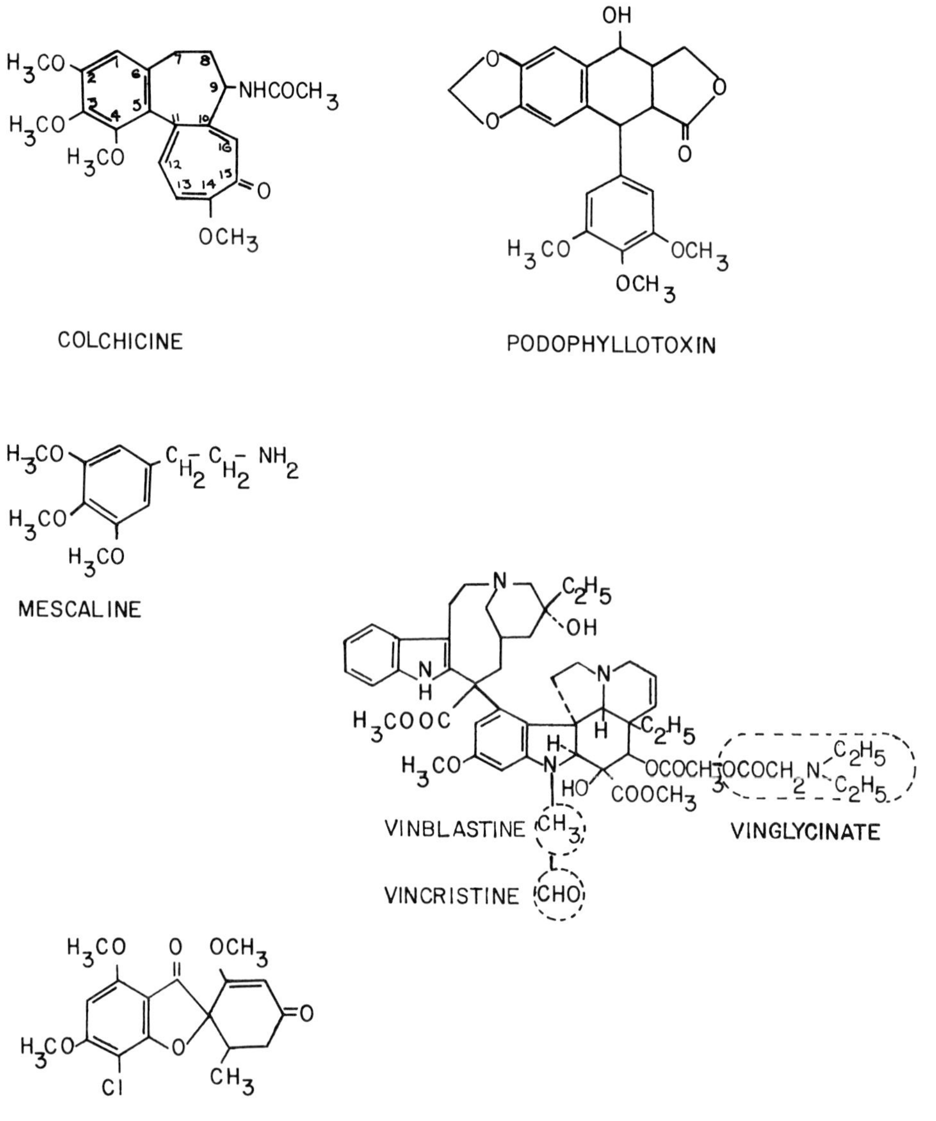

Figure 15.1 Specific spindle poisons.

specific than colchicine. The inhibition of the incorporation of uridine into RNA and the aggregation of ribosomes are the most notable effects. Nevertheless, the agents can cause sensory disturbances and motor nerve damage at 0.1–0.2 mg/kg weekly while the leukocyte count stays above 4000/mm^3. An overdose can cause leukopenia, which clears up about 1 week after the cessation of treatment. Despite the *Allium* test results, vinblastine has a more pronounced effect on tumor inhibition, but is more toxic in rats than vincristine. In rodents and in humans, bone marrow suppression is a problem.

Podophyllotoxin, obtained from *Podophyllum* species, is one of several toxic substances in plants formerly used as purgatives. In binding to tubulin it uses

Table 15.1 Threshold Concentrations for Spindle Poisons as Determined by the
Allium Test

Agent	Specific inhibitive threshold (moles/ml)	Agent	Mitodepressive threshold (moles/ml)
Colchicine	1.25×10^{-7}	Ethanol	3.4×10^{-4}
Colcemid	2.5×10^{-7}	Diethyl ether	1.3×10^{-4}
Vinblastine	2.2×10^{-8}	Chloroform	7.4×10^{-6}
Griseofulvin	2.5×10^{-8}	Ethylene glycol	7.0×10^{-4}

Source: Data from Deysson, Int. Rev. Cytol. 24 (1968), 99.

Note: *Allium* test—onion root tips are immersed in a dilution series of the test substance. After 24 hr they are fixed and stained for microscope examination, which discloses contracted chromosomes and disappearance of the spindle.

the colchicine site, and in combination experiments the two agents compete for the site. Podophyllotoxin causes side effects at moderate doses, possibly because its ability to inhibit nucleoside transport is 20-fold higher than that of colchicine. The psychomimetic agent mescaline binds to purified tubulin and inhibits division in cultured human cells. Its molecular structure resembles an abbreviated version of colchicine. Maytansine isolated from *Maytenus* plants is effective against mouse tumors and is more potent than *Vinca* alkaloids in the inhibition of cleavage in marine eggs. With persistent research the list of specific mitotic inhibitors will continue to grow. There are already 350 known indole alkaloids from only three plant families, and the biochemistry of marine invertebrates is in its infancy.

A mold metabolite, griseofulvin, obtained from *Penicillium griseofulvin*, has been employed as an antifungal agent. Administered in doses of up to 2 mg daily by mouth it is relatively nontoxic in man, but depression of hematopoiesis and spermatogenesis has been reported in animals given higher doses. In 10^{-5}–10^{-6} M solutions griseofulvin destroys the spindles in marine eggs, grasshopper embryos, plant meristems (Table 15.1), and cultured vertebrate cells. Griseofulvin either binds at another (third) site on tubulin, or may have a completely different mode of action from the agents discussed thus far.

Another mode of action has been discovered for phenyl carbamate herbicides. Cytological studies on dividing plant cells treated with isopropyl *N*-phenyl carbamate (IPC) or related compounds disclosed blocked metaphases and arrested anaphases accompanied by enlarged polyploid nuclei and multinucleate cells. Instead of dissolution of microtubules, IPC disorients intact microtubules. In cells treated with 10 ppm IPC the microtubules lose their parallel alignment and orient in radial arrays as if micropoles developed. Scattered papers in the literature give accounts of carbamate damage to animal cells, including minnow oogonia and human fibroblasts.

15.2.2. Nonspecific Agents

Microtubule-specific action is an example of "selective toxicity,"[1] in which small changes in molecular structure are important for biological activity of the

---

[1] Albert, A. Selective Toxicity, fifth edition. London: Chapman & Hall, 1973.

agents. No such correlation exists for the depressants or cell "narcotics" that interfere with dividing cells. Here lipid/water partition coefficients correlate well with the depression of cellular activity, and the effect is readily reversible when the concentration of the agent falls. Among the common organic compounds that can cause mitotic disorganization are ethanol, diethyl ether, chloroform, benzene, and naphthalene. In Table 15.1 note that much higher concentrations are needed to reach a mitodepressive threshold compared to specific spindle poisons. In animals the lipophilic agents pose more of a problem in lung and liver toxicity than the specific spindle poisons. However, in chronic benzene exposure of humans an important toxic manifestation is injury to the blood-forming cells.

In this account we have considered only the agents that interfere with cells entering division. The time course of the cell cycle leading to the onset of division can be influenced by a variety of inhibitors, especially those that interfere with nucleic acid, protein, and ATP synthesis. These matters are considered in Chapter 14.

15.2.3. Cytochalasins

Cell responses completely different from spindle repression are caused by a group of fungal metabolites known as cytochalasins. There are three major effects caused by six compounds of similar structure: an inhibition of cytoplasmic division without interference with division of the nucleus, resulting in binucleate and large multinucleate cells; the inhibition of cell movement; and the induction of nuclear extrusion. The six compounds, by convention designated A through F, are not equally effective at identical concentrations. Their effects on division are probably due to interference with cell filaments. However, binding to cell membranes may be involved in their inhibition of glucose transport, hormone secretion, and phagocytosis.

15.3. Chromosome Damage

15.3.1. Methods of Detection

Usually chromosomes are present as compact structures only during cell division. Therefore, observations of structural changes are made by microscopic examination of metaphase or anaphase figures in stained preparations. A major exception to midmitotic viewing is afforded by the exceptional polytene structure in the nondividing cells of specialized tissues of larval Diptera. In all types of cells, staining with preferential dyes is used to bring out contrasts between cell components. Dyes with specificity for DNA are particularly useful. The preparation may be fixed either before or during the staining process. Fixation employs preservatives that render the cell structures firm and capable of undergoing subsequent treatments with a minimum of distortion.

Squash preparations and smears of cell populations, or whole mounts of thin layers of tissue, provide an optimum opportunity for cytological analysis. Tissue slices are less desirable because true fragments may be difficult to distinguish from cut pieces. In plants, microsporocytes, microspores, nuclei of germinating pollen grains, and root tip cells have been studied extensively in species with a small number of large chromosomes. For visualizing human chromosomes, the culture of peripheral blood leukocytes has become the procedure of choice. This technique is also used in other vertebrates, as well as the culturing of other types of cells. Amphibian epidermis and tail tips lend themselves to whole mounts. Preparations appropriate to invertebrate studies include teased testes, whole mounts of oocytes and cleavage embryos, and spread preparations of larval tissues.

Phase contrast microscopy and the autoradiography of radioactive nucleotides incorporated into DNA have added dimensions to cytology which will not be discussed here.

Chromosome aberrations are of three main types, involving pieces of chromosomes, whole chromosomes, and sets of chromosomes. The third type, polyploidy, was considered in Section 15.2.1. Our concern here is with individual chromosomes.

15.3.2. Effective Agents

The maintenance and replication of the genetic materials of a cell are active processes that can be disturbed by alterations in their intimate environment. Any toxicant presented to cultured cells in near lethal concentration may damage their chromosomes. Under these conditions many different types of compounds have been able to break chromosomes. Relatively few agents are effective in vivo and at low concentrations. These agents include analogs of DNA components and antibiotics that inhibit DNA synthesis, but the most potent are the alkylating agents.

Sulfur and nitrogen mustards, the alkylating agents that provided the first convincing evidence of chemically induced point mutations (Auerbach and associates), also induced deletions, inversions, and translocations. These terms refer to loss of a chromosome segment (deletion), reversal of a segment (inversion), and the shifting of a segment from its normal position (translocation). The segment may be translocated in the same chromosome or it may become attached to a nonhomologous chromosome.

The consequences of these aberrations are various. Loss of chromosomal material results in a deficient genome, which is usually lethal, possibly when heterozygous and invariably when homozygous. Inversions and translocations lead to pairing difficulties in meiotic prophase. This in turn may suppress crossing over or, if not, cell lethality can result from crossing over within the inversion. Another possibility, if offspring are viable, is the "position effect," in which a change in expression of one or more genes accompanies the change in position with respect to neighboring genes. Space limitations prohibit more detailed explanations, which can be found in cytogenetics texts.

In comparison with the effects of X-rays, there was a "shortage" of large rearrangements (Table 15.2) and a relative "excess" of small ones in the sulfur mustard–treated material. Initially these results were interpreted as indicating a difference in the production of lesions. Recent evidence suggests that mustard-induced breaks tend to remain open longer than those caused by X-rays. Typically, the resulting large deletions cause death in early development of any zygote receiving such an inheritance. Thus, potential offspring can be eliminated by "dominant lethals" before the stage at which cytological analysis can be accomplished in *Drosophila*.

Table 15.2   Comparison Between the Large Rearrangements Recovered After
Equivalent Gene-Mutation Doses of X-ray and Mustard Gas Treatments
of Adult Male Drosophilia (Calculated for 10,000 Chromosomes)

Dose (percent of sex-linked lethals)	Deletions		Translocations	
	X-ray	Sulfur mustard	X-ray	Sulfur mustard
5	25	2	203	19
10	63	28	561	85

Source: Adapted from Auerbach, Mutation Research. New York: Halstead Press, 1976, p. 258.

Another difference from X irradiation was an evident tendency for delayed effects and unstable aberrations from alkylating agents. The presence or absence of oxygen, so important for the indirect action of ionizing radiations, was found to be insignificant as an attendant feature of the action of alkylating agents. Furthermore, the sites at which chromatids were involved in aberrations had a nonrandom distribution after treatment with alkylating agents. No localization of radiation-induced aberrations has been obtained with X-rays.

Initially it was supposed that only polyfunctional alkylating agents were able to induce chromosome aberrations. Then Loveless demonstrated that monofunctional representatives of each of the classes could induce chromosomal aberrations in *Vicia*. However, higher doses were necessary, and in this sense confirmed the greater effectiveness of bi- and polyfunctional alkylators. This dose-related aspect has subsequently been verified in insects and mammals.

Until techniques for culturing mammalian cells were developed, plant root tip studies dominated the literatures. The root tips are easy to handle and available all year around, but more important is the ease with which root tips or tissue cultures can be exposed directly to a chemical agent of interest. A chemical that produces aberrations in plant root tips usually causes chromosomal changes in animal cells, but the type of effect may be different in the two materials. Figure 15.2 contrasts the types and frequencies of chromosomal aberrations in onion root tips and in Chinese hamster cell cultures produced by 2-hr treatments with caffeine (a methylated purine). The metaphases in onion roots contained a high frequency of subchromatid and chromatid exchanges, whereas the hamster cells showed a high percentage of breaks. Tritiated thymidine was used to demonstrate the difference in stage sensitivity. G_2 was most sensitive in onion root tips, and S phase was vulnerable in hamster cells.

However, compounds mutagenic in vitro are not necessarily effective in vivo. In mouse or man, organism morphology and metabolism are important complications. An agent's distribution in the body and its penetration to gametogenic cells, the functioning of activation and inactivation reactions, and the efficiency of excretion are considerations in a complex situation. For example, caffeine causes no significant increase in aberrations in the meiotic chromosomes of male mice when administered either by injection or in the drinking water for a long period. On the other hand, positive results are obtained consistently when alkylating agents are used. Ethyl methanesulfonate (EMS), methyl methanesulfonate (MMS), nitrogen mustard, ethyleneimines, and other alkylators act promptly after intraperitoneal injection.

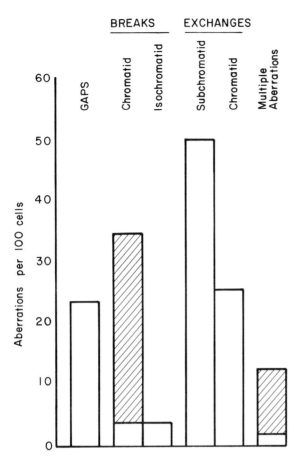

Figure 15.2 Contrast between the type and frequency of chromosome aberrations produced by 2×10^{-2}M caffeine in onion root tips (unshaded) and in hamster cell cultures (shaded bars). Bars are superimposed. Fixation was at the time of peak frequency of aberrations.
SOURCE: *Based on Kihlman's data, Chemical Mutagens (A. Hollaender, ed.) 2(1971), 510.*

Two tests are commonly used: the spermatocyte test, and the F_1 translocation test. Deviation from the characteristic meiotic configurations of spermatocyte chromosomes are featured in both approaches. In the first case, cells undergoing first maturation division are examined when a suitable time interval has elapsed after treatment. In the second test, cytological analysis is used to confirm the presence of translocations indicated by the semisterility of first-generation offspring.

15.3.3. Mode of Action

The mode of action is best understood for alkylating agents. In the physiological conditions of living tissues the alkylating compounds produce positively charged carbonium ions, which combine with electron-rich or negatively charged centers in the cells. For most types of alkylators the production of the carbonium ions is rapid and independent of the receptive center. This is known as first-order nucleophilic substitution. A second-order reaction, such as that occurring with methylsulfonyloxy esters, is mediated by the nucleophilic center.

The N-7 position is more susceptible to alkylation than any other site on the nucleotide bases comprising the DNA molecule. Pulsed treatments during interphase indicate that maximum sensitivity is attained in the S phase. The chromosomal DNA is probably more protected at other stages of the cell cycle. For an aberration to appear at the next division post treatment, alkylation of the DNA must occur during presynthesis but not so early that there is time for excision. Two possible courses of events are conceivable: (a) the alkylation of DNA, or (b) the alkylation of DNA precursors. The former has been given more credence in recent years.

In attempts to visualize how a DNA alkylation can escalate from the molecular level to the structural chromosome defect visible under the light microscope at midmitosis, two types of events have been postulated. Molecular cross-linkage could cause an arrest of synthesis. That is, the break would reflect an inability to synthesize a segment in the region of a cross-linkage. Alternatively, the break might come from an abortive attempt at repair involving only the steps of DNA excision. In these matters the final answer awaits definitive elucidation of the ultrastructure of the eukaryote chromosome and the associated molecular biochemistry. Similarly, it is not clear how incorporation of a base analog into the chromosomal DNA renders the structure more fragile, unless by halted synthesis or aborted repair.

15.4. Gene Mutation

15.4.1. Modification of the Genetic Code

By definition, gene mutation is an event localized to as small a specific site as a single nucleotide in the DNA sequence. This ultimate alteration was inferred as the explanation of the molecular defect responsible for the sickle cell trait in humans. Figure 15.3 exemplifies the reasoning by which (a) the demonstration of an electrophoretic variant in a peptide fragment, traced to (b) the substitution of a single amino acid, points to (c) a change in a three-letter "code word" (coding triplet or codon). The DNA sequence of nucleotides taken three at a time

Figure 15.3 A diagram of the first six of the 141 amino acids comprising the beta chain of adult human hemoglobin. The sickle cell variant S differs from normal by only one amino acid in position six. The phenotypic change can be explained by the replacement of a single nucleotide within the critical trinucleotide sequence of the genetic code. Arrows indicate the direction of transcription and translation.

DNA	CTC or CTT (3'⟶5')
mRNA codon	GAG or GAA (5'⟶3')
Normal	Val.- His.- Leu.- Thr.- Pro.- Glutamic acid – – – – – – – –141 amino acids
S Variant	1 – 2 – 3 – 4 – 5 – Valine – – – – – – – – – – – –141 amino acids
mRNA codon	GUG or GUA (5'⟶3')
DNA	CAC or CAT (3'⟶5')

specifies the amino acid sequence that comprises the β polypeptide chain of hemoglobin. By substituting one nucleotide for another in a three-nucleotide codon, a different amino acid may be specified, as in the above case, or more seriously in other examples, protein synthesis may be terminated at the altered codon.

In actuality the molecular basis of point mutation was worked out on viruses and bacteria, where there is no problem of a chemical penetrating to the living unit containing the genetically important nucleic acid. Furthermore, the haploid condition of the microbial forms of life simplify detection of genetic changes. In diploid organisms, mutations are usually recessive and require inbreeding schemes or other special crosses to reveal them. In Hymenoptera the parthenogenetically produced male insects are genetically haploid and provide a useful test system. In higher plants techniques have been developed to produce artificial haploids, or diploids from haploid cells.

Usually the mutant condition is less desirable than the standard, which is the consequence of a long process of natural selection. Newly arisen mutations causing slight changes in the morphology and physiology of highly evolved organisms are more common than marked effects in the individuals surviving to maturity. Therefore, the investigator's ingenuity and faculties of perception are taxed even by the progeny of experimental crosses designed to reveal mutations. The development of techniques to detect electrophoretic variants or other molecular alterations has improved the objective classification of phenotypic traits.

15.4.2. Methods of Detection

15.4.2a. Higher Organisms

In diploids, the detection of lethal or visible mutation typically takes either of two approaches: (a) all loci on a chromosome are investigated, or (b) changes at a few specific loci are scored. The all-loci approach utilizes either the hemizygous X in the digametic sex or employs a breeding scheme to render one of the autosomes homozygous. Muller introduced the study of treated X chromosomes in his historical demonstration of X-ray–induced mutations in fruit flies. For many years this technique predominated.

Stocks homozygous for recessive genes at specific loci must be maintained for the alternative approach. Despite opportunities for self-fertilization in higher plants, Stadler (who obtained the first convincing evidence in plants) favored the specific-locus approach. For example, he maintained an *a/a* strain of corn to use in tests crosses that revealed *A* to *a* color changes in irradiated *A/A* plants. More complex strains have since been derived. In mice, Russell found it difficult to maintain a tester strain homozygous for more than 7 recessive genes at as many loci on 5 of the 40 mouse chromosomes. In *Drosophila*, 6 mutant loci per long second and third chromosome appears to be a practical limit. Poor fecundity, fertility, and viability accompany the accumulations of homozygous recessive genes. In principle, when treated wild-type organisms are mated with the tester strain, the progeny will have a wild-type phenotype unless a mutation occurred at one of the marker loci.

In human genetics, pedigree analysis has been the time-honored approach. The lineages of European royalty are especially well documented and revealed the absence of father-to-son transmission of X-borne sex-linked traits. Among other things revealed was the probable mutation to hemophilia in the germ line of Queen Victoria. This provided a reoccurrence of the gene for hemophilia A, the classic type known since prehistoric time because of the practice of circumcision. The Talmud, as early as the second century AD, exempts future boys in families where death has occurred because of excessive bleeding following the operation.

Detection is not an experimental problem with agents potent enough to induce dominant lethals. The dominant lethal assay is usually performed by mating treated males with untreated females that can be replaced after each mating. In oviparous organisms early death of the embryo can be verified in unhatched eggs. In laboratory mammals the females are killed shortly before term in order to examine the uterus for live fetuses, dead fetuses, and resorption sites (deciduomata). In comparison with control values, an increase in the incidence of fetal death and resorption sites provides a measure of induced dominant lethal mutation. A decrease in the number of implantations suggest preimplantation loss, which can be due to other causes such as a spermacidal effect.

A mere decrease in litter size is an inadequate basis for a conclusion about sperm inactivation as opposed to zygotic death. On this point, decisive experiments can be performed only in animals lacking a block against development of *un*fertilized eggs, as is normal for wasps and mites, in which one class of offspring is normally produced by parthenogenesis. Thus a comparison of the proportion of uniparental to biparental offspring reflects the failure or success in fertilization. In wasps, when sperm are inactivated an increase in the number of sons produced from unfertilized eggs accompanies a decrease in biparental offspring (Figure 15.4). Induced dominant lethality kills biparental offspring without changing the number of sons. Furthermore, when investigated cytologically many of the supposed dominant lethal gene mutations proved to be associated with chromosomal aberration.

15.4.2b. Microbial Tests Modified by Mammalian Influences

A major problem in detecting mutation in mammals is the relative insensitivity of the mammalian test systems. The populations required to rule out low levels of effects are so large that the expenditure of time and funds make it impractical. Microorganisms provide the most sensitive tests of mutagenicity without posing the problem of adequate sample size, but the simpler tests ignore activation and detoxification mechanisms that occur in intact animals.

Host-mediated assay. In this approach a mammal undergoing treatment with a chemical agent is injected with an indicator microorganism in which mutation frequency can be measured. After sufficient time has elapsed, the microorganisms are withdrawn from the host and cultured on media that will reveal newly arisen mutant types. Comparisons are made between the direct action of the compound and its action in the host-mediated assay.

Gabridge and Legator developed the test with *Salmonella typhimurium,* which cannot be kept in the rodent peritoneal cavity more than 3 hr. Malling and de Serres use the ad-three test system of *Neurospora crassa,* which can remain in an animal for 18 hr.

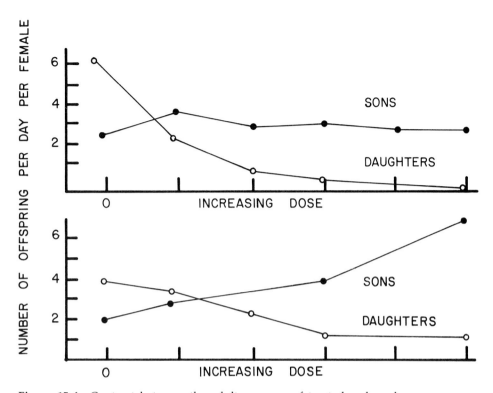

Figure 15.4 Contrast between the adult progeny of treated males when sperm carry induced dominant lethals (above), or when sperm are inactivated (below) in an insect whose male offspring come from unfertilized eggs. In braconid wasps, much of the radiation damage to sperm chromosomes kills potential daughters (above), but topical applications of polyfunctional alkylating agents can decrease the number of zygotes formed (below).

Tests employing body tissues or fluids. A logical adjunct to the host-mediated assay are tests that include mammalian blood or urine as conditioners. A further step is the use of tissue homogenates to provide an in vitro activating system.

B. N. Ames and associates have developed a sensitive test system combining rat liver cellular fraction for mutagen activation and special *Salmonella* strains for mutagen detection. Each strain contains a mutation in the histidine operon, caused by a known type of DNA damage, which results in a dietary require-ment for histidine. There is also a deletion that has eliminated the DNA excision repair system to increase the recovery of induced changes. An even further improvement was the derivation of a lipopolysaccharide-defective type; these bacteria are highly permeable to toxic agents.

In molten top agar, the microsomal fraction of a liver homogenate is added to a solution of the compound to be tested, mixed with the bacterial strain, and poured on the surface of the test plates containing only a trace of histidine. The His$^+$ revertant colonies are counted after 2 days of incubation at 37°C. The small amount of histidine allows all bacteria to undergo several divisions, but only the mutants can produce colony-size populations.

15.4.2c. Tests with Cultured Mammalian Cells

Some investigators consider the microbial systems genetically too foreign to mammalian genomes to serve adequately in the estimation of mutagenic risk for eukaryotes. Instead they have developed specific-locus assay systems for cultured mammalian cells. Chu and collaborators used Chinese hamster cells to demonstrate that the X-linked hypoxanthine guanine phosphoribosyltransferase (HGPRT) locus lends itself to the detection and quantitation of forward mutational events because the enzyme specified at this locus is responsible for cell sensitivity to purine analogs. The drugs are enzymatically converted to nucleotides that cause cell death after their incorporation into nucleic acids. Thus, in media containing a purine analog, HGPRT-competent cells are selected against, while HGPRT-deficient cells survive. An alternative pathway for the generation of purine nucleotides makes survival possible. Reverse mutation experiments require a different selection medium that contains mcthotrexate to prevent purine synthesis.

Clive decided to exploit an alternative specific locus after demonstrating the difficulties of working at the low cell densities required by an HGPRT line of mouse lymphoma cells. His locus, designated TK, specifies thymidine kinase, which normally phosphorylates thymidine, but also converts 5-bromodeoxyuridine (BUdR) to the monophosphate, which can be incorporated into DNA with lethal consequences. TK-deficient mutants lack the enzyme and suffer no ill effects from BUdR. Selection media are employed with the TK system in a fashion similar to that with the HGPRT system.

There are two TK-competent genotypes (TK +/+ and TK +/−), and a single TK-deficient homozygote (TK −/−). The heterozygous TK +/− genotype is used for tests of induced forward mutations: TK +/− to TK −/−. The reverse of this experiment serves to determine reversion rates.

15.4.3. Molecular Events

Gene mutation has occurred when a heritable change has become established in the genetically important DNA molecule. The loss of large portions is dominantly lethal; the loss of small segments is recessive. In the case of single nucleotides it may not be the loss itself that is serious, but the change in reading frame when the encoded information is transcribed into mRNA.

During the past decade, tautomeric shifts have served as the generally accepted explanation of the submolecular steps leading to point mutation; that is, by tautomerism, pairing errors arise through the transition of the pairing relationship of one purine base into the pairing form of another purine, or of a pyrimidine into another pyrimidine. The resulting changes in the nucleotide code are termed transitional errors. The alternative possibility, in which a purine is substituted for a pyrimidine, or vice versa, is called transversion. Replication of the DNA sequence must occur if the errors produced by tautomeric shifts are to appear in the DNA molecules. As shown in Figure 15.5, mistakes in copying mechanisms (copy errors) can occur after base analogs with ambiguous pairing relationships are incorporated into DNA. Other types of nucleotide changes are listed below.

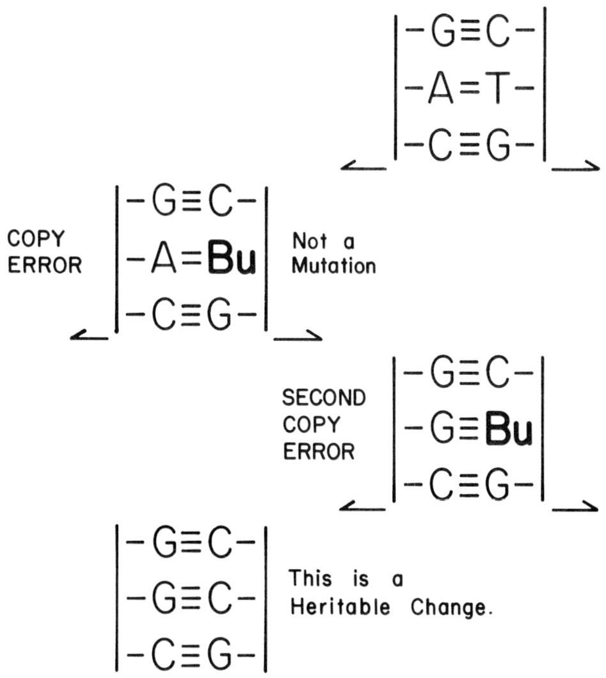

$$
\begin{array}{c}
\left| \begin{array}{c} -G\equiv C- \\ -A=T- \\ -C\equiv G- \end{array} \right|
\end{array}
$$

COPY
ERROR
$$
\left| \begin{array}{c} -G\equiv C- \\ -A=\textbf{Bu} \\ -C\equiv G- \end{array} \right|
$$
Not a
Mutation

SECOND
COPY
ERROR
$$
\left| \begin{array}{c} -G\equiv C- \\ -G\equiv \textbf{Bu} \\ -C\equiv G- \end{array} \right|
$$

$$
\left| \begin{array}{c} -G\equiv C- \\ -G\equiv C- \\ -C\equiv G- \end{array} \right|
$$
This is a
Heritable Change.

Figure 15.5 Diagram of the steps leading to mutation according to the tautomerism theory. Arrows indicate replication. Bu represents 5-bromouracil.

Recently, emphasis has turned from tautomeric shifts to explanations based upon error-prone pathways of repair of nucleotide defects. After enzymatic excision of the defective region, gaps in the sequence are filled in reference to the template of a sister chromatid or even some other length of nucleotides. The exotic strands may not be easily copied, or they may be copied inaccurately. This type of scheme more easily accounts for transversions and frame shifts.

15.4.4. Types of Chemical Mutagens

15.4.4a. Destructive

A classification on the basis of submolecular alteration provides three main types of mutagens: destructive, additive, and substitutive. Among the destructive agents are compounds as simple as hydrogen peroxide, which causes point mutations in viruses and microbes. Although used extensively in bleaching textiles and wood pulp and in converting oils into the epoxides used in plastic industries, exogenous hydrogen peroxide is not considered an important mutagen for higher organisms since it does not penetrate to the gametogenic cells.

Nitrous acid, which is mutagenic in phage, bacteria, and fungi, can deaminate adenine to form the purine hypoxanthine with pairing properties like those of guanine. It can also deaminate cytosine to produce the pyrimidine uracil. Both types of events can lead to heritable changes in the nucleotide code. In man, its mutagenic potential in gametes is discounted; the danger lies in the potential carcinogenicity of the nitrous acid produced by the reaction of nitrite salts with stomach acids. Sodium nitrite has been widely used as a preservative for meat, fish, and cheese. The toxic level of nitrates and nitrites in the acute poisoning of birds, ruminants, and human infants has been established. In addition, the formation of organic nitroso derivatives from the reaction of nitrous acid with secondary and tertiary amines causes concern. Cancer of the digestive tract is a delayed effect involving the genetic machinery of the somatic cells. No penetration of nitrous acid from the lumen of the digestive tract to the gametogenic cells of the gonads is implied.

15.4.4b. Additive

In their mutagenic action, alkylating agents add alkyl groups to the DNA nucleotides. Initially, the sites of major chemical reaction were identified as the N^7 position of guanine, the N^1 and N^3 positions of adenine, and the N^3 position of cytosine and thymine. Subsequently, other important sites were reported for adenine and guanine (see Singer's tables).[1] However, in higher organisms, sulfhydryl groups, ionized acid groups, nonionized amino groups, and other components of the tissues compete for alkyl groups before an alkylating agent penetrates or is transported to the gametogenic cells in the gonad. Even within the cells the highly reactive agents alkylate proteins and nucleic acid precursors in addition to the various nucleic acids. It is remarkable that some alkylating molecules reach the DNA of the precursor cells of sperm and eggs. Types are shown in Figure 15.6.

Nevertheless, when alkylating agents are added to the diet of chickens and mammals, enough reactive molecules reach the gonads to destroy gametogenic cells. If injected intraperitoneally or intravenously, an alkylator travels more directly. For example, the number of sperm ejaculated by rabbits declined to an aspermic nadir 10–11 weeks after a single injection of any one of three different alkylating agents. Presumably some of the sperm ejaculated before and after the aspermic period carried induced point mutations. Unfortunately, there are few published accounts of experiments on chemical mutagenesis in the mammalian organism, despite the 1949–1952 reports of visible point mutations obtained in mice treated with nitrogen mustard in Auerbach's laboratory. On the other hand, all types of alkylating agents have been demonstrated to be mutagenic in higher plants, insects, and cultured mammalian cells, as well as in microbes. The purpose of this text will not be served by an attempt to summarize the volumes of information on the induction of mutations in the biochemical traits of microbes. Our concern is with higher organisms.

For animals, quantitative dose–effect curves for chemical mutagens cannot yet be plotted with assurance. Dosage itself is a problem at the cellular level, and the interpretation of results is further complicated by the induced mosaicism of the gonad cells. Qualitatively, visible mutations have been produced at a few specific loci in mice and in considerable numbers at many loci in *Drosophila*. In this intensively investigated insect, nitrogen mustard, MMS, EMS, triethylene melanine (TEM), and other alkylators have been used to obtain congeries of

---

[1] Singer, B. Chemical effects of nucleic acid alkylation. Prog. Nucleic Acid Res. Mol. Biol. 15 (1975), 219.

Sulfur mustards	$S(CH_2CH_2Cl)_2$	mustard gas
Nitrogen mustards	$HN(CH_2CH_2Cl)_2$	nitrogen mustard (HN_2)
Epoxides	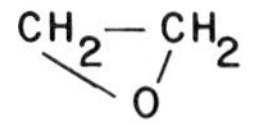 $CH_2\!-\!CH_2$ $\diagdown O \diagup$	ethylene oxide (EO)
	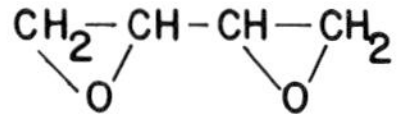 $CH_2\!-\!CH\!-\!CH\!-\!CH_2$ $\diagdown O \diagup \qquad \diagdown O \diagup$	diepoxybutane (DEB)
Ethylene imines	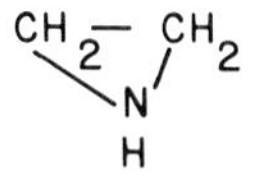 $CH_2\!-\!CH_2$ $\diagdown \underset{H}{N} \diagup$	ethyleneimine (EI)
Alkyl alkanesulfonates	$C_2H_5OSO_2CH_3$	ethyl methane-sulfonate (EMS)
	$CH_3OSO_2CH_3$	methyl methane-sulfonate (MMS)
Dialkyl sulfates	$SO_2(OC_2H_5)_2$	diethylsulfate (DES)
β-lactones	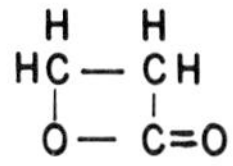 $\underset{O\,-\,C=O}{\overset{H\quad H}{HC-CH}}$	β-propiolactone
Diazo compounds	$CH_3N=N$	diazomethane
Nitroso compounds	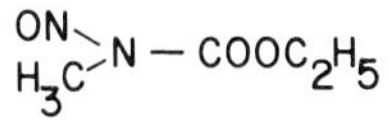 $\underset{H_3C}{\overset{ON}{\diagdown}}N\!-\!COOC_2H_5$	N-nitroso-N methyl urethane (NMU)
	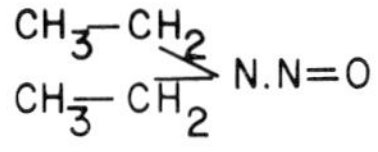 $\underset{CH_3-CH_2}{\overset{CH_3-CH_2}{}}N.N=O$	diethylnitrosamine (DEN)
	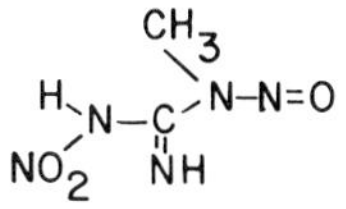 $\underset{NO_2}{\overset{H}{\diagdown}}N\!-\!\underset{NH}{\overset{CH_3}{C}}N\!-\!N=O$	N-methyl-N'-nitro-N-nitrosoguanidine

Figure 15.6 The chemical structures of the important types of alkylating agents. A great variety of compounds have been synthesized containing one or more of these groups in the molecular structure.

mutants in various complex loci to enable intracistronic recombination analysis. In these studies the mutagen is employed as a tool in the study of genetic mechanisms by investigators not particularly concerned with the agent's mode of action.

In studies with cultivated plants, in which selected new mutants are of economic importance, the empirical approach has also been successful, and many of the foremost agronomists have also given attention to mode of action. The ease of treating seeds and pollen under controlled conditions contributes greatly to the situation.

Unlike the results for chromosome breakage, monofunctional agents have proved to be more effective than polyfunctional types in causing gene mutation (Table 15.3). Thus far, sulfonates appear to be the most effective mutagens for plants. The broad spectrum of chlorophyll mutations is shown in Figure 15.7. Other traits in other plants respond similarly. For example, in the common bean *Phaseolus vulgaris* L., mutations to white, yellow, brown, deep brown, and gray brown can be recovered from nearly every replication of 200–300 seeds treated with EMS. Gamma irradiation and nonsulfonate agents induce only one or two types of color mutants in the same sample size. In peanuts diethyl sulfate has induced mutations of leaflets, chlorophyll, habit and size, fertility, pods, and testa. Four kinds of plants have featured most prominently in analytical research into the mode of mutagenic action: barley, peas, wheat, and arabidopsis.

In speculative human genetics, particular concern has been expressed about agents such as nitrosoguanidine and EMS, which are highly mutagenic but relatively nontoxic to somatic tissues. Nitrosoguanidine is chemically related to the nitrosamines, -amides, and -ureas that can result from biological nitrosation. In this way, nitrites and nitrous acid from preserved foods again become a matter for concern. They also occur as synthetic derivatives in the battery, rubber, rocket fuel, and polymer industries. Because they serve as highly reactive molecular "building blocks" in the chemical industries, other alkylating agents are in large-scale production. Ethyleneimine and derivatives are shipped in tonnage lots for use in paper processing and textile finishing in addition to the above mentioned industries. Also in demand is ethylene oxide, which is produced in excess of 1 million tons per year. Alkylating agents have been employed in smaller quantities as insect chemosterilants and in cancer chemotherapy; these applications can lead to the extinction of nontarget organisms or damage to nontarget tissues, respectively.

Additive in a different sense are the acridine dyes long used in histological techniques to stain nucleic acids. These dyes can insert between neighboring base pairs of DNA. They are good mutagens for phage and *E. coli* but are poor

Table 15.3 Maximum Percentage of Chlorophyll Mutants per Mutated Spike in Barley

Agent	Bifunctional		Monofunctional	
Mustards	Nitrogen	1.7	2-Chlorethyl dimethylamine	15
	Sulfur	0.3		
Epoxides	Diepoxybutane	1.3	Ethylene oxide	9.4
Methane sulfonates	Myleran	5.1	Propyl	26
			Methyl	16
Ethylenimine	TEM[a]	1.5	EI	33

Source: Based mainly on the data of Gustafsson and Ehrenberg. See references in Loveless, Genetics and Allied Effects of Alkylating Agents. Pennsylvania State University Press, 1966.

Note: Hundreds of loci are involved in the barley chlorophyll system. A parallel situation may occur for sex-linked recessive lethals in *Drosophila*, where Fahmy found 11.6% of mutations with MMS.

[a] Polyfunctional.

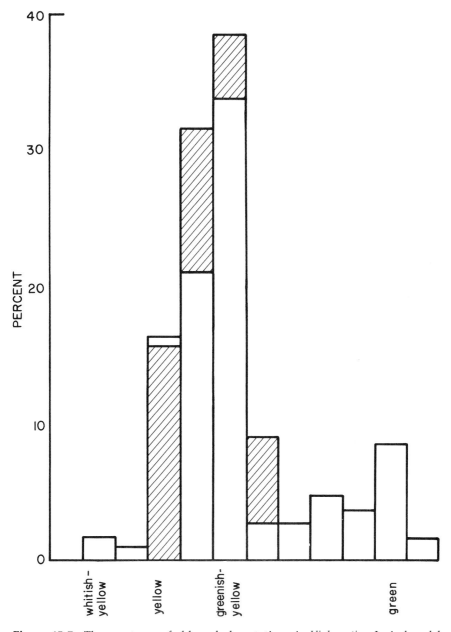

Figure 15.7 The spectrum of chlorophyl mutations in *Viola sativa* L. induced by two different agents: EMS = unshaded and EI = shaded bars. Bars are superimposed. Eleven distinct color classes are represented in the percentage of the total mutants obtained. SOURCE: *Based on data of L. Zannone, Radiation Botany 5 (Suppl.), 210.*

mutagens for eukaroytic cells. Nevertheless, recessive lethals and visible mutations were obtained using pyronin in early *Drosophila* feeding and injection experiments. For humans these dyes are used primarily as topical antiseptics, but in veterinary medicine their usage has been extended to intravenous injection for acute mastitis and septicemia.

15.4.4c. Substitutive

The analogs of nucleotide bases comprise a category of mutagens that can be termed substitutive. An analog is a compound whose molecular structure is very similar to some natural component, so that it can take the place of a normal component in a molecule or molecular complex. Halo, amino, aza, and thio forms of purines and pyrimidines have been synthesized. These drugs, developed for cancer therapy, were the rational result of the recognized importance of DNA and the bacteriostatic success of sulfanilimide, an analog of *para*-aminobenzoic acid. Those incorporated into DNA include BUdR, 5-fluorodeoxyuridine, 2-aminopurine, and 6-mercaptopurine.

BUdR and other halo-uracil derivatives can replace all the thymidine in DNA when synthesis occurs under conditions of thymidine depletion. The sequence of events that results in mutation via tautomerism is shown digrammatically in Figure 15.5. Note that the initial change is not heritable; a base change in normal nucleotides must be built into the DNA molecule before the process has completed itself. Furthermore, mutations affect only one strand and its progeny. A chemical consideration is that tautomeric shifts can occur more frequently in the base analogs than in the normal bases. Furthermore, the existence of "hot spots'" with a high frequency of mutagenic change suggest that neighboring bases play a role; i.e., its position in the nucleotide sequence rather than the base analog alone determines mutagenic effectiveness. This implicates the DNA replication or repair processes as possibly playing a role.

15.4.5. Comparative and Quantitative Results

Most of the research to date has tended to answer a qualitative question: Does a particular compound induce mutations with a particular test system? Furthermore, only a limited choice of agents have been tested. The fundamental purpose of mutagen screening is to obtain data relevant to humans. For extrapolation to man, data from a system closest to man seems desirable. Therefore, results with mammals are of great interest, but even with mice "visible" mutation research is costly and time consuming. Instead of days or weeks, it can take years to obtain data for an adequate sample of offspring. Even then, the available data are not encouraging. Table 15.4 summarizes results from three laboratories. Each worked with a different type of compound but all used the seven-locus tester stock derived by Russell at the Oak Ridge National Laboratory. The original control frequency of spontaneous mutation was 5.3×60^{-5}. Although these alkylating agents had proved effective in breaking chromosomes, the yield of mutations from the specific locus test was not impressive. Indeed, Cattanach considers only the TEM results positive for the premeiotic gonial cells. Despite smaller samples, postmeiotic frequencies were higher for three of the five agents. Another study estimated that the mutation yield from 248 mg EMS/kg is equivalent to that from 100 rads X irradiation assessed by the specific-locus test on mouse spermatozoa.

More impressive results have been obtained with cultured mammalian cells, in which penetration to the cell is not a problem. A 2-hr exposure to 3.16×10^{-3} M EMS induced a mutation frequency at the TK locus identical to that from an acute dose of 600 rads X irradiation. However, mutation rates differ from locus

Table 15.4 Chemically Induced Recessive Mutations at Seven Loci in Spermatogenic Cells of Mice

Agent	Premeiotic cells		Postmeiotic cells	
	Frequency ($\times 10^{-4}$)	Sample size	Frequency ($\times 10^{-4}$)	Sample size
TEM	4.5	11,144	17.6	1701
EMS	0	14,393	5.6	3579
MMS	1.2	16,547	8.5	2344
PMS[a]	3.1	6,394	0	1250
IMS[b]	1.4	7,178	0	517

Source: Frequencies calculated from a summary by Cattanach, Chem. Mutagens 2 (1971), 538.

[a] Propyl methanesulfonate.

[b] Isopropyl methanesulfonate.

to locus. Exposure to 10^{-2} M EMS produced 2×10^{-3} mutations per locus per generation at the TK locus (TK +/− to TK −/−), whereas the mutation frequency at the HGPRT locus was only 10% of that value. Nevertheless, linear dose–response curves were obtained over a survival range of 0.3–100% of control values for the HGPRT locus of Chinese hamster ovary cells as well as HGPRT and TK loci of mouse lymphoma cells (strain L 5178Y) using 144–168-hr expression times. At shorter expression times (48–72 hr) curves were nonlinear.

Therefore, comparable results were obtained for two different cell types in three laboratories. Unfortunately, few agents have been investigated this thoroughly, and only two loci are available for study. This was demonstrated persuasively in 1977 at the Comparative Chemical Mutagenicity Workshop (Research Triangle Park, N. C.) Despite adequate representation from Europe the group reviewing mutagenicity studies on cultured mammalian cells had to rely too heavily on one laboratory's data, based at best on only two loci. These data characterized a majority of the 12 mutagens considered. At least 8 other known mutagens had never been tested. For those mutagens studied by several laboratories, results suffered from "remarkably diverse deficiencies." Although a popular agent for research, EMS did not fare well in the rankings. It placed near the middle in induced mutation frequency at the 10% survival dose, but low in mutagenic potency and near the bottom in effective concentration. Mutagenic potency is determined by the number of induced mutants per 10^6 survivors per micrograms mutagen per milliliter per hours treated.

The Workshop also evaluated data on reference mutagens obtained by 30 different test systems. However, only a few agents could be examined across all test systems: EMS, MMS, cyclophosphamide, and TEM. The lowest effective dose obtained from different tests varied greatly. Because of this wide range, Clive and Spector had to calculate risk factor on a geometric basis for their overall summary.

When mutation was considered in the broad sense to include chromosome aberrations as well as point mutations, three in vivo mammalian systems were classed among the nine best risk-estimating tests: oncogenicity, and germinal and somatic cytogenetics. In the same category were the in vitro mammalian cell systems, cytological studies, and changes in specific loci. The relative importance of genomal architecture in estimating the mutagenic risk to mammals was most convincingly demonstrated by how well three plant systems (barley, soybean, and *Vicia faba*) fared in comparison with bacterial systems.

15.5. Matters for Human Concern

The human gene pool is the primary resource of mankind, and it is extremely important to guard its genetic quality. Experiments on the population genetics of lower animals have demonstrated a genetic disadvantage from increasing the mutational load. A population tends to reach a balance between the input of "spontaneous" mutations and their elimination by selection. An increase of induced mutations disturbs the balance. Then a trend toward attaining another equilibrium begins, which culminates in a higher incidence of debility and mortality. Death or nonreproduction of individuals carrying the gene in a homozygous condition (for autosomal recessives) is the price paid. X-Linked recessives are expressed in the heterogametic sex, the male in humans. Codominant gene expression occurs in heterozygotes, and individuals may survive but with impaired efficiency.

Natural selection opposes the spread of deleterious mutants in populations. Until recently the human gene pool was a culmination of billions of years of provisional mutation and evolutionary selection. Now, however, advances in medicine are counteracting natural selection by enabling the survival of individuals handicapped in their genetic endowment. At the same time, our technology provides an environment rich in new organic compounds of unknown mutagenic potency. At present the consequences of this complex situation are only speculative, but no predictions are optimistic. The "genetic disease" burden of more than 2000 known examples of mendelian inheritance suggests that the human gene pool is already overloaded.

Monitoring the human population for a change in mutation rate can merely indicate whether there is a change. The cause would not be identified. It is very difficult to determine the particular agent responsible for an increase. Even the relative influences of chemical versus physical agents is uncertain. Ionizing radiation is the most important physical mutagen, and medical and dental technology is the source of more than 75% of the genetically significant dose from man-made sources.

In a drug-oriented society also committed to food additives and cosmetics, there persists a disquieting possibility that some widely used compound with small toxic effect may be a potent mutagen and/or carcinogen. Workers in industry and agriculture experience occupational exposure to toxicants at levels above those typical for the general population. A haunting thought is that only the so-called "supermutagens" are being identified and that the test systems available are unable to detect a number of weaker mutagens. Part of the problem stems from the concept of induced presumptive lesions that may or may not develop into true mutations as a result of molecular misrepair or other action of human cellular physiology. We are not yet in a position to state quantitatively the magnitude of the health hazards.

15.6. Concluding Remarks

This chapter has been written during a period in which most of the research has been directed toward developing tests for identifying mutagens and carcinogens. Efforts toward improving test protocols have not been accompanied by comprehensive studies of point mutations in mammals. An enormous number of old and new agents remain to be tested. Even the Ames test has been utilized more for identifying potential carcinogens, accompanied by the premise that most mutagens function as carcinogens (see Chapter 16). Section 15.4 on gene mutation is particularly indecisive and Section 15.5 addresses itself to some of the causes of anxiety.

Genetic defects are now realized to have an ever-increasing importance in medical practice. The catalog of genetic variations in man has grown to nearly 1000 pages of fine print, but this does not mean we know what caused them. The term spontaneous mutation is a confession of ignorance. In addition, chromosomal defects are constantly being discovered in man. The first human autosomal aberration recognized was the triploid condition of chromosome 21. Following the realization that a phenotypic syndrome (Down's) may signal a karyotypic change, other trisomys were identified as well as other gross chromosomal aberrations. Several hundred types have been characterized form humans, but again causation is problematic. The more common examples have been known for centuries. Long before radiation or chemical mutations were appreciated, Down's syndrome was known and postulated to represent a throwback to the Mongolian invasion of Europe. Thus we may appreciate that an age-old problem has taken on quite a different aspect. A variety of different kinds of agents have been identified here. One hopes that experimental results extrapolative to humans will be forthcoming in the next few years.

Suggested Reading

General

Albert, A. Selective Toxicity, fifth edition. London: Chapman & Hall, 1973.

Brown, A. W. A. Genetics of insecticide resistance in insect vectors. In Wright, J. W., Pal, R. (Eds.). Genetics of Insect Vectors of Disease. Amsterdam: Elsevier, 1967, pp. 505–552.

Grosch, D. S. Effects of Toxicants on Reproductive Performance. Essays Toxicol. 7 (1976), 1.

Moriarty, F. The sublethal effects of synthetic insecticides on insects. Biol. Rev. 44 (1969), 321.

Schein, P. S. The prediction of clinical toxicities of anticancer drugs. In Pharmacological Basis of Cancer Chemotherapy. 1974 Symposium at M. D. Anderson Hospital. Baltimore: Williams & Wilkins, 1975, 383–400.

Spindle Poisons

Borisy, G. G., Taylor, E. W. The colchicine binding to sea urchin eggs and the mitotic apparatus. J. Cell Biol. 34 (1967), 535.

Deysson, G. Antimitotic substances. Int. Rev. Cytol. 24 (1968), 99.

Eigsti, O. J., Dustin, P., Jr. Colchicine in Agriculture, Medicine, and Biology. Ames, Iowa: Iowa State University Press, 1955.

Harrison, C. M. H., Page, B. M., Keir, H. M. Mescaline as a mitotic spindle inhibitor. Nature 260 (1976), 138.

Hepler, P. K., Jackson, W. T. IPC affects spindle microtubule orientation in dividing endosperm cells of *Haemanthus catherenae* Baker. J. Cell Sci. 5 (1969), 727.

Kihlman, B. A. Actions of Chemicals on Dividing Cells. Englewood Cliffs, N. J.: Prentice Hall, 1966.

Wilson, L., Bryan, J. Biochemical and pharmacological properties of microtubules. Adv. Cell Mol. Biol. 3 (1974), 22.

Chromosome Breakage

Evans, H. J. Population cytogenetics and environmental factors. In Jacobs, P. A., Price, W. H., Law P. (Eds.). Human Population Cytogenetics. Pfizer Medical Monograph 5, Edinburgh: Edinburgh University Press, 1970.

Falconer, D. S., Slyzynski, B. M., Auerbach, C. Genetical effects of nitrogen mustard in the house mouse. J. Genet. 51 (1952), 81.

Kihlman, B. A. Biochemical aspects of chromosome breakage. Adv. Genet. 10 (1961), 1.

Loveless, A. Genetic and Allied Effects of Alkylating Agents. University Park: Pennsylvania State University Press, 1966, Chapter 1.

Shaw, M. W. Human chromosome damage by chemical agents. Ann. Rev. Med. 21 (1970), 409.

Sieber, S. M., Adamson, R. H. The clastogenic, mutagenic and carcinogenic effects of various antineoplastic agents. In Pharmacological Basis of Chemotherapy, 27th (1974) Annual Symposium on Fundamental Cancer Research. Baltimore: Williams & Wilkins, 1975, pp. 401–468.

Vogel, F., Rohrhorn G. (Eds.). Chemical Mutagenesis in Mammals and Man. Heidelberg: Springer, 1970.

Gene Mutation

International Atomic Energy Agency, Radiation Botany, Supplement to Vol. 5 (1965) Symposium on the Use of Induced Mutations in Plant Breeding. Vienna.

Ames, B. N., Durston, W. E., Yamasaki, E., Lee, S. E. Carcinogens are mutagens: A simple test system combining liver homogenates for activation and bacteria for detection. Proc. Natl. Acad. Sci. U.S.A. 70 (1973), 2281.

Auerbach, C. Mutation Research. London: Chapman and Hall, 1976.

Auerbach, C., Kilbey, B. J. Mutation in eukaryotes. Ann. Rev. Genet. 5 (1971), 163.

Clive, D., Spector, J. F. S. Laboratory procedure for assessing specific locus mutations at the TK locus in cultured L5178Y mouse lymphoma cells. Mutat. Res. 31 (1975), 17.

Drake, J. W. The Molecular Basis of Mutation. San Francisco: Holden-Day, 1970.

Drake, J. W., Kock R. E. (Eds.). Mutagenesis/Benchmark Papers in Genetics, Vol. 4. Dowden, Hutchinson & Ross, distributed by Halsted Press, New York, 1976.

Fishbein, L., Flamm, W. G., Falk, H. L. Chemical Mutagens. New York: Academic Press, 1970.

Holleander, A. (Ed.). Chemical Mutagens, An Open End Series from Volume 1. New York: Plenum Press, 1971.

Hirono, Y., Smith, H. H. Mutations induced in Arabiodopsis by DNA nucleoside analogs. Genetics 61 (1969), 191.

Loveless, A. Genetic and Allied Affects of Alkylating Agents. University Park: Pennsylvania State University Press, 1966.

Prakash, L. (Ed.). Molecular and Environmental Aspects of Mutagenesis. Springfield, Ill.: Thomas, 1974.

Singer, B. Chemical effects of nucleic acid alkylation. Prog. Nucleic Acid Res. Mol. Biol. 15 (1975), 219.

Sobels, F. (Ed.). Mutation Research (a journal). 1 (1964) to 52 (1978).

Human Concern

de Grouchy, J., Turleau, C. Clinical Atlas of Human Chromosomes. New York: Wiley, 1977.

Hartl, D. L. Our Uncertain Heritage: Genetics and Human Diversity. Philadelphia: Lippencott, 1977.

Levitan, M., Montague, A. Textbook of Human Genetics. London: Oxford University Press, 1971.

McKusick, V. A. Mendelian Inheritance in Man: Catalogs of Autosomal Dominant, Autosomal Recessive and X-Linked Phenotypes, fourth edition. Baltimore: John Hopkins University Press, 1975.

Stern, C. Principles of Human Genetics, third edition. San Francisco: Freeman, 1973.

Handler P. (Ed.). U. S. National Academy of Sciences Committee. Biology and the Future of Man. New York: Oxford University Press, 1970. (See particularly Chapter 20, also entitled "Biology and the Future of Man."

David J. Holbrook, Jr.

16

Chemical Carcinogenesis

16.1. Introduction

It has been established that a high proportion of human cancers are attributable to environmental agents—mainly environmental chemicals, but also viral and physical agents. It is unclear to what extent genetic factors may contribute to individual susceptibility to chemically induced carcinogenesis. However, the estimate that perhaps three-fourths of human cancer is due to environmental chemicals serves to emphasize the importance of further research on the carcinogenic hazards of these agents. In a series of reviews of the carcinogenicity of approximately 300 substances by panels of the International Agency for Research on Cancer, 21 substances are listed as carcinogenic in humans and an additional 150 as carcinogenic in experimental animals. Others have claimed that 30 identified compounds are definite human carcinogens. Much of the current research effort is directed toward the identification of carcinogenic agents among environmental substances, industrial chemicals, and drugs and the development of methodology to predict the carcinogenicity of a tested substance.

The distribution of potential carcinogens in the environment is essentially ubiquitous. Water sources may contain carbon tetrachloride and other chlorinated compounds or metallic salts that may be potentially carcinogenic. Laboratory and industrial solvents such as benzene and carbon tetrachloride may also be carcinogenic. Nitroso compounds may represent another important type of potential carcinogens. The nitroso compounds are produced by the reaction of nitrites with a wide variety of secondary or tertiary amines; an acidic medium, such as that within the stomach, increases the likelihood of the reaction. The nitrites may be present in the diet (e.g., in certain processed meats) or may be formed from nitrates (especially in vegetables) by oral bacteria. Alternatively, during the cooking of food, the nitrites can react with the amines to yield nitrosamines. Approximately three-fourths of the total 100–120 nitroso compounds tested are carcinogenic to experimental animals. Certain foods may also be contaminated with the aflatoxins, potentially carcinogenic compounds produced by some *Aspergillus* strains. Epidemiological investigations in several human populations have suggested an association of increased incidence of human hepatic tumors with increased dietary contamination by aflatoxins. Various polynuclear aromatic hydrocarbons, such as the carcinogen ben-zopyrene, are formed in the combustion of organic substances such as fossil fuels. Exposure of some employees to the polynuclear aromatic hydrocarbons often exceeds 0.25 μg/day and may exceed 50 μg/day in a few instances.

16.2. Mechanism of Chemical Carcinogenesis and Role of Somatic Mutation

16.2.1. Initiation and Promotion

The overall process of carcinogenesis can be divided into at least two stages. The first, *initiation,* involves the interaction of the carcinogen (i.e., the reactive species) with a normal cell to produce a potentially cancerous or precancerous cell. If repair or cell death does not occur, carcinogenic initiation may be a rapid and irreversible process, but such an altered cell may remain dormant for a long interval before the expression of a tumor. The second major stage, *promotion,* involves the subsequent proliferation of the precancerous cells. The administra-tion of certain agents, namely promoters (or cocarcinogens) after, or even long after, initiation leads to the observed neoplasm. The promoters include croton oil, the classic model, and various phorbol esters, the active ingredients of croton oil. The specific actions of promoters have not been established. However, a large number of the promoters induce cellular proliferation and thus may lead to the premitotic replication of DNA which continues to have unre-paired, damaged sites. The use of the damaged DNA as a template, in turn, increases the opportunity for the fixation of altered genetic information (muta-tion fixation) during the DNA replication and/or DNA postreplication repair, since the latter may constitute an error-prone repair system. The process of carcinogenesis is a relatively rare event within a tissue. Typically, treatment with a carcinogen results in the covalent reaction of the carcinogen (or its metabolites) with components in most of the cells within a tissue. Eventual tumor formation typically occurs at only a few foci (i.e., from only a few cells) within the tissue although most cells were originally damaged to some limited extent.

16.2.2. Proposed Mechanisms of Chemical Carcinogenesis

Miller and Miller[1] have enumerated possible mechanisms of chemical car-cinogenesis, categories of genetic mechanisms that produce heritable changes in the information in the genome, and categories of epigenetic mechanisms, i.e.,

---

[1] Miller, J. A., Miller C. E., *in* Chemical Carcinogenesis Part A (T'so, P. O. P., and DiPaolo J. A., Eds.). New York: Marcel Dekker, 1974.

those which include changes in transcription associated with repression and expression (derepression). "There is at present no firm basis on which to decide that . . . [either a genetic or epigenetic model] . . . is an accurate description of carcinogenesis by any specific chemical."

The direct modification of DNA by intrinsically reactive or metabolically activated ultimate carcinogens is well established. The role of DNA in the storage of genetic information makes the direct modification of the DNA theoretically consistent with a carcinogen-induced somatic mutation. Most of the carcinogens produce mutations in one or more test systems, and most (but not all) of the known mutagens are carcinogenic. Such observations do not unequivocally establish a causal relationship. Some of the uncertainty is due to the lack of specificity in the covalent reaction of the reactive species of the carcinogens; such species react with any suitable site—with macromolecules such as DNA, RNA, proteins, polysaccharides, and lipids, and with low molecular weight substances. What role, if any, do the reactions with macromolecules other than DNA have on the initiation event(s) in carcinogenesis?

Mammalian DNA polymerases normally exhibit a high degree of fidelity—the ability to incorporate the proper complementary nucleotide as dictated by the template DNA strand. A carcinogen-induced loss of such fidelity would lead to the synthesis of erroneous segments of the DNA that may or may not be critical to the controlled mitotic fate of the cell. Carcinogens may cause indirectly heritable changes in the DNA—i.e., a genetic mechanism of carcinogenesis—by means other than a primary, direct modification of the DNA. For example, there may be an interaction of the reactive species of a carcinogen with some component involved in the synthesis of the DNA polymerase molecule, e.g., the RNA polymerase responsible for the synthesis of the mRNA of DNA polymerase or any component involved in translation of the mRNA (rRNA, mRNA, tRNA, or any of the regulatory or structural proteins of the ribosome). The product DNA polymerase molecule with a slightly altered amino acid sequence may possess polymerization ability but lack the high degree of fidelity of the normal DNA polymerase molecule. Once such an error-prone process is started in DNA replication, accentuation of error accumulation may be manifested as malignant progression. In support of this proposal, it has been found that DNA polymerase from human leukemic cells exhibits a relatively error-prone polymerization in comparison to the DNA polymerase from normal lymphocytes.

In a like manner, the alteration in polypeptide synthesis by the carcinogenic reactive species may lead to the formation of a regulatory protein with a slightly altered primary structure and a resultant deficiency in its regulatory capacity. If such a regulatory protein is involved directly or indirectly in the repression or derepression of certain regions of the genome, carcinogenesis may be initiated by an epigenetic mechanism of differentiation without an alteration in the DNA. It has been concluded that observations on experimental liver cell tumors are compatible with the concept that *both* a genetic mechanism and an epigenetic mechanism participate. The initial event by the reactive species of a carcinogen is probably a somatic mutation to produce an altered but noncancerous cell; the subsequent sequence of events that yields the cancerous cells appears to be aberrant or interrupted differentiation.

16.3. Chemical Nature and Reactivity

16.3.1. Electrophilic Reactive Species

No common structural feature is evident among the organic carcinogens. Most organic carcinogens have the capacity to react covalently with various tissue macromolecules. Certain compounds, including many of the methylating, ethylating, and other alkylating agents, are intrinsically reactive. In other cases, the organic carcinogens must undergo one or more enzymatic reactions for the conversion of an unreactive compound to a reactive species. In either case, the reactive species of almost all organic carcinogens contains an electrophilic (relatively electron-deficient) atom that can react nonenzymatically and covalently with any available nucleophilic (electron-rich) atom of a target molecule. In contrast to the *electrophilic* reactive species of carcinogens, the organic carcinogens do not appear to be converted to reactive *nucleophilic* species capable of reacting with electrophilic sites of macromolecules.

The covalent reaction with sites on the nucleic acids will be discussed further in Section 16.4.4. The sulfur atoms of cysteine and methionine, and sites on histidine and tyrosine are especially reactive sites within proteins. The exact molecular reactions that are crucial in the initiation of a neoplastic response have not been established. It is presumed that the reactive species of carcinogens initiate the neoplastic response by reaction with DNA, RNA, and/or protein, i.e., the macromolecules involved in carrying or expressing genetic information. Because of the cellular role of DNA and the availability of information, most of the subsequent discussion emphasizes the covalent reaction of the reactive species with DNA.

16.3.2. Intrinsically Reactive Carcinogens

The structures of representative intrinsically reactive carcinogens have been presented in Figure 15.6.

The alkyl alkanesulfonates, namely methyl and ethyl methanesulfonates, and related compounds such as dimethyl sulfate are intrinsically reactive and methylate or ethylate macromolecules. Likewise, certain model nitroso compounds such as N-methyl- and N-ethyl-N-nitrosourea and N-methyl-N'-nitro-N-nitrosoguanidine, without prior metabolic activation, alkylate macromolecules. Lactones (e.g., β-propiolactone) and β-chloroethyl derivatives also react with macromolecules without prior enzymatic activation. Nitrogen mustard and sulfur mustard, the two examples of β-chloroethyl derivatives presented (Figure 15.6), are both bifunctional alkylating agents. Consequently, if each chloroethyl group reacts, the DNA can undergo *intra*molecular cross-linking by attachment at two sites within the same strand of DNA, or *inter*molecular cross-linking by reacting with one site in each DNA strand to form a bridge between the complementary strands. Alternatively, nitrogen mustard may cause cross-linking between DNA and its associated protein.

16.3.3. Organic Carcinogens that Undergo Metabolic Activation

The majority of the organic carcinogens are not reactive as such but must undergo enzymatic reactions to form the electrophilic species. In most cases, the mixed-function oxidase system of the endoplasmic reticulum or the outer nuclear membrane participates in the metabolic activation. The term "procarcino-gen" (or "precarcinogen") is applied to the nonreactive parent compound, the term "proximate" carcinogen to any intermediate compound involved in the overall metabolic activation, and the term "ultimate" carcinogen to the final product which is reactive with tissue macromolecules. The term ultimate car-cinogen is used to refer to either the final identifiable compound, such as an epoxide, or to a hypothetical reactive species such as a carbonium ion.

Figure 16.1 Representatives of carcinogens that require metabolic activation to form reactive species.

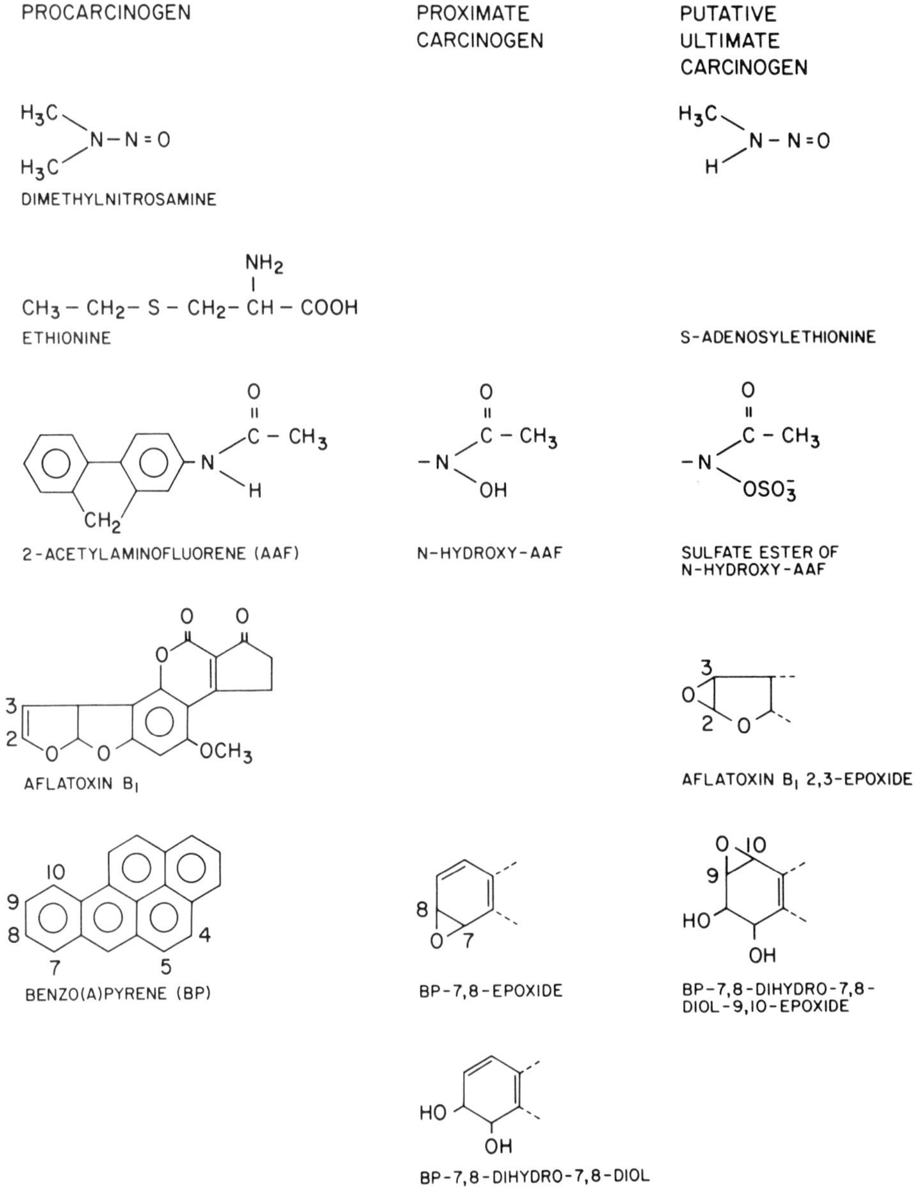

The structures of some representative procarcinogens, proximate carcinogens, and ultimate carcinogens are presented in Figure 16.1. Dimethylnitrosamine and diethylnitrosamine undergo demethylation and deethylation reactions, respectively, catalyzed by the mixed-function oxidases to yield unstable monoalkylnitrosamines. The latter compounds then undergo nonenzymatic degradation to carbonium ions, which results in the alkylation of tissue macromolecules. Ethionine, an analog of methionine, undergoes an activation that does not involve the mixed-function oxidases; the ultimate carcinogen, S-adenosylethionine, ethylates target macromolecules, especially tRNA. One of the most extensively studied carcinogens is 2-acetylaminofluorene, an aromatic amine. The amine undergoes hydroxylation catalyzed by the mixed-function oxidase to yield a proximate carcinogen, the N-hydroxy derivative. Sulfotransferase in the cytosol yields one of the probable ultimate carcinogens, the sulfate ester of the N-hydroxy-2-acetylaminofluorene. N-Acetoxy-2-acetylaminofluorene, the acetate ester, is commonly used as a model compound for the ultimate carcinogen of the parent aromatic amine. Aflatoxin B_1 is a naturally occurring carcinogen that is produced by a few strains of the fungus *Aspergillus*. Aflatoxin B_1 is converted by a mixed-function oxidase to the 2,3-epoxide derivative, the probable ultimate carcinogen. In the case of several carcinogenic polynuclear aromatic hydrocarbons, the ultimate carcinogen appears to be a reactive diol epoxide. The metabolism of benzo[a]pyrene and benz[a]anthracene yield a large number of products including the dihydrodiol non-K region epoxides 7,8-dihydro-7,8-dihydroxybenzopyrene 9,10-epoxide (Figure 16.1) and 3,4-dihydro-3,4-dihydroxybenzanthracene 1,2-epoxide, respectively. In these and other examples of the polynuclear aromatic hydrocarbons, the ultimate carcinogen possesses, on a saturated angular benzo ring, a highly reactive epoxide which forms a part of a *bay* region (Figure 16.2). The bay regions correspond to the regions between positions 10 and 11 of benzo[a]pyrene and positions 1 and 12 of benz[a]anthracene. Epoxides in the K region, once considered to be the ultimate carcinogens, are probably not involved in the carcinogenicity of benzo[a]pyrene and benz[a]anthracene.

Figure 16.2 Representative polynuclear aromatic hydrocarbons and their bay region and K region molecular sites.

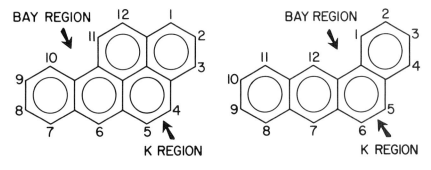

BENZO [a] PYRENE   BENZ [a] ANTHRACENE

16.4. Covalent Reaction of Organic Carcinogens with DNA and Other Macromolecules

16.4.1. Intact Cellular Systems

The administration of organic carcinogens to the experimental animals or the incubation with cultured cells commonly results in the covalent reaction of the carcinogen with cellular macromolecules. A vast number of organic carcinogens have been demonstrated to react covalently with DNA in vivo. The types of compounds include the polynuclear aromatic hydrocarbons, aromatic amines, aminoazobenzene derivatives, nitroso compounds, and others.

In studies of the covalent reaction of carcinogens with cellular macromolecules, the emphasis is usually placed on the covalent reaction with DNA on the basis of the theoretical importance of DNA in maintaining a heritable error. RNA, protein, and lipid also contain molecular sites that are susceptible to reaction, and the covalent binding to these molecules has been studied in vivo for carcinogens such as ethionine, carbon tetrachloride, dimethylnitrosamine, and methyl methanesulfonate. The possible importance and significance of the covalent reaction of a carcinogen with a regulatory macromolecule (protein or RNA) other than DNA as the initiating event in carcinogenesis should not be ignored.

16.4.2. Reactions In Vitro

16.4.2a. Isolated Microsomes

In a number of instances, the metabolic activation of a carcinogen to a DNA-reactive product by the microsomal mixed-function oxidase system can be achieved in vitro. The studies are conducted by incubation of the radioactive carcinogen, isolated microsomes, NADPH, and exogenous DNA (either as free DNA or as chromatin). Reisolation of the DNA after incubation permits the measurement of the covalent reaction with the DNA. The carcinogens that undergo activation by isolated microsomes to yield DNA-reactive metabolites include benzopyrene, other polynuclear aromatic hydrocarbons, diethylstilbestrol, aflatoxin B_1, and N-hydroxyarylamines. The covalent reaction of benzopyrene and other polynuclear aromatic hydrocarbons to DNA is markedly increased if the hepatic microsomes are isolated from rats previously pretreated with 3-methylcholanthrene. The pretreatment also increases the microsomal aryl hydrocarbon hydroxylase activity.

The enzymatic hydrolysis of the DNA permits the separation and identification of some of the modified deoxyribonucleosides, and thus identification of the molecular site on the DNA susceptible to covalent reaction. When comparable studies are conducted with the synthetic and carcinogenic hormone diethylstilbestrol, eight low molecular weight modified deoxyribonucleosides are separated from the enzymatically hydrolyzed DNA. In studies with benzopyrene, most of the covalently attached adduct is present in only two products.

16.4.2b. Isolated Nuclei

Isolated nuclei also contain cytochrome P-450, presumably in the outer nuclear membrane, and are capable of the metabolism of certain xenobiotics. The incubaton of a radioactive carcinogen, isolated nuclei, and NADPH may bring about the covalent reaction of a reactive metabolite with the DNA of the endogenous chromatin. Isolated hepatic nuclei from normal rats are capable of converting six carcinogenic polynuclear aromatic hydrocarbons (including benzopyrene, 3-methylcholanthrene, and 7,12-dimethylbenzanthracene) and one noncarcinogenic polynuclear aromatic hydrocarbon (anthracene) to metabolites that react covalently with the DNA of the endogenous chromatin. The induction of the nuclear mixed-function oxidase system by pretreatment of the rats with 3-methylcholanthrene increases the covalent reaction of the metabolites of the carcinogenic hydrocarbons with the nuclear DNA in vitro.

Once a reactive species has been formed from a carcinogen, it potentially may have a number of fates. If the product is highly reactive, it will react rapidly with water, low molecular weight substances, or macromolecules within the same cell, or even within the same cellular compartment in which it was formed. At the other extreme, a weakly reactive product may migrate from the cell in which it was formed to other cells (or tissues) before reacting with a suitable site. Although it has long been recognized that microsomes can convert many nonreactive carcinogens to reactive metabolites, it is commonly found that reaction occurs with microsomal protein or lipid, i.e., with substances in close proximity to the mixed-function oxidase system. Since the mixed-function oxidase of the outer nuclear membrane is capable of forming the DNA-reactive metabolites, the role of the nuclear system may be of greater significance because of the shorter migration that a reactive species must traverse to reach the DNA of the chromatin. Thus, the nuclear system may be especially relevant to an initiating event in carcinogenesis. The association of histones and nonbasic chromosomal proteins with the DNA of chromatin may alter the extent and the molecular sites of the DNA that are susceptible to the formation of covalent adducts.

16.4.3. Metabolism of Xenobiotics in Relation to Covalent Reactions and Carcinogenesis

As discussed in Chapter 4, cytochrome P-450 exists in multiple forms that differ in catalytic properties. Pretreatment of rodents with certain inducers of mixed-function oxidases typically increases the enzymatic conversion of nonreactive carcinogens to reactive metabolites capable of covalent binding to DNA or other macromolecules. The induction of xenobiotic metabolism by pretreatment with 3-methylcholanthrene increases the aryl hydrocarbon hydroxylase in hepatic microsomes and in nuclei. There is a marked increase in the ability of the induced microsomes or nuclei to convert benzopyrene and other polynuclear aromatic hydrocarbons to metabolites that react covalently with DNA in vitro. In contrast, the treatment with phenobarbital, another inducer of mixed-function oxidases, does not appreciably alter either the nuclear level of aryl hydrocarbon hydroxylase or the ability to convert benzopyrene to DNA-bound metabolites.

However, induction of the mixed-function oxidase system and the resultant increased metabolism of a carcinogen do not always lead to an increased covalent reaction of the metabolites with DNA and other macromolecules. Pretreatment of rats with phenobarbital increases the microsomal hydroxylation of four sites on the carcinogen 2-acetylaminofluorene. Although the metabolism of the carcinogen is increased, there is a decrease in vivo in the covalent reaction of metabolites with hepatic DNA and a decrease in hepatic and extrahepatic tumors in rats treated concurrently with phenobarbital and 2-acetylaminofluorene. In the case of this carcinogen, there are multiple steps from the procarcinogen to the ultimate carcinogen. Although the initial step in the metabolism is increased by pretreatment or concurrent treatment with phenobarbital, there is an apparent alteration in the subsequent steps in metabolism. The alteration leads to an increased formation of the glucuronide conjugate, which is perhaps noncarcinogenic in the liver, and a decreased formation of the sulfate ester, which is probably the ultimate carcinogen in the liver. Although the glucuronide metabolite may not be carcinogenic in the liver because of its rapid exit, subsequent reactions of this metabolite in the urinary bladder may account for the carcinogenicity of arylamines in the latter tissue.

Alterations in the total metabolism of a carcinogen may not always result in like alterations in the carcinogenicity or the covalent reaction of metabolites with DNA. For example, the short-term administration of pregnenolone-16α-carbonitrile, a hormonally inactive steroid, decreases the acute toxicity and the N-demethylation in vivo of the carcinogen dimethylnitrosamine but does not significantly alter the total methylation of hepatic DNA in vivo. In contrast, the decrease in dimethylnitrosamine metabolism upon treatment with aminoacetonitrile is accompanied by a reduction in the toxicity and hepatocarcinogenicity of dimethylnitrosamine.

The ability of a substance to react covalently with DNA is not a specific property of carcinogens. Substances that are not hepatocarcinogens are capable of causing DNA damage and its subsequent repair in rat liver. Isolated nuclei are capable of the conversion of both carcinogenic and noncarcinogenic polynuclear aromatic hydrocarbons to metabolites that react covalently with the DNA of the endogenous chromatin. If damage to DNA is the prerequisite to carcinogenesis, other factors such as persistence of the damage and the efficiency of the repair processes must contribute to the fate of the affected cell.

The identity of and the reactive site on the metabolically activated carcinogens are topics of active investigation. In most proposals the ultimate reactive species of the polynuclear aromatic hydrocarbons is an epoxide and, in well-studied instances, specifically a diol epoxide. The polynuclear aromatic hydrocarbons can undergo microsomal metabolism to yield epoxides at locations broadly classified as K region and non-K region sites (Figure 16.2). In the case of benzopyrene (specifically the benzo[a]pyrene isomer), the sequence of reactions converting the procarcinogen to the probable ultimate carcinogen, a diol epoxide, consists of the following steps (Figure 16.1): (a) oxygenation of the 7,8 double bond of benzopyrene to yield the 7,8-epoxide by means of the mixed-function oxidase; (b) hydration of the 7,8-epoxide by epoxide hydratase (also called epoxide hydrase) to yield the 7,8-dihydro-7,8-dihydroxy derivative; and

(c) in a second reaction by a mixed-function oxidase, oxygenation at the 9,10 double bond to yield the putative major ultimate carcinogen, the 7,8-dihydro-7,8-dihyroxybenzopyrene 9,10-epoxide. Appreciable evidence indicates that it is the latter dihydrodiol non-K region epoxide which is the major reactive species that binds covalently to cellular DNA. Benzopyrene is also metabolized to a large number of other products, including the 4,5 epoxide, the K region epoxide. The probably ultimate carcinogen of benz[a]anthracene is also a diol epoxide, namely 3,4-dihydro-3,4-dihydroxybenz[a]anthracene 1,2-epoxide.

The principal route of oxidative metabolism of polynuclear aromatic hydrocarbons is effected by the microsomal mixed-function oxidase system (aryl hydrocarbon hydroxylase) of the endoplasmic reticulum and the nuclear envelope. Upon formation of the initial epoxide (or arene oxide), the epoxide can react nonenzymatically with tissue macromolecules, rearrange nonenzymatically to phenolic derivatives, be converted to dihydrodiols by microsomal and nuclear epoxide hydrase or nonenzymatically, or be converted to glutathione conjugates by the glutathione S-transferases of the cytosol or nonenzymatically.

The relative importance of the various epoxides in carcinogenesis and covalent reaction with DNA may be dictated in part by the susceptibility of each type of epoxide to inactivation by epoxide hydrase and glutathione transferases. The various epoxide derivatives of benzopyrene differ appreciably in their susceptibilities to hepatic epoxide hydrase and to hepatic glutathione S-transferases. The dihydrodiol non-K region epoxides of benzopyrene and benzanthracene are very poor substrates for epoxide hydrase. The dihydrodiol epoxides may also be intrinsically more reactive because one of the neighboring hydroxyl groups forms an intramolecular hydrogen bond and thereby accelerates the reaction of the epoxide with nucleophiles. The dihydrodiol epoxides with a stereochemistry that permits such intramolecular hydrogen bonding are 100–500 times more reactive with a model thio compound than other stereoisomers.

16.4.4. Molecular Sites of DNA and RNA Susceptible to Covalent Reactions

A large number of sites on DNA and RNA are susceptible in vivo (or in cultured cells) to methylation or ethylation by intrinsically reactive alkylating substances, such as methyl or ethyl methanesulfonate, dimethyl sulfate, N-methyl-N-nitrosourea, and N-methyl-N'-nitro-N-nitrosoguanidine, or by metabolically activated alkylating agents such as dimethylnitrosamine. Under almost all circumstances the most reactive site on DNA or RNA is the N^7 position of guanine. The following additional sites on DNA undergo alkylation: the N^1, N^3, and N^7 of adenine; the N^3 and oxygen on C-6 of guanine; the N^3 of cytosine; and the oxygen on C-4 of thymine (Figure 16.3). Alkylation on the N^3 or N^7 position of purines is not at the sites that participate in hydrogen bonding of complementary bases. In contrast, alkylation at the oxygen on C-6 of guanine, the N^3 of cytosine, or the oxygen on the C-4 of thymine is at the sites that normally participate in base pairing (Figure 16.3) and thus are potentially critical in a possible induced base mispairing. In addition, DNA can also undergo alkylation of the phosphates to yield phosphotriesters.

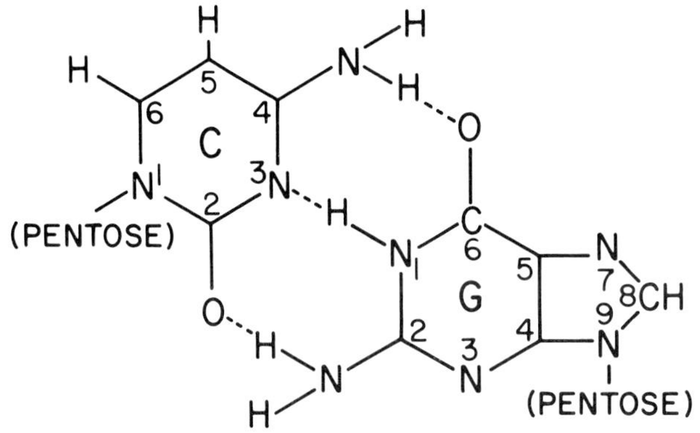

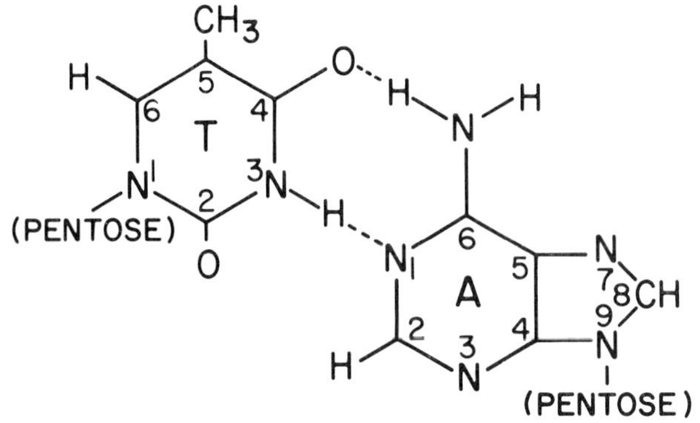

Figure 16.3 Complementary base pairs and molecular sites involved in hydrogen bonding.

The sites of attachment to DNA by the larger aryl groups of aromatic carcinogens also vary, but fewer sites on the DNA appear to be susceptible to covalent attachment. The sites typically are identified by incubation of the radioactive carcinogen with cultured cells or with a mixture of hepatic microsomes and free DNA, enzymatic hydrolysis of the DNA, and chromatography to separate the nucleoside adduct. In such studies the principal adduct formed from the aflatoxin B_1 metabolite is attached to the N^7 of guanine (approximately 90%). In contrast, the metabolites of polynuclear aromatic hydrocarbons (e.g., benzopyrene) react preferentially with the amino group of guanine, and the metabolites of aromatic amines and amides (e.g., 2-acetylaminofluorene) react preferentially with the C-8 of guanine.

16.5. Metal Carcinogenesis

16.5.1. Metallic Cation Interactions

Cancers are induced in various experimental animals by salts of at least eight metals, including beryllium, cadmium, cobalt, chromium, iron, nickel, lead, and zinc. In addition, epidemiological investigations have indicated that carcinogenesis in humans is associated with exposure to compounds of arsenic, cadmium, chromium, and nickel. Salts of beryllium and lead also are implicated as possible human carcinogens. There are instances in which various metallic salts exhibit actions consistent with chromosome damage in cultured mammalian cells. Likewise, mutations are induced in bacterial test systems by some, but not all, carcinogenic metallic salts.

Various carcinogenic metallic cations inhibit DNA replication and RNA synthesis and cause nucleotide mispairing in polynucleotides. Certain carcinogenic and noncarcinogenic metallic cations exhibit binding to polynucleotides at various specific molecular sites, especially purines and thymine, in addition to interacting with the anionic phosphate groups. In addition, as discussed below (Section 16.5.2), most of the carcinogenic metallic cations induce mispairing during nucleotide polymerization by viral reverse transcriptase, a nominal RNA-directed DNA polymerase. However, some of the carcinogenic metallic cations appear to produce the nucleotide miscoding by complex formation with the viral polymerase rather than with the polynucleotide template. The observations on carcinogenic metallic cations in enzymatic and physical studies are consistent with potential mechanistic roles in metal-induced carcinogenesis.

16.5.2. Metallic Cation–Induced Miscoding of Viral DNA Polymerases

Nucleotide mispairing during reactions catalyzed by DNA polymerase may have a role in tumor development and aging. The nucleotide miscoding by a DNA polymerase is detected by the measurement of the incorporation in vitro of a radioactive deoxyribonucleoside phosphate into DNA in the presence of a synthetic template that does not contain a nucleotide complementary to the radioactive nucleotide; e.g., by the measurement of the incorporation of the moieties of radioactive dCTP in the presence of poly(dA-dT) template or radioactive dATP in the presence of poly(dC) · oligo(dG) template–primer. The detection of the incorporation of mispaired nucleotides during polymerization is enhanced if the polymerase lacks an associated exonuclease activity which might excise noncomplementary nucleotides after incorporation.

Certain metallic cations induce nucleotide mispairing by viral reverse transcriptases (nominally RNA-directed DNA polymerases). Various carcinogenic metallic cations, such as Be^{2+}, Cd^{2+}, Mn^{2+}, and Ni^{2+}, cause an increased error frequency during polymerization by the DNA polymerase of avian myeloblastosis virus. In contrast, a number of putative noncarcinogenic metallic cations, including Ca^{2+} and Mg^{2+}, do not produce nucleotide mispairing during polymerization. In the case of the carcinogenic cation Be^{2+}, studies suggest that the Be^{2+}-facilitated errors occur due to the formation of a polymerase–Be^{2+} complex rather than a template–Be^{2+} complex. Although there may be some disagreement about the assignment of a few of the metallic cations to carcinogenic or noncarcinogenic categories, of the approximately 30 metallic cations tested, almost all of the carcinogenic cations induce nucleotide miscoding by the viral DNA polymerase. In contrast, the noncarcinogenic cations do not induce nucleotide miscoding. The measurement of metallic cation–induced miscoding during polymerization of deoxyribonucleotides is suggested as a potential screening method for metallic carcinogens and mutagens.

16.6. DNA Repair

16.6.1. DNA Repair Processes in Mammalian Cells

Two general types of mammalian DNA repair, namely DNA excision repair (or DNA repair synthesis) and postreplication repair, are involved in the removel of most covalently attached adducts from cellular DNA. Photoreactivation, a third type of DNA repair in mammalian cells, may be involved in the removel of pyrimidine dimers produced in DNA exposed to ultraviolet radiation although the pyrimidine dimers are also removed by excision repair and postreplication repair.

16.6.1a. DNA Excision Repair

Excision repair, which can occur throughout the cell cycle, consists of a series of steps, including the following: (a) an endonuclease-catalyzed incision and/or an initial hydrolysis of a phosphodiester bond in the damaged DNA chain; (b) the excision or removal of the damaged site and the adjacent nucleotides by an exonuclease; (c) the nucleotide polymerization by a DNA polymerase to re-place the excised nucleotides of the damaged chain; and (d) the closing of the nick in the repaired strand by DNA ligase to re-form the double-stranded structure. Excision repair appears to be a relatively error-free process. Excision repair can be initiated by damage to DNA such as alkylation, arylation, the production of pyrimidine dimers by ultraviolet radiation, or the production of apurinic or apyrimidinic sites.

There are at least two modes of DNA excision repair, and they may be characterized as either "short-patch" or "apurinic" repair, or as "long-patch" or "nucleotide" excision repair. The enzymatic systems may be markedly different. The short-patch repair is accompanied by the removal and replacement of only a few (perhaps three to four) nucleotides. Short-patch repair is initiated by DNA damage by alkylation with methylating and ethylating agents and by ionizing radiation, which produces predominantly single-strand breaks. The endonuclease involved in the short-patch repair may recognize apurinic or apyrimidinic sites, which may occur after the enzymatic or nonenzymatic removal of abnormal bases. There exist in bacterial cells, and apparently in mammalian cells, certain glycosylases (also called N-glycosidases) that hydrolyze the β-glycosyl bonds (traditionally termed N-glycosidic bonds) between the C-1 of deoxyribose and the nitrogen of an abnormal purine (e.g., 3-methyladenine) or an abnormal pyrimidine (e.g., uracil) within the DNA strand. Alternatively, the alkylation of purines at the N^3 or N^7 position labilizes the glycosyl linkage, and nonenzymatic depurinations may occur to yield apurinic sites. In either case, the endonuclease then acts by recognition of the apurinic or apyrimidinic site.

The long-patch repair results in the removal and replacement of the damaged site and up to 100 adjacent nucleotides. The long-patch repair is initiated by damaged sites or adducts which produce large distortions in the double helix, e.g., pyrimidine dimers produced by ultraviolet radiation or nucleoside adducts with large ring systems, such as the metabolites of 2-acetyl aminofluorene or polynuclear aromatic hydrocarbons. A different *group* of endonucleases probably are active against damaged DNA containing large distorted regions, and the long-patch repair process may reflect several distinct activities that depend on the nature of the DNA-damaging event. Various cell types differ in the *relative* ability to repair pyrimidine dimers and adducts of acetylaminofluorene derivatives, each characterized by the long-patch repair process. The capabilities of the various cell types may differ due to the relative activities of several incision endonucleases, which exhibit specificity for a different type of damaged site.

16.6.1b. Postreplication Repair

Postreplication repair occurs only during the S phase, or DNA replication phase, of the cell cycle. The typical model of postreplication repair contains the following sequence of events: (a) After damage to the DNA by ultraviolet radiation (yielding pyrimidine dimers) or carcinogen–adduct formation, the cellular DNA undergoes replication. (b) The replicative polymerase, as it encounters a large damage site on the template strand, cannot use the site as template. (c) The result, then, is a newly synthesized DNA that contains gaps of up to 1000 nucleotides and/or shorter gaps. In either case, the single-strand molecular weight of the newly synthesized DNA in damaged cells is appreciably less than in normal cells using undamaged DNA template. (d) In the DNA-damaged cells, the gaps and nicks in the newly synthesized DNA eventually are filled by chain elongation (that is, postreplication repair) during the S phase and are ligated, even though some damaged sites still remain in the template strand of the DNA. Because the repair polymerase must utilize a damaged DNA template, it is probable that the newly synthesized DNA strand contains errors introduced during the nucleotide polymerization; thus, postreplication repair may reflect an error-prone repair.

16.6.1c. Removal of Alkylated Bases

The methylation or ethylation of DNA results in alkylation at the N^3 and N^7 of the purines (predominantly on the N^7 of guanine) and at other sites (Section 16.4.4; Figure 16.3). The rates of removal of the alkylated sites from DNA by nonenzymatic processes and by enzymatic repair processes differ markedly depending on the molecular site of alkylation. In addition, various tissues differ markedly in their ability to remove specific alkylated bases (Section 16.6.2). The alkylation of purines at N^3 or N^7 labilizes the β-glycosyl bond with the deoxyribose, and nonenzymatic depurination may occur and result in the introduction of an apurinic site. In contrast, methylation of guanine on the oxygen at C-6 does not labilize the glycosyl bond. In most mammalian and bacterial systems, the relative rates of the removal of methylated bases are 3-methyladenine > O^6-methylguanine > N^7-methylguanine. A portion of the removal of the N^3- and N^7-methylpurines probably occurs through a nonenzymatic depurination followed by the initiation of a short-patch excision repair process by hydrolysis of the phosphodiester bond by an apurinic-specific endonuclease. The removal of certain methylated or other abnormal bases may also be initiated by the base-specific glycosylases, which results in the presence of an apurinic or apyrimidinic site on the DNA. *E. coli* contain glycosylases specific for 3-methyladenine and for uracil (i.e., derived from the deamination of cytosine in DNA). The latter type of enzymatic activity also occurs in mammalian cells. Mammalian tissues may contain glycosylases and/or other enzymatic activities that function in the removal of O^6-methylguanine from DNA.

16.6.2. Persistence of DNA Damage in Relation to Carcinogenesis

It is not known to what extent the histones and other chromosomal proteins protect the DNA from reactive substances. It is obvious, however, from the repression of certain genes that chromosomal proteins prevent access of various enzymes to the DNA. It is anticipated that the enzymes of the relatively error-free DNA excision repair likewise have limited access to damaged DNA— perhaps access only to the derepressed regions. However, the lack of excision repair of damaged DNA sites in the repressed regions (i.e., those not available to the RNA polymerases for transcription) probably will not interfere with the normal functions in a nonmitotic cell. The unrepaired DNA sites within the chromatin, inaccessible to repair enzymes, assume a more critical role upon the initiation of replicative DNA synthesis. The newly synthesized DNA then may undergo an error-prone postreplication repair accompanied by muta- tion fixation. Such mutation potentially may then lead to cell death or a so- matic cell mutation and carcinogenesis. Thus, the persistence of certain types of DNA damage theoretically is of importance in the process of carcinogene- sis.

The production of DNA strand breaks and their persistence, in some cases, appear to correlate with carcinogenicity or organotropic (i.e., organ-specific) carcinogenicity. In one comparative study, all chemical carcinogens tested in- duced single-strand breaks in rat liver DNA in vivo, and 5 of 13 tested hepatocarcinogens induced double-strand breaks. The DNA strand breaks produced by the hepatocarcinogens were not completely repaired by 14 days. In contrast, the DNA damage induced by 3 chemotherapeutic agents was repaired within 4 hr, and 9 noncarcinogenic hepatotoxic agents did not induce any measurable strand damage in hepatic DNA. It is suggested that a hepatocar- cinogen induces either double-strand breaks or single-strand breaks that require a long time for repair. If the damaged, unrepaired DNA is replicated during that interval, the single-strand breaks may become double-strand breaks, which potentially have more harmful consequences. In a second study, in which the organotropic actions of the carcinogens 4-nitroquinoline 1-oxide and dimethylnitrosamine were compared, it was found that the production of DNA strand breaks (measured by centrifugation on alkaline sucrose gradients) correlated with the sites of tumor induction. Furthermore, no DNA damage was induced by the noncarcinogenic 4-aminoquinoline 1-oxide. In a third study in the pancreas, two carcinogenic substances and one noncarcinogen induced strand breaks in pancreatic DNA shortly after administration. The DNA strand breaks by the noncarcinogen were repaired relatively rapidly, but the DNA damage by the carcinogenic substances persisted for 1 or 4 weeks. It is suggested that the relative persistence of strand breaks may be an accurate indicator of the organotropic carcinogenic potential in the pancreas.

The rates of removal of alkylated purines from *hepatic* DNA are 3-alkyladenine > O^6-alkylguanine > 7-alkylguanine after treatment with methylating and ethylating agents (see Section 16.6.1c). O^6-alkylguanine is of probable importance in base mispairing; in addition, the relative extent of its formation by different compounds appears to correspond to the carcinogenic potency of the compounds. The organotropic specificity of monofunctional al- kylating carcinogens appears to depend, in part, on the differential capacities of the tissues to remove O^6-methylguanine from the tissue DNA.

Tissues may exhibit highly differential sensitivities to the carcinogenic action of various substances. Factors that may participate in the organotropic effect of a carcinogen include the following: (a) the extent of entrance of the carcinogen (or its metabolites) into the target and nontarget tissues; (b) the ability of the tissue to convert a nonreactive carcinogen to a reactive metabolite; (c) the presence of agents (such as epoxide hydrase or glutathione and glutathione S-transferases) that decrease the likelihood of the reaction of the active species with a critical macromolecule; (d) the extent and molecular site of reaction with the DNA (or another sensitive and critical tissue component); and (e) the ability to repair the functionally critical, damaged sites within the cell before an irreversible process occurs leading to cellular transformation. Studies on the carcinogenicity of, and covalent reaction with DNA by, the N-alkyl-N-nitrosoureas are directed at some of the appropriate factors.

The principal target organ of the carcinogenicity of N-methyl- or N-ethyl-N-nitrosourea is the nervous system; in contrast, the intact liver is resistant to the carcinogenicity of the nitrosoureas. These compounds are intrinsically reactive, and the reactive species are formed by the nonenzymatic decomposition of the respective nitrosourea derivatives. Consequently, the difference in the organotropic carcinogenicity of the nitrosourea derivatives is not due to a difference in metabolic activation to yield reactive species. The organotropic carcinogenic action of the N-alkyl-N-nitrosoureas and perhaps other methylating and ethylating carcinogens appears to depend on the differential capacity of various tissues to remove O^6-alkylguanine from the DNA. Following the administration of N-ethyl-N-nitrosourea, the O^6-ethylguanine is removed from the DNA of liver, a nontarget tissue, with a half-life of 36 hr, whereas the same ethylated guanine is removed from the DNA of brain, a target tissue, with a half-life of 229 hr. In contrast, the half-lives of N^3-ethyladenine in brain and in liver are very short and nearly equal, and the half-lives of N^7-ethylguanine do not differ appreciably in the two tissues. Comparable observations on the removal of O^6-methylguanine from DNA of brain and liver are made after the administration of N-methyl-N-nitrosourea. Since O^6-methylguanine in polynucleotides results in base mispairing, the decreased rate of repair in the target tissue is consistent with a potential role of the decreased repair in carcinogenesis.

16.6.3. Assay of Chemical Carcinogens in Mammalian Systems

An appreciable effort has been made to develop and to assess the reliability of various short-term tests for carcinogens. The importance of the development of such screening systems resides in the necessity for the *provisional* safety assessment of the multitude of industrial and environmental chemicals and for the initial selection of the chemicals in need of further, more time-consuming studies. Some of the screening systems are based on bacterial mutations or on transformation of cultured mammalian cells. The properties of genetic poisons are discussed in Chapter 15. The present discussion of the assay of chemical carcinogens will be limited to two systems that are associated with DNA damage and repair, namely, the detection of strand breaks in DNA and unscheduled DNA synthesis. The metallic cation–induced miscoding by viral DNA polymerase, proposed as an assay for metallic carcinogens, is presented elsewhere (Section 16.5.2).

16.6.3a. DNA Damage Measured by Centrifugation on Sucrose Gradients

One of the most commonly used techniques to detect DNA damage by a potential carcinogen is the measurement of the size of single-strand fragments of DNA on an alkaline sucrose gradient. The formation of single- or double-strand breaks within cellular DNA potentially can occur by direct action of a DNA-damaging agent or radiation, by enzymatic or nonenzymatic depurination or depyrimidination of a substituted or abnormal base followed by a nuclease specific for an apurinic or apyrimidinic site, or by the activity of an incision endonuclease. Two additional sites, namely apurinic (or apyrimidinic) sites and phosphotriester groups, also may be observed as single-strand breaks only upon centrifugation in alkaline gradients. Depending upon conditions (alkali concentration, temperature, and duration), the apurinic sites and phosphotriesters are hydrolyzed in alkaline solutions—e.g., during tissue lysis or centrifugation in alkaline sucrose gradients—and the sites are then detected as DNA strand breaks. The procedure typically includes the following steps:

1. The DNA is prelabeled by the incorporation of radioactive thymidine into the DNA during replication. In order to prevent overloading of the sucrose gradients, only a small amount of DNA (1 μg/10–14 ml gradient) can be applied; radioactive DNA generally is used because the quantity of DNA is too small to be measured conveniently by methods other than its radioactivity. The use of larger centrifuge tubes, zonal rotors, and/or a fluorometric assay for DNA permits the application of centrifugation on sucrose gradients to tissues that cannot be prelabeled with radioactive thymidine, e.g., human tissues.

2. At an appropriate interval after exposure to a potentially DNA-damaging substance, a sample of tissue is subjected to the lysing solution, which contains a detergent such as sodium dodecyl sulfate and a metal ion complexing agent such as EDTA in a very alkaline (pH 12–12.3) salt solution. The mixture brings about cellular disruption and releases the DNA. The ability to release the cellular DNA in this manner obviates the need for isolation of the DNA preparatory to its centrifugation.

3. The lysing mixture is applied to the top of a gradient prepared from 5% and 20% sucrose solutions containing NaCl and NaOH (pH 12–12.3). The high pH of the lysing medium and the sucrose gradient solutions causes the DNA to undergo alkali-induced denaturation. Consequently, the centrifugation characteristics reflect single-stranded DNA and the introduction of single-strand breaks in the damaged DNA.

4. Centrifugation conditions (relative centrifugal force and duration) are selected such that the undamaged, high molecular weight, single-stranded DNA sediments far into the gradient but the damaged, lower molecular weight DNA sediments to a lesser extent.

5. The gradients are fractionated, and the relative amount of DNA in each fraction is quantitated from the radioactivity.

6. With appropriate standardization, it is possible to estimate the molecular weight of the DNA in gradients of control and toxicant- or carcinogen-treated cells and the number of breaks introduced in the DNA (i.e., the sum of the breaks endogenous to the cellular DNA and those formed from apurinic sites and/or phosphotriesters because of the alkali lability of such sites).

It is also possible to measure the formation of double-strand breaks by the use of a lysing medium containing detergent, metal-complexing agent, and NaCl at neutral pH and a subsequent centrifugation on a neutral pH sucrose gradient. Among the carcinogens that induce double-strand breaks are certain derivatives of 2-acetylaminofluorene.

The centrifugation technique has a number of advantages and disadvantages. Some of the evident advantages are as follows: (a) the method often can be used to distinguish a carcinogen from a noncarcinogen in vivo; (b) organotropic or tissue-specific carcinogenesis can be detected; (c) the DNA damage and repair can be measured quantitatively, although it is difficult to distinguish between certain types of damage, e.g., between strand breaks in the endogenous DNA and the alkali-labile sites; (d) the technique encompasses the entire process of excision repair, including the final ligation step; and (e) the method can be applied to those compounds that require metabolic activation in order to form the DNA-reactive species. The disadvantages are that it is generally necessary to prelabel the DNA with a radioactive precursor and the DNA strand breakage is not observed with all types of DNA damage and/or tested carcinogens.

16.6.3b. Unscheduled DNA Synthesis

Normal nonmitotic cells, such as peripheral lymphocytes or cultured cells in a plateau phase, exhibit little thymidine incorporation into DNA. However, if the cells are subjected to an appropriate DNA-damaging toxicant, the nucleoside phosphates of thymidine (and the other deoxyribonucleosides) are incorporated during the polymerization stage of excision repair.

The technique can be applied to most nonmitotic cells such as lymphocytes. After exposure to the DNA-damaging toxicant, the cells are incubated for several hours with radioactive thymidine. Hydroxyurea, which is noted as an indirect inhibitor of semiconservative DNA replication but not of nucleotide polymerization during excision repair, is included in the incubation medium to suppress most of the low-level DNA replication observed in lymphocytes and other essentially nonmitotic cells. The thymidine incorporation then is measured either from the macromolecular radioactivity or by autoradiographic techniques.

The advantages of the technique are that it can be applied readily to human cells since the exposure of the cells to a DNA-damaging agent and to the radioactive thymidine are conducted in vitro with isolated cells, and the DNA repair can be evaluated in individual nuclei to reveal variations within a cell population when the procedure is conducted by autoradiographic techniques. The disadvantage of the technique is that it does not measure the completeness of repair since it measures only a portion of the overall excision repair process and does not include the activity of the ligase. Moreover, it cannot be applied to rapidly proliferating cells since the thymidine incorporation during semiconservative DNA replication is many-fold greater than during excision repair.

Suggested Reading

Carcinogenesis—Theoretical and General Aspects

Farber, E. The pathology of experimental liver cell cancer. In Cameron, H. M., Linsell, D. A., Warwick, G. P. (Eds.). Liver Cell Cancer. Amsterdam: Elsevier 1976, pp. 243–277.

Loeb, L. A., Springgate, C. F., Battula, N. Errors in DNA replication as a basis of malignant changes. Cancer Res. 34 (1974), 2311.

Miller, E. C., Miller, J. A. Hepatocarcinogenesis by chemicals. Prog. Liver Dis. 5 (1976), 699.

Miller, J. A., Miller, E. C. Some current thresholds of research in chemical carcinogenesis. In Ts'o, P. O. P., DiPaolo, J. A. (Eds.). Chemical Carcinogenesis, Part A. New York: Marcel Dekker, 1974, pp. 61–85.

Preussmann, R. Chemical carcinogens in the human environment. Problems and quantitative aspects. Oncology 33 (1976), 51.

Trosko, J. E., Chu, E. H. Y. The role of DNA repair and somatic mutation in carcinogenesis. Adv. Cancer Res. 21 (1975), 391.

Weisburger, E. K. Mechanisms of chemical carcinogenesis. Ann. Rev. Pharmacol. Toxicol. 18 (1978), 395.

Covalent Reaction of Carcinogens with DNA

Croy, R. G., Essigmann, J. M., Reinhold, V. N. Wogan, G. N. Identification of the principal aflatoxin B₁-DNA adduct formed *in vivo* in rat liver. Proc. Natl. Acad. Sci. U.S.A. 75 (1978), 1745.

Irving, C. C. Interaction of chemical carcinogens with DNA. Methods Cancer Res. 7 (1973), 189.

Rajewsky, M. F. Augenlicht, L. H., Biessmann, H., Goth, R., Hülser, D. F., Laerum, O. D. and Lomakina, L. Y. Nervous-system-specific carcinogenesis by ethylnitrosourea in the rat: Molecular and cellular aspects. In Hiatt, H. H., Watson, J. D., Winsten, J. A. (Eds.). Origins of Human Cancer, Book B. Cold Spring Harbor, N.Y.: Cold Spring Harbor Laboratory, 1977, pp. 709–726.

Sarma, D. S. R., Rajalakshmi, S., Farber, E. Chemical carcinogenesis: Interactions of carcinogens with nucleic acids. In Becker, F. F. (Ed.). Cancer: A Comprehensive Treatise, Vol. 1. New York: Plenum Press, 1975, pp. 235–287.

Singer, B. The chemical effects of nucleic acid alkylation and their relation to mutagenesis and carcinogenesis. Prog. Nucleic Acid Res. Mol. Biol. 15 (1975), 219.

Chemistry and Metabolism of Carcinogens

Freudenthal, R., Jones, P. W. (Eds.). Carcinogenesis—A Comprehensive Survey, Vol. 1, Polynuclear Aromatic Hydrocarbons: Chemistry, Metabolism, and Carcinogenesis. New York: Raven Press, 1976.

Weisburger, J. H., Williams, G. M. Metabolism of chemical carcinogens. In Becker, F. F. (Ed.). Cancer: A Comprehensive Treatise, Vol. 1. New York: Plenum Press, 1975, pp. 185–234.

Metal-Induced Carcinogenesis

Sirover, M. A., Loeb, L. A. Infidelity of DNA synthesis *in vitro:* Screening for potential metal mutagens or carcinogens. Science, 194 (1976), 1434.

Sunderman, F. W., Jr. Carcinogenic effects of metals. Fed. Proc. 37 (1978), 40.

DNA Repair

Cleaver, J. E. Methods for studying excision repair of DNA damaged by physical and chemical mutagens. In Kilbey, B. J., et al. (Eds.). Handbook of Mutagenicity Test Procedures. Amsterdam: Elsevier, 1977, pp. 19–48.

Hart, R. W., Trosko, J. E. DNA repair processes in mammals. Interdisciplinary Topics Gerontol., 9 (1976), 134.

Lehmann, A. R., Bridges, B. A. DNA repair. Essays Biochem. 13 (1977), 71.

Lieberman, M. W. Approaches to the analysis of fidelity of DNA repair in mammalian cells. Intern. Rev. Cytol. 45 (1976), 1.

Pegg, A. E., Hui, G. Formation and subsequent removal of O⁶-methylguanine from deoxyribonucleic acid in rat liver and kidney after small doses of dimethylnitrosamine. Biochem. J. 173 (1978), 739.

Testing of Carcinogens in Mammalian Systems

Bridges, B. A. Short term screening tests for carcinogens. Nature 261 (1976), 195.

Cox, R., Damjanov, I., Abanobi, S. E., Sarma, D. S. R. A method for measuring DNA damage and repair in the liver *in vivo*. Cancer Res. 33 (1973), 2114.

Laishes, B. A., Koropatnick, D. J., Stich, H. F. Organ-specific DNA damage induced in mice by the organotropic carcinogens 4-nitroquinoline 1-oxide and dimethylnitrosamine. Proc. Soc. Exp. Biol. Med. 149 (1975), 978.

Sarma, D. S. R. Chemical interaction measurements. In Golberg, L. (Ed.). Carcinogenesis Testing of Chemicals. Cleveland: CRC Press, 1974, pp. 95–100.

Stoltz, D. R., Poirier, L. A., Irving, C. C., Stich, H. F., Weisburger, J. H., Grice, H. C. Evaluation of short-term tests for carcinogenicity. Toxicol. Appl. Pharmacol. 29 (1974), 157.

William E. Donaldson

17

Trace Element Toxicity

17.1. Definition of Trace Elements

Several elements are required for the nutritional well-being of animals and humans. Nutritionists generally classify these elements into two broad categories: (a) The macroelements (calcium, phosphorus, sulfur, magnesium, sodium, potassium, and chlorine), which are required in the diet in substantial quantities; and (b) the micro- or trace elements, which are required in the diet in small to minute amounts. The trace elements recognized currently as dietary essentials are cobalt, copper, fluorine, iodine, iron, manganese, molybdenum, selenium, and zinc. Chromiun and tin are thought to be dietary essentials also, but the evidence is less extensive than for the other elements listed.

A dietary deficiency of any ot the trace elements will produce specific symptoms because each element serves a specific function(s). The body has the ability to tolerate excesses of the trace elements, but this ability is limited. If the dietary level of a trace element is greater than the body's ability to cope with it, toxicity symptoms will develop.

Trace element toxicity can also develop as a result of environmental exposures other than diet. For example, industrial uses of selenium can lead to selenium intoxication in workers exposed during manufacturing processes. Industrial and other enviornmental exposures can be a problem with nonnutritive as well as nutritionally required trace elements. The toxicity of cadmium, lead, and mercury, as well as the toxicity of the nutritionally required trace elements, will also be discussed in this chapter.

17.2. Trace Element Interactions

The nutritional interactions of trace elements have been known for years. Several hypotheses have been put forward to explain these interactions, and in particular cases, each hypothesis has validity. However, it appears that there is no single explanation for all the interactions observed.

Some elements interact on the basis of the similarity of their electronic configuration and valence. Zinc is an element that is essential to the function of several enzymes. Because the electronic structure of cadmium is similar to that of zinc, cadmium interferes with the function of zinc-containing enzymes by substituting for zinc in the enzyme structure. The cadmium-substituted enzymes are not as active as the native, zinc-containing enzymes, and therefore function is impaired. Several instances of trace element interactions of this type have been verified, including interactions of mercury and arsenic, zinc and copper, and copper and molybdenum.

Other types of interactions are known to exist. Concern was recently expressed over high levels of mercury found in tuna and swordfish. The high levels of mercury always occurred in conjunction with concomitantly high levels of selenium. Selenium and mercury are antagonistic, and marine animals appear to counteract any toxic manifestations of mercury by absorbing stoichimetric amounts of selenium. As a consequence, neither the mercury nor the selenium content of these marine animals poses a health threat to animals or humans that consume them. Those cases of mercury toxicity that have occurred as the result of eating contaminated fish have been associated with dumping of high levels of mercury into a local habitat in which only limited amounts of selenium were present.

Dietary mercury and selenium antagonize one another by an as yet undefined mechanism. It is known that certain mercury and selenium compounds react to form insoluble complexes. Such complexes may be formed in the gut or in the tissues, effectively obviating the toxicity of both elements.

Manganese can interfere with the absorption of iron from the gut. The mechanism of iron absorption is complex and involves several proteins with the capacity to bind iron. It may be that manganese competes with iron for binding sites on these proteins.

17.3 Nutritionally Required Trace Elements That Exhibit Toxicity

17.3.1. Cobalt

Normal foods and beverages do not contain enough Co to produce toxicity. However, misuse of trace mineral supplements in animal feeds or overconsumption of mineral supplements by humans can cause problems with Co as well as with other trace elements. Symptoms of Co toxicity include depressed weight and appetite, anemia, polycythemia, hyperplasia of the bone marrow, reticulocytosis, and increased blood volume.

Although not normally a problem, several cases of heart failure in heavy beer drinkers have been attributed to Co toxicity. In these cases, Co was added to beer in concentrations of 1.2–1.5 ppm to improve the foaming quality of the beer. The victims of congestive heart failure drank approximately 12 liters of beer daily, which would provide an intake of approximately 8 mg cobalt sulfate per day. It is difficult to accept Co as the sole source of the toxicity since 300 mg/day of Co salts have been used therapeutically to treat anemias without cardiotoxic effects. It has been postulated that high alcohol intake coupled with low protein and thiamine intakes interacted with Co to produce the toxicity.

17.3.2. Copper

Monogastric animals tolerate relatively high Cu levels in the diet without manifestations of toxicity, although toxicity is evident if the levels are high enough. In contrast, ruminants are very susceptible to Cu toxicity. Sheep can develop liver Cu concentrations of over 1000 ppm at dietary Cu levels of 10–15 ppm. Increasing the dietary molybdenum level can counteract Cu toxicity in the presence of inorganic sulfate, since molybdenum is a Cu antagonist that reduces Cu retention. High dietary levels of zinc and iron interfere with Cu absorption.

Symptoms of Cu toxicity include loss of weight, anemia, and jaundice associated with hemolysis. The hemolysis is related to a sudden release of liver Cu stores. Hemoglobinemia and hemoglobinuria are also present.

The level of Cu required to produce toxicity in humans is not known. Humans are probably more resistant than ruminants to the effects of excess Cu. High Cu intakes have been reported as the result of soft water corrosion of Cu pipes used for drinking water supplies, but overt toxicity has not been observed as a result of consumption of such water. Industrial exposure to Cu has been reported to produce toxicity.

Biochemical parameters of Cu toxicity include high serum asparate aminotransferase and ornithine carbamyltransferase activities, which are indicative of general tissue damage. Prior to the hemolytic crisis in sheep resulting from excessive Cu intake, there is an increase in the activities of serum lactate dehydrogenase, glutamic oxalacetic transaminase, and glutamic pyruvic transaminase.

Wilson's disease is a rare, autosomal recessive trait that results in excessive accumulation of Cu in the liver and certain areas of the brain. High Cu intake is not a prerequisite for Cu accumulation to occur. The disease can be fatal within a few years of appearance of symptoms if not treated. Treatment consists of the administration of chelating agents, of which penicillamine is the most effective. Chelating agents mobilize the tissue Cu and promote urinary excretion. The biochemical lesion in Wilson's disease is unknown, but Cu absorption from the gut is enhanced and biliary excretion is reduced.

17.3.3. Fluorine

Fluorosis is a cumulative toxicity syndrome that can occur in humans as a result of industrial exposure, drinking water of high F content, or consumption of large amounts of "tea." Tea is one of the few plants that can concentrate F, and levels as high as 100 ppm are common. Marine fish can contain up to 10 ppm F. Fluorosis also occurs in livestock as a result of the consumption of phosphate supplements that are high in F. Symptoms are similar to those observed in humans.

Fluoride accumulates in human bones with increasing age despite low F intake. Three stages of F accumulation in bone are recognized: In the first, less than 2500 ppm F accumulates. Levels in excess of 2500 ppm do not occur in humans with normal intakes even in advanced age. No pathological changes occur at these levels. The F content can be beneficial since the F sequestered by bone can impart greater strength. In the second stage, with 2500–5000 ppm F, the bone exhibits chalky white areas with some loss of bone strength. Finally, at concentrations of over 5000 ppm F severe fluorosis occurs, which is characterized by progressive pain and stiffness in the joints and spinal column. Excessive calcification occurs, and the spine becomes one continuous column of bone. There is also calcification of ligaments and tendons. Loss of appetite, emaciation, and death follow.

Mottling of tooth enamel is the first observable sign of excessive F intake. Chalky white areas appear in the enamel. Yellow and brown staining also occurs, and the enamel surface eventually becomes pitted. The amount of F tolerated in the drinking water before tooth mottling is observed varies depending upon intake from other sources. Normal F intake in the United States is approximately 0.5 mg daily. Under these conditions mottled teeth are not observed at 1 ppm in the drinking water. Mild mottling is observed at 2–3 ppm, and moderate mottling is seen at 5–6 ppm in the drinking water.

Fluorides inhibit glycolysis but have no effect on oxygen consumption. Pronounced hyperglycemia and glucosuria are induced in rabbits by sodium fluoride. The hyperglycemia is reversible by insulin. Fluoride ion inhibits cholinesterase and several phosphatases and interferes with the metabolism of arginine and glutamine. Fluoroacetate is a metabolic poison by virtue of its strong inhibition of the tricarboxylic acid cycle. Fluoroacetate combines with oxalacetic acid to form fluorocitric acid, which blocks tricarboxylic acid cycle activity and causes citric acid to accumulate in the tissues.

17.3.4. Iodine

Goiter is endemic in areas where the iodine content of the soil is low. The so-called "goiter belt" of the American Midwest and the island of Tasmania are two examples. The incidence of goiter has been reduced markedly in these areas by the inclusion of iodine compounds as additives to dietary staples such as salt and bread. In most areas, the soil contains sufficient iodine so that goiter induced by iodine deficiency is not a problem.

Humans can be exposed to toxic levels of iodine from several sources. In addition to the iodine contained in foods to which the element is added, iodine is found in large quantities in marine fish and seaweed. Iodine is used in medicines and as an antiseptic agent in several food processing industries. Although toxic levels of iodine may not be encountered from a single source, the effects are cumulative. The effects of excess iodine can be particularly severe in those individuals suffering from goiter because of previous iodine insufficiency. The enlarged thyroid incorporates the excess iodine into organic compounds that produce thyrotoxicosis.

Excessive iodine intake can produce goiter and thyrotoxicosis in normal individuals also. In some coastal areas of Japan, the population consumes large quantities of seaweed. Iodine intakes reach up to 80 mg iodine daily with high levels of urinary excretion. Goiter is endemic in this population since the safe daily intake of iodine is 1 mg with potentially harmful effects at 2 mg daily.

17.3.5. Iron

Toxic reactions from excessive Fe intake are rare in humans and animals. Although Fe is rather abundant in the food supply, the body possesses an elaborate mechanism for limiting Fe absorption from the digestive tract. Most of the

Fe in the body is recycled so that Fe absorption is low except in cases of Fe loss, as from excessive bleeding or certain pathological conditions.

Hemochromatosis is a condition in humans in which the regulation of Fe absorption is faulty. Iron accumulates in most of the body tissues and especially in the liver and pancreas. Hemochromatosis often occurs after Fe overload. Such overload can result from repeated blood transfusions, long-term intake of medicinal Fe, and high Fe intake in alcoholics as the result of the high Fe content of many alcoholic beverages. Hemochromatosis is common in Bantus of South Africa due to a chronic overload of dietary Fe. The overload results from contamination of food with Fe from cooking vessels and from high consumption of Kaffir beer, which can contain up to 120 mg Fe/liter. The symptoms of hemochromatosis, other than high Fe content of tissues, are enlarged liver, impaired liver function, and increased pigmentation of the skin. The condition can precipitate diabetes and cardiac failure.

Acute Fe poisoning is rarely seen in adults. It is more common in children under 5 years of age, especially in the 1–2-year-old age group. Iron poisoning is almost always the result of consumption by children of Fe medication intended for adults. Such medication is attractive to children because it resembles candy and has a sugar-containing coating. The average human lethal dose is 200–250 mg/kg body weight. Within 30 min of massive Fe intake, vomiting occurs. The vomit is bloody in 80% of the cases. At about 10–12 hr the victim becomes drowsy and lethargic, and bloody diarrhea is observed in 40% of the cases. The initial episode is followed by either complete recovery or a sudden relapse at approximately 20 hr after ingestion. The relapse is characterized by fever, pneumonitis, shock, coma, and convulsions, and death may follow. If the victim survives 3–4 days, recovery is rapid. Laboratory findings in acute Fe poisoning are metabolic acidosis, hyperbilirubinemia, and deranged blood coagulation. Post mortem examination shows hemorrhagic necrosis of the gastrointestinal tract, Fe deposits in the mucosa and liver, damage to mitochondria, and elevated citrate and lactate concentrations in liver cells.

Massive oral doses of Fe (150–250 mg/kg body weight) are required to produce toxicity in experimental animals. Iron is absorbed as Fe^{2+} and is oxidized to Fe^{3+} for transport. When the Fe^{3+} concentration in blood exceeds the binding capacity of the Fe transport proteins, Fe^{3+} is precipitated as $Fe(OH)_3$. The excess H^+ released as a result of the hydroxide precipitation results in metabolic acidosis; blood pH values as low as 6.7 have been observed. Ferric iron complexes accumulate in the liver and inhibit glucose-6-phosphatase and oxidative enzymes such as succinic acid dehydrogenase. Impaired liver function causes elevated blood levels of lactic and citric acids.

Iron injections into preweanling pigs are commonly employed to correct anemia. The injections seldom cause problems; however, they can be fatal in vitamin E– or selenium-deficient pigs.

17.3.6. Manganese

The toxicity of Mn is relatively low. The concentration of Mn in most foods is low enough that excessive intake from dietary sources is improbable. Manganese can interfere with Fe absorption. It is possible that Mn competes with Fe for binding sites on the ferroproteins involved in Fe absorption and transport.

In livestock, excessive Mn intake depresses hemoglobin formation and Fe concentration in several tissues.

Manganese toxicity occurs in workers in Mn mines. The toxicity develops as a result of deposition of Mn oxides in the lungs. Manganese is absorbed from the lungs over a long period. The toxicity results in psychiatric disturbance followed by paralysis with trembling.

Oral ingestion of Mn salts induces gastrointestinal irritation, which accounts for most of the toxic effects of this element, such as interference with Fe absorption. Excess Mn impairs renal function, and a decrease in renal ATPase and increases in renal acid phosphatase and DNAase activities are observed. Manganous ion can cause agglutination and hemolysis of erythrocytes.

17.3.7. Molybdenum

This element has a very low order of toxicity in all species except cattle. The amounts of Mo in human diets is low enough to preclude excessive intake.

In cattle, severe diarrhea results from grazing in pastures with a high Mo content. Pastures with moderate Mo content will produce molybdenosis if the Cu content of the pasture is low. Molybdenosis can be controlled by oral or intravenous administration of copper sulfate. The nature of the Mo:Cu antagonistic interaction is unknown. High oral intake of Mo inhibits the activities of ceruloplasmin, sulfite oxidase, cytochrome oxidase, glutaminase, and cholinesterase.

17.3.8. Selenium

Probably more is known about Se toxicity than the toxicity of any other element because widespread areas exist in which the Se content of the soil is high. Selenosis, especially of livestock grazing these areas, is common and of considerable economic importance. Moreover, the etiology of this type of selenosis has been recognized for a considerable time.

The chemistry of Se is similar to that of S, and the two elements are antagonistic. Inorganic S is more antagonistic to inorganic Se than it is to organic Se. Selenium is required in the diet of most species studied at a level of approximately 0.1 ppm. Chronic toxicity is observed at 3–4 ppm, acute toxicity is observed at 10 ppm.

The symptoms of selenosis vary somewhat depending upon the species involved. In all species, growth retardation and anorexia occur. Anemia is also a common symptom. In horses, cattle, and pigs, there is hair loss and a sloughing of hooves. Severe liver damage with necrosis and hemorrhaging are common in rats and chicks. In humans, the first sign of Se intoxication from industrial exposure is a garlic-type smell on the breath. In fact, physicians involved with industrial medicine in factories that handle Se rely on periodic smelling of workers' breath to detect incipient selenosis. A trained nose can detect a subtle difference between true garlic and Se. The garlic odor is produced by dimethylselenide, a metabolite resulting from the biomethylation of inorganic Se. Rats excrete trimethylselenide in the urine; however, some species, such as the chicken, produce the di- but not trimethyl forms.

The interactions of Se with Hg and S have been mentioned. Selenium also interacts with arsenic, but the mechanism is not fully understood. Arsenic reduces Se toxicity but does not necessarily reduce the Se content of tissues. It has been suggested by some that Se promotes dental caries and is a carcinogen, but the data are open to question. In fact, some studies suggest that Se may be helpful in the prevention of cancer in humans.

Organic forms of Se such as selenomethionine and selenocystine are present in plants. This was also thought to be the case in animal tissues. However, recent experiments suggest that Se, as selenite, binds to the S atoms of methionine and cystine rather than replaces S.

Selenite is an inhibitor of many oxidase enzymes. It probably interacts with the sulfhydryl groups of such enzymes to inhibit activity. Selenite is a competitive inhibitor of fatty acid synthetase, a sulfhydryl-dependent enzyme. Selenite inhibition of fatty acid synthetase can be alleviated by the addition of sulfhydryl compounds in vitro. However, at certain ratios of enzyme, selenite, and sulfhydryl compounds, sulfhydryl compounds can potentiate the selenite inhibition.

Selenosis in human populations that reside in areas of high Se content in soil is rare. Although certain garden vegetables such as cabbage, broccoli, kale, and cauliflower can take up significant quantities of Se, most garden vegetables do not. Much of the Se in vegetables can be lost in cooking. Refining of such materials as seleniferous wheat removes much of the Se. These facts, combined with the fact that many dietary items could come from outside the area of high-Se soils, may account for the rarity of selenosis from dietary sources in humans. Certain plants tolerate high Se levels and can take up significant amounts of Se from the soil. These indicator plants, which thrive in high-Se soils to the exclusion of less tolerant plants, are primarily responsible for selenosis in grazing animals.

17.3.9. Zinc

The levels of Zn encountered in human and animal diets are relatively low, whereas Zn tolerance is relatively high. Rats tolerate up to 2500 ppm Zn without toxic effects. Pigs and chickens show no toxicity with high dietary Zn intakes. The toxic level of dietary Zn for humans is unknown. However, the Zn content of human diets seldom exceeds 15–20 ppm. Use of Cu rather than galvanized pipes for water supplies reduces Zn intake further. Furthermore, there is some evidence for a metabolic interaction of Cu and Zn.

Symptoms of Zn toxicity in animals are impaired growth, anorexia, anemia, internal hemorrhages, arthritis, and, with high enough intakes, death. The reduced growth and food consumption appear to be related primarily to diet palatability. Zinc toxicity has been reported in humans after prolonged consumption of water from galvanized pipes and cooking vessels. The symptoms included irritability, muscle pain, anorexia, and nausea.

17.3.10. Chromium

It is difficult to assess the toxicity of Cr for humans or animals because of deficiencies of analytic methodology and reagent contamination with Cr. Human intake of Cr from food averages less than 1 mg daily. Toxicity in animals has been reported with 50 ppm Cr in the diet. The toxicity of Cr(VI) appears to be greater than that of Cr(III) because of differences in absorption. Chromium toxicity results in poor growth and liver and kidney damage. Chromate dust has been reported to be carcinogenic in humans. Hexevalent Cr can enter erythrocytes and bind to the globin moiety of hemoglobin. Trivalent Cr binds to the β-globulins of serum and to siderophilin. Unlike most other metals, Cr levels in tissues decline with age except in the lung.

17.3.11. Tin

Unequivocal evidence of poisoning from Sn is not available. The Sn content of foods is low, and the major source of Sn contamination of food, from tin cans, has been eliminated by newer technology such as coating of cans with lacquer and crimping of soldered seams. Tin is absorbed poorly, and this poor absorption is probably the principal reason for the low toxicity. Like Cr, Sn concentration in tissues decreases with age.

17.4. Nonnutritive Trace Elements as Environmental Contaminants

17.4.1. Cadmium

Although Cd is found in foods, the levels are too low to be of any toxicological significance. Cadmium has many industrial uses, for example in electroplating, in low-melting alloys, in low-friction, fatigue-resistant bearing alloys, in solders, in batteries, in pigments, and as a barrier in atomic fission control. Therefore, it is to be expected that low to moderate Cd content of the environment is widespread. Since chronic exposure to even low levels of trace elements can lead to health problems, Cd is of particular concern to those concerned with environmental quality.

Industrial exposure is the most prevalent cause of chronic and acute Cd toxicity. Chronic toxicity is manifested in humans by anosmia as a result of olfactory nerve damage, kidney dysfunction, and emphysema. Cadmium has also been implicated as a possible cause of lung cancer. The Cd content of tobacco leaves is significant, but there is no experimental evidence linking Cd in tobacco to emphysema and lung cancer. It has also been suggested that Cd may play a role in the production of arteriosclerosis, hypertension, and cardiovascular disease, but the data are limited and contradictory. It is worth noting that the body burden of Cd in smokers is 1.5–2 times than that of nonsmokers.

Acute Cd toxicity in humans often leads to pneumonitis ranging from severe to fatal. Vomiting, diarrhea, and prostration are also symptoms of acute Cd poisoning.

In laboratory animals, Cd produces reduced growth, kidney and liver damage, brain hemorrhages, skeletal decalcification, and testicular necrosis. Rats develop hypertension as a result of Cd ingestion. It is not clear whether the hypertension results primarily from kidney damage (which involves lesions in the renal arterial system, glomeruli, and the tubular system) or from the fact that low concentrations of Cd increase pressor response to norepinephrine. The latter result has been demonstrated in isolated arterial strips, and it should be noted that higher concentrations of Cd have the opposite effect.

Increased intake of Zn can ameloriate or prevent the toxic manifestations of

Cd, and, conversely, if the nutritional Zn status is borderline or deficient, Cd toxicity is magnified. The Zn : Cd interrelationship is a reflection of competition for absorption and binding sites as well as competition for incorporation into Zn-containing metaloenzymes.

The main biochemical finding in Cd toxicity is proteinuria as a result of renal damage. It has been postulated that the proteinuria results from Cd transport to the proximal tubules by metallothionein (a low molecular weight Zn- and Cd-binding protein). In the tubules Cd acts upon enzymes that are responsible for reabsorption. Although the significance of the finding is unknown, tryptophan is not found in the low molecular weight proteins of serum and urine from Cd-treated monkeys. There is a marked increase of retinol-binding protein in the urine of humans with tubular proteinuria.

Cadmium affects the activities of several enzymes. Enhanced activity of δ-aminolevulinic acid dehydratase, pyruvate dehydrogenase, and pyruvate decarboxylase have been noted, while depressed activity of δ-aminolevulinic acid synthetase, alcohol dehydrogenase, arylsulfatase, and lipoamide dehydrogenase result from Cd intoxication.

Cadmium has been shown to interact with phospholipids such as phosphatidylserine and phosphatidylethanolamine. These interactions may be responsible for the toxic effects of Cd on membranes.

17.4.2. Mercury

There is no known nutritional requirement for Hg, and most of the Hg present in foods results from environmental contamination. Because it has many uses, there are numerous opportunities for contamination of food, air, and water with Hg. Elemental Hg is used in thermometers, barometers, diffusion pumps, Hg vapor lamps, electrical switches, dental fillings, paints, batteries, catalysts, and the manufacture of chlorine. Mercury salts are used as medicine, paint pigments, explosive detonators, and in the manufacture of paper. Organic Hg compounds are used as fungicides for seed treatment and in the manufacture of certain types of plastic.

The body's ability to eliminate Hg is limited, and therefore Hg is a cumulative poison. Reduced elimination appears to result from a high affinity of the tissues for Hg rather than poor excretion, since excretion kinetics are first order. Mercury can be absorbed through the gastrointestinal and respiratory tracts and through the skin. Elemental and organic Hg compounds are volatile, and only small quantities are needed to saturate the atmosphere. Both elemental and organic Hg compounds pass the blood–brain barrier, and thus can induce central nervous system symptomology. Methyl Hg compounds are particularly dangerous since tissue retention is even longer than for other forms of Hg. As a consequence, elemental and organic Hg compounds need to be handled with extreme caution.

Symptoms of Hg intoxication are varied. They range from excessive salivation and diarrhea to tremors, ataxia, irritability, dizziness, moodiness, and depression. Acute exposure to elemental Hg by inhalation results in pulmonary edema and the symptoms closely resemble influenza. If not immediately fatal, recovery is usually complete. Chronic exposure can lead to symptoms of central nervous system involvement. The character of the Mad Hatter in *Alice in Wonderland* is derived from the fact that hat makers often suffered from neurological disorders resulting from the use of mercuric nitrate to treat felt. Mercury poisoning has also been observed in dental technicians and industrial workers.

Cases of severe Hg poisoning of humans have been described in detail. These include suicide attempts in which mercuric chloride was swallowed. Necrotic areas develop in the mouth, esophagus, and stomach. After a short period of apparent recovery, severe kidney damage ensues, which, if not treated immediately, is fatal. The proximal convuluted tubules are damaged, but the glomeruli are not affected. Nervous symptoms do not occur, but there is some conversion to organic forms. Methyl Hg toxicity was described in a young man who was exposed in an industrial laboratory over a period of several months. There was a gradual loss of eye focus, shortening of attention span, slurred speech followed by an inability to speak at all, impaired mental processes, and tremors. The symptoms grew progressively worse until exposure to methyl Hg was ended. The young man survived but never recovered fully despite intensive therapy.

Mercury poisoning occurred in a farm family from eating meat from a pig contaminated with Hg. The animal had received feed containing grain that had been intended for planting and that had been treated with an organic Hg compound as a fungicide. The children were affected most severely, and there was also damage to the fetus of the pregnant mother. Fetal damage is usually manifested some time after the birth of an apparently healthy baby.

Several epidemic-type outbreaks of organic Hg poisoning have been described in the literature. These have occurred in Pakistan, Guatemala, and Iraq as a result of human consumption of seed grains treated with organic Hg. Minamata disease occurred in Japan as a result of local inhabitants consuming fish and shellfish from Minamata Bay, into which a local plastics factory had been dumping methyl Hg.

Mercury compounds are highly reactive and can interact with various chemical groupings of proteins and nucleic acids. The binding of Hg to sulfhydryl groups of membrane proteins causes an inactivation of membrane ATPase and a blockage of glucose transport into the cell. Mercury also reacts with phosphoryl groups of membranes, sulfhydryl, amino, and carboxyl groups of enzymes, and phosphoryl groups and bases of nucleic acids.

Enzymes that are sulfhydryl dependent are inactivated by Hg, but activity can be restored upon removal of Hg. Mercury is a potent inhibitor of lactate dehydrogenase and fatty acid synthetase. Metabolism of pyruvate in the brain is markedly inhibited by Hg as a result of the reaction of Hg with lipoic acid, pantetheine, and CoA. The derangement of brain pyruvate metabolism mimics the effects of dietary thiamine deficiency.

Mercury has been reported to bind more tightly to metallothionein than either Cd or Zn. It can also react with disulfides to form the S-Hg-S bond in proteins.

Mercuric ion concentrates selectively in lysosomes with a concomitant increase of lysosomal acid phosphatase activity. It has been suggested that much of the cellular toxicity of Hg results from lysosomal damage and the consequent release of hydrolytic enzymes.

17.4.3. Lead

Exposure to Pb takes many forms, in addition to that of industrial hazards. Although Pb intake from paints, water pipes, tin cans, and insecticides has decreased, exposure to other forms of Pb such as in motor vehicle exhausts and tobacco smoke has either stabilized or increased. Intake of Pb paint by children is still a problem in poor urban neighborhoods where Pb-containing painted surfaces still remain. Lead poisoning has been reported in the southern United States as a result of consumption of non-tax-paid, distilled alcoholic beverages commonly known as moonshine whiskey. Old auto radiators, which contain Pb, Cd, and Zn, are often used to distill illegal whiskey. Storage of acidic foods in cans in which solder is exposed or in crockery with Pb-containing glazes has also been reported to result in increased Pb concentration in the food.

Symptoms of Pb poisoning include abdominal pain, anemia, and lesions of the central and peripheral nervous systems. The lesions of the central nervous system cause behavioral problems. The anemia is characterized by a larger than normal number of erythrocytes and is of the hypochromic, microcytic type.

The principal biochemical effect of Pb intoxiciation in humans and animals is defective hemoglobin synthesis. Lead inhibits Fe incorporation into protoporphyrin, which results in lower heme concentrations and higher protoporphyrin concentrations in erythrocytes. Excretion of coproporphyrin is increased, and the Fe content of the blood plasma and bone marrow is elevated. Lead also interferes with an earlier step in heme synthesis by inhibiting δ-aminolevulinic acid dehydratase, which converts δ-aminolevulinic acid to porphobilinogen. The resulting increase of δ-aminolevulinic acid in blood and urine is a sensitive indicator of plumbism. In advanced Pb poisoning, synthesis of the globin moiety of hemoglobin is also inhibited.

The Na, K-APTase of red cell membranes is inhibited by Pb. Serum levels of transaminases and aldolase are increased by Pb exposure, while the serum levels of alkaline phosphatase and cholinesterase are decreased. Lead can also inhibit enzymes with a single, functional sulfhydryl group, but the effect of Pb on sulfhydryl groups is not as marked as that of Hg or Cd.

Lead interferes with tryptophan metabolism, probably by inhibiting monoamine oxidase (MAO). The inhibition of MAO by tetraethyl Pb blocks serotonin catabolism in the brain, and the increased serotonin levels may account for some of the psychological and nerve function impairment.

Suggested Reading

Brown, S. S. (Ed.). Clinical Chemistry and Chemical Toxicology of Metals. Amsterdam: Elsevier, 1977.

Committee on Food Protection, Food and Nutrition Board, National Research Council. Toxicants Occurring Naturally in Foods, second edition. Washington, D. C.: National Academy of Sciences, 1973.

Gerstner, H. B., Huff, J. E. Clinical toxicology of mercury. J. Toxicol. Environ. Health 2 (1977), 491.

Luckey, T. D., Venugopal, B., Hatcheson, D. Heavy Metal Toxicity, Safety, and Hormology. New York: Academic Press, 1975.

Nordberg, G. F. (Ed.). Effects and Dose–Response Relationships of Toxic Metals. Amsterdam: Elsevier, 1976.

Symposium on biological and pharmacological effects of metal contaminants. Fed. Proc. 37 (1977), 15.

Arun P. Kulkarni and
Ernest Hodgson

18

Hepatotoxicity

18.1. Introduction

Man, in his living and working environment, ingests, inhales, and absorbs many chemicals that can impose stress, either subtle or obvious, on numerous biochemical mechanisms. The liver, being the primary site for biotransformation of foreign compounds, is particularly vulnerable to these chemical assaults. Activation of xenobiotics to highly reactive intermediates occurs to such an extent that many of these chemicals are transformed to hepatotoxins, and as such are involved in the etiology and pathogenesis of liver disorders, both carcinogenic and noncarcinogenic. This chapter is restricted to noncarcinogenic responses, of which fatty liver and necrosis are the two most common.

18.2. Fatty Liver

A fatty liver is defined biochemically by a lipid content greater than 5% by weight and histochemically by the presence of an excess of stainable fat. Fatty infiltration in the liver is a common pathological condition resulting from disrupted lipid metabolism. Many xenobiotics, nutritional imbalances, and some diseases cause such abnormal accumulation of fat. In most cases, the lipid that accumulates is composed exclusively of triglycerides.

18.2.1. Triglyceride Cycle

Knowledge of the normal operation of the triglyceride cycle is essential for an understanding of the various mechanisms proposed for the development of fatty liver. Figure 18.1 illustrates this cycle. In brief, albumin-bound free fatty acids are constantly mobilized from adipose tissue and pass, via the blood stream, to the liver, where they are either oxidized or resynthesized to triglycerides. The triglycerides, along with phospholipids, cholesterol, cholesterol esters, and car-

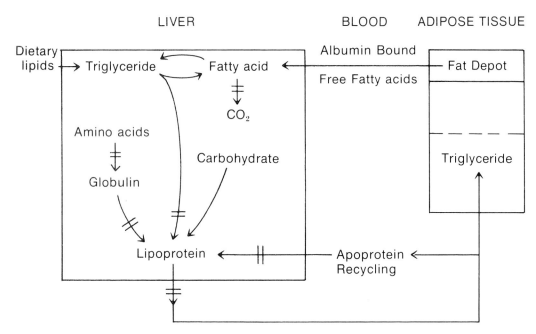

Figure 18.1 Triglyceride cycle in relation to fatty liver genesis. The scheme shows the transport of free fatty acids from fat depot to liver and the return of surplus as triglyceride. Also shown are the metabolic blocks (‡) in hepatotoxicity.

bohydrate, are then combined with carrier globulin to yield very low density lipoprotein (VLDLP). It is in this form that the liver secretes triglycerides into the blood. In addition to this pathway, an auxiliary mechanism exists in which the liver recycles apoprotein used in the production of VLDLP. The enzymes necessary for the synthesis of fatty acids and proteins also exist in the liver. In addition to depot fat, fatty acids may arise from dietary lipids, from carbohydrates, or from amino acids. The level of triglycerides in the liver at any particular time, therefore, reflects a balance between the rates of exogenous supply and endogenous fatty acid synthesis on the one hand, and the rates of free fatty acid oxidation and triglyceride secretion from the liver on the other.

18.2.2. Mechanisms of Fatty Liver Production

Although lipid accumulation is a common parameter in all fatty livers, the underlying biochemical events may differ widely with various causative agents. Several mechanisms have been proposed but there have been few decisive conclusions.

18.2.2a. Oversupply of Free Fatty Acids to the Liver

This seems to be a major mechanism in fatty liver induced by carbon tetrachloride, ethionine or phosphorus. These agents trigger lipolysis in the adipose tissue and cause a dramatic increase in circulating free fatty acids (FFA). Under these conditions all the enzymes of the triglyceride cycle are saturated and triglycerides accumulate in the liver. Presumably, the rate-limiting step is the synthesis of VLDLP for transport from the liver. Mobilization of depot fat from adipose tissue is under the control of the pituitary–adrenal axis, the stimulation of which triggers massive release of catecholamines, leading to liberation of large quantities of FFA. Physical stress such as noise or hypoxia as well as the chemical stress of DDT, nicotine, or hydrazines also stimulate this system. This hormonal mechanism is said to be operative in the genesis of fatty liver in starved animals given a large dose of ethanol, but it appears to be of minor importance in the oversupply of FFA in carbon tetrachloride poisoning.

18.2.2b. Interference with the Triglyceride Cycle

Any interference with the synthesis of apoprotein or phospholipid, and possibly of fatty acid, cholesterol, cholesterol esters, or the carbohydrate moiety of VLDLP may be implicated in the genesis of fatty liver. This type of liver lesion has been extensively studied and includes that evoked by ethionine, carbon tetrachloride, orotic acid, phosphorus, cerium acid salts, puromycin, and other agents.

Increased synthesis and esterification of hepatic fatty acids. Several studies in vitro and in vivo have shown that alcohol causes a shift in the redox potential with a concurrent rise in hepatic NADH. A concomitant stimulation of synthesis, chain elongation, and esterification of FFA to form triglycerides has also been observed. However, the significance of these findings is doubtful since pretreatment with pyrazole, a known inhibitor of alcohol dehydrogenase, does not always prevent fatty liver formation.

Decreased fatty acid oxidation. Because fatty acids are a major source of energy for the liver, interference with their oxidation via the tricarboxylic acid cycle may play a major role in the genesis of some forms of fatty liver. In fact, several studies have established the fact that this metabolic route is severely impaired following alcohol administration, the key events being the inhibition of citrate synthetase and isocitrate dehydrogenase due to the alcohol-induced change in the redox potential.

Decreased apoprotein synthesis. The normal hepatic endoplasmic reticulum is very active in protein synthesis and also participates in VLDLP assembly. In ethionine-intoxicated female rats, a dramatic drop in the hepatic ATP level is observed. Ethionine acts as an adenosyl trap, and its toxicity is reversed by treatment with adenine. Based on these observations, the chain of events was thought to be low ATP leading to depressed apoprotein synthesis, reduced VLDLP level, and triglyceride accumulation. Electron microscopic examination of livers from animals treated with either ethionine or carbon tetrachloride shows a pronounced detachment of ribosomes from the endoplasmic reticulum. The intoxicated animals also exhibit a marked depression in their capacity to incorporate ^{14}C-amino acids into liver proteins. Thus, in ethionine poisoning, a low ATP level causes a block in mRNA synthesis, leading to ribosome breakup and diminished apoprotein synthesis. In the case of carbon tetrachloride, it has been claimed that microsomal lipid peroxidation is linked to the inhibition of protein synthesis, polyribosomal dispersion, and fatty liver genesis. If this hypothesis, involving inhibition of protein synthesis, is generally applicable, all inhibitors of protein synthesis would be expected to produce fatty livers. Although puromycin treatment does cause fatty liver, doses of cycloheximide that inhibit protein synthesis do not. Likewise, actinomycin D, which blocks mRNA synthesis, does not cause fatty infiltration in hepatocytes.

Decreased very low density lipoprotein synthesis and secretion. An inadequate supply of choline and other components limits VLDLP synthesis. This, and possible abnormalities induced in the phospholipid-rich cell membranes, may result in impaired lipid metabolism leading to triglyceride accumulation. Interestingly, it is not apoprotein synthesis but a failure in VLDLP assembly that probably constitutes the key biochemical derangement responsible for fatty liver development in orotic acid and yellow phosphorus poisoning. Impairment of the contractile system has also been considered as a possible contributory factor in the genesis of fatty liver. It is generally considered that contraction of intracellular contractile proteins is governed by local cAMP levels. At high concentrations, contraction is restricted, hindering the intracellular movement of VLDLP and its components, while at low levels the opposite effects are produced. During the early hours of carbon tetrachloride poisoning, cAMP and the cAMP/cGMP ratios increase significantly, possibly creating blockage in the intracellular movement of VLDLP.

In carbon tetrachloride and orotic acid hepatotoxicity, the hepatic secretory mechanism whereby triglycerides are transported from the liver for general circulation is severely and rapidly depressed. Although defective operation of the secretory mechanism contributes to fatty liver genesis, this effect may be related to lipoprotein synthesis.

Inhibition of the auxiliary mechanism. The normal operation of the liver VLDLP secretory process requires an intact auxiliary mechanism, which recycles the apoprotein moiety from the plasma for lipoprotein resynthesis in the liver. A block in this pathway may also contribute to excessive fat infiltration in the carbon tetrachloride–poisoned liver. In addition to this direct effect, a similar response is also exerted by low hepatic potassium ion content. In ethionine poisoning, low ATP levels cause hepatocytes to lose potassium, ultimately resulting in a 50–70% reduction in the rate of serum apoprotein transfer across the liver cell membranes. This defect can be reversed quickly when potassium levels are restored by the administration of adenine.

Lipid peroxidation. The role of lipid peroxidation in ethanol-induced fatty liver has been a subject of debate. Interpretations are complicated by differences in experimental design, dose, duration of treatment, nutritional status of the animals, and other factors. Evidence for ethane evolution in ethanol-treated animals and protection from ethanol-induced fatty liver by antioxidants has been presented. In general, in acute ethanol poisoning, mitochondria show more damage and accumulate more conjugated dienes than do microsomes, while prolonged treatment causes high lipid peroxidation in microsomes. However, in choline-deficient animals and those poisoned with orotic acid, lipid peroxidation is not considered to be the primary reason for the initiation of fatty liver. Yellow phosphorus poisoning is very similar to that from carbon tetrachloride, in that the conjugated dienes appear quickly in the endoplasmic reticulum, whereas mitochondria are affected later.

18.3. Liver Necrosis

Liver necrosis, strictly defined, signifies only the death of hepatocytes. The underlying biochemical lesion is the inhibition of one or more essential metabolic processes in the hepatocyte, such as severe inhibition of RNA, DNA, and/or protein synthesis resulting from nuclear and endoplasmic reticulum damage, disruption of mitochondrial energy generation and control, damage to lysosomes causing autolysis, depletion of ATP and uridine 5-triphosphate, or drastic shifts in the Na^+ and K^+ balance between hepatocytes and blood. Any of these events may contribute to cell death. Liver necrosis is an advanced and usually irreversible stage of degeneration and is characterized by the presense of cell fragments or dead hepatocytes without nuclear staining. Due to a lack of suitable methods to detect the precise moment of cell death, our present knowledge of the mechanisms of cell death is less than complete. A large number of chemicals induce liver necrosis, and, depending upon the time elapsed since exposure to the hepatotoxicant, necrosis may be either localized or involve the entire liver.

18.3.1. Mechanism of Liver Necrosis

18.3.1a. Mitochondrial Damage

Mitochondrial destruction was first believed to be the primary event in the genesis of liver necrosis induced by carbon tetrachloride. Uncoupling of oxidative phosphorylation in mitochondria occurs rather early and leads to a significant ATP depletion. However, more drastic ATP depletion is observed in ethionine poisoning without any liver necrosis. The possibility that Ca^{2+} acts as a killing agent was suggested on the basis of a very early rise in liver Ca^{2+} seen in carbon tetrachloride poisoning. In vitro, mitochondria take up excess Ca^{2+} from the incubation medium, eventually causing irreversible membrane changes and destruction of the mitochondria. The changes in hepatic Ca^{2+} levels are typical only of carbon tetrachloride poisoning and are not detected with other necrogenic agents such as thioacetamide and pyrrolizidine alkaloids. Since the endoplasmic reticulum is affected much earlier in carbon tetrachloride poisoning, damage to mitochondria is now considered less crucial in the genesis of necrosis.

18.3.1b. Lysosomal Enzymes

The release of latent enzymes due to lysosomal damage has been suggested as a mechanism of cell death. However, this response is also observed in ethionine poisoning without necrosis. Lysosomal enzymes cannot be considered of primary importance in initiating cell death since, with many hepatotoxicants, their liberation occurs at a very late stage of poisoning.

18.3.1c. Inhibition of Protein Synthesis

Protein synthesis is inhibited by agents causing damage to the endoplasmic reticulum and nucleus, thus blocking RNA, DNA, and protein synthesis. Although impaired liver regeneration and an inadequate supply of vital enzymes may be necrogenic, discrepancies often exist between the time of inhibition of protein synthesis and the onset of necrosis. For example, amanitin blocks RNA polymerase II in the nucleus within a few minutes, whereas necrosis does not appear until several hours later. With carbon tetrachloride, cell death occurs much earlier, but inhibition of protein synthesis is not so profound. Furthermore, pretreatment with cycloheximide affords protection against necrosis evoked by carbon tetrachloride and other poisons. These observations clearly suggest that impairment of protein synthesis is not the primary biochemical lesion causing cell death.

18.3.1d. Binding to Macromolecules

In recent years, it has become increasingly clear that hepatic xenobiotic metabolism in vivo does not always lead to the formation of chemically inert or easily excretable products, but may yield reactive alkylating, arylating, or acylating derivatives capable of covalent binding to tissue macromolecules. Those entities with relatively low reactivity tend to bind to specific tissue receptor sites, first combining reversibly to form a complex, which in turn rearranges to form a covalently bound conjugate. Highly reactive entities, on the other hand, bind indiscriminately to intracellular components such as protein, lipid, glycogen, RNA, DNA, and many smaller molecules.

Presumably, as soon as a covalent complex is formed, it triggers one or more mechanisms that cause functional impairments. The resulting damage may be localized and specific, such as destruction of cytochrome P-450 in the endoplasmic reticulum, or in severe cases it may lead to cell death. Investigations on halogenated benzenes, furosemide, acetaminophen, α-methyl dopa and other hepatotoxins have clearly shown a direct correlation between the magnitude of covalent binding and the incidence and severity of liver necrosis.

Although quantitation of covalent binding seems to be a simple measure of hepatotoxicity, great caution should be exercised as several factors govern the ultimate toxic effects of such chemicals. In any event, covalent binding is not the primary cause of cell death, although it is intimately related to it.

18.3.1e. Lipid Peroxidation

Lipid peroxidation is a unique form of cellular injury implicated in the genesis of the liver necrosis evoked by hepatotoxicants such as carbon tetrachloride and yellow phosphorus. It is multiphasic and involves initiation, propagation, and termination reactions (Figure 18.2). The hydrogen atoms on methylene carbons separating double bonds in polyenoic fatty acids are highly susceptible to free radical attack. The abstraction of hydrogen from unsaturated fatty acids during this attack yields free radicals of lipids, and this represents the initiation of lipid peroxidation. The mechanism of initiation of lipid peroxidation is still not fully understood. Its promotion by oxygen, singlet oxygen, hydroxyl radical,

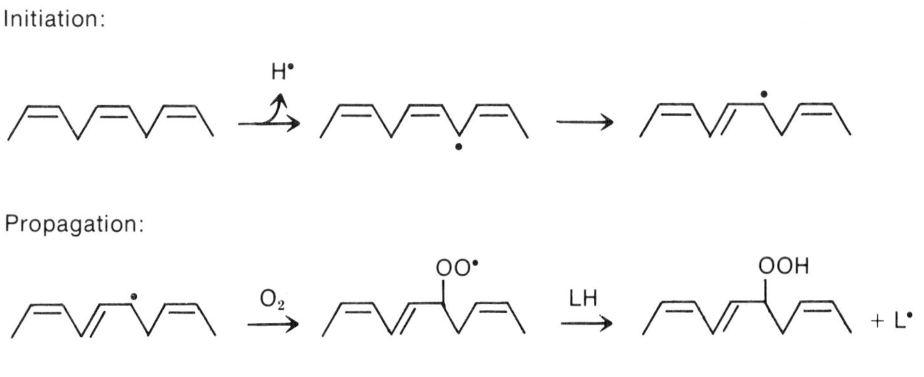

Initiation:

Propagation:

Termination:

$$L^\bullet + L^\bullet \rightarrow \text{nonradical products}$$
$$L^\bullet + LO_2^\bullet \rightarrow \text{nonradical products}$$
$$LO_2^\bullet + LO_2^\bullet \rightarrow \text{nonradical products}$$

LH = polyunsaturated lipid; $L^\bullet$ = lipid radical; $LO_2^\bullet$ = lipid peroxy radical

Figure 18.2 Initiation, propagation, and termination reactions in lipid peroxidation.
SOURCE: *Bus and Gibson, Rev. Biochem. Toxicol. 1 (1979) 125.*

superoxide anion, or some form of perferryl ion have all been proposed by some and disputed by others. Free radicals generated during the metabolism of various chemicals have also been suggested as initiators.

The free radicals generated from fatty acids are unstable and undergo a series of transformations, including shifting of double bonds to give the diene configuration. The free radicals react rapidly with molecular oxygen to form organic peroxy free radicals. The peroxy free radicals from one fatty acid chain abstract methylene hydrogen of a neighboring unsaturated fatty acid, yielding one hydroperoxide and one new radical. This autocatalytic chain reaction represents the propagation step in which there is a linear spread of lipid peroxidation. The unstable hydroperoxides decompose to form additional free radicals. When substrate is depleted, termination reactions are initiated, yielding nonradical products that stop the lipid peroxidation process.

Subcellular membranes rich in unsaturated fatty acids are the obvious targets of lipid peroxidation, resulting in the loss of both structural integrity and function in the affected organelles. In addition to this localized damage, the breakdown products of lipid peroxides, such as aldehydes, migrate far from their production site and may cause damage at distant loci. Several lipid peroxides are known for their extremely high toxicity. However, recent findings that stable products of lipid peroxidation, and not the binding of the $\cdot CCl_3$ radical, may be responsible for the major damage caused in carbon tetrachloride poisoning (as evidenced by lysis of red blood cells) support this view.

The evidence against the lipid peroxidation hypothesis in carbon tetrachloride hepatotoxicity includes the fact that, unlike α-tocopherol and phenothiazines, promethazine (a potent antioxidant) is not much more effective than such nonantioxidant stabilizers as diphenylhydramine. Chloramphenicol antagonizes carbon tetrachloride hepatotoxicity in vivo by inhibiting lipid peroxidation. However, it fails to restore cytochrome P-450 levels. Some unexpected results reported recently are noteworthy. Pretreatment with pyrazole or aminotriazole partially protected liver by inhibiting either $CCl_4 \rightarrow CCl_3$ conversion or lipid peroxidation. Although neither of these processes were affected by ethyl (2-diethylaminoethyl)-2-phenyl-2-ethylmalonate, they effectively prevented liver injury by reducing the susceptibility of hepatocytes, if given prior to carbon tetrachloride but not later. The ability of SKF-525A, cysteine, and cystamine to reduce the extent of carbon tetrachloride–induced necrosis when given as late as 12 hr after carbon tetrachloride is surprising. The investigators consider that the beneficial effects of these compounds is produced by exerting an effect on some processes that must be critical for cell death.

Furthermore, in view of the prooxidant property of carbon tetrachloride, other related halogenated hydrocarbons that also produce liver necrosis have been examined for their prooxidant capacity. In contrast to carbon tetrachloride, 1,1-dichloroethylene and chloroform failed to stimulate lipid peroxidation either in vivo or in vitro. Ethylene dibromide, although it causes triglyceride accumulation with the appearance of conjugated dienes in vivo, does not act as a prooxidant in vitro. Similarly, thioacetamide and halothane, which produce liver necrosis in vivo, fail to stimulate lipid peroxidation in vitro.

Lipid peroxidation, which had come to be considered a universal concomitant of cellular injury, does not seem to be involved in many cases. There are several possibilities that should be taken into account before the dismissal of the lipid peroxidation hypothesis, however. Lack of evidence for conjugated dienes in vivo may indicate only that the products of lipid peroxidation are metabolized further at a rate too rapid to permit their accumulation and detection by the tests employed. The new technique in which in vivo rates of lipid peroxidation are examined by monitoring the evolution of ethane seems to offer a better solution to this yet unsolved problem. Changes in glutathione peroxidase and antioxidant activities of the tissues, which considerably modify in vivo lipid peroxidation rates, must also be examined before meaningful conclusions can be drawn.

18.4. Compounds Causing Liver Damage

A wide range of naturally occurring and synthetic chemicals are known to be hepatotoxicants. A few of these are listed in Table 18.1. The plant species yielding hepatotoxins include *Lantana camara, Sassafras albidum,* more than 200 species of *Crotalaria,* and a large number of species of the genera *Senecis, Heliotropium, Cyanoglossum,* and *Trichoderma.* In addition to the alkaloids from these plants, the hepatotoxic effects of tannins, phallotoxin, and amatoxin from poisonous mushrooms are also known. Several metabolic products of bacteria and fungi cause similar liver injury. Cases of hepatotoxicity caused by some inorganic chemicals, including phosphorus, colloidal gold, selenium, lead, uranium nitrate, ferrous sulfate, and cobalt salts, have been reported infrequently in humans and farm animals.

In addition to these, several industrial solvents and raw materials, organophosphorus pesticides, and other agents have been implicated in

Table 18.1 Examples of Hepatotoxic Agents

Drugs	*Natural products*
Acetaminophen	Furosemide
Diphenyl hydantoin	Furans
Iproniazid	Amanitin
Chlorpromazine	Colchicine
Isoniazid	
Phenothiazines	*Antibiotics*
Sulfonamides	Tetracycline
Methyl dopa	Erythromycin
Anabolic steroids	Terramycin
Halogenated chemicals	*Other chemicals*
Carbon tetrachloride	Ethionine
Trichloroethylene	Ethanol
Chloroform	Carbon disulfide
Bromotrichloromethane	Inorganic phosphorus
Halothane	Organophosphates
Bromobenzene	Cobalt salts
Lindane	Organic and inorganic selenium compounds

hepatotoxicity (Table 18.1). The list of drugs that are potential hepatotoxins is large and continues to grow almost daily. Several therapeutic agents used as anesthetics, tranquilizers, antidepressants, anticonvulsants, antimicrobial agents, or antituberculosis drugs, as well as some prescribed in cardiovascular, nervous, endocrine, rheumatic, and neoplastic diseases have been found to

Based on the mechanisms of injury, hepatotoxicants have been classified either as intrinsic or host idiosyncratic (see Zimmerman[1] for detailed classification and examples). The type of injury inflicted by agents of either group may be either cytotoxic (leading to necrosis) or cholestatic (producing fatty liver), or mixed. Intrinsic toxicants may be subdivided into direct and indirect classes.

The direct toxicants are cytotoxic agents that damage other organs besides the liver. In the liver, their attack tends to involve all of the subcellular organelles. Typically, they require brief exposure, and dose-dependent injury can be observed with experimental reproducibility and a high incidence rate in a variety of animal species. Examples of this class include carbon tetrachloride, chlorinated hydrocarbons, and some metals. They all cause necrosis usually, accompanied by steatosis.

Indirect hepatotoxins bring about dose-dependent liver injury by creating malfunctions in specific metabolic routes. Thus, in contrast to direct toxicants, they are selective in action. Not only do they require longer exposure, but the results are less reproducible. Hepatocyte injury may lead to either necrosis or fatty liver. Ethanol, tetracyclins, puromycin, cancer therapeutic agents, urethane, tannic acid, C-17-alkylated anabolic and contraceptive steroids belong to this class.

---

[1] Zimmerman, H. J. Hepatic injury caused by therapeutic agents. In Becker, F. F. (Ed.), The Liver: Normal and Abnormal Functions, Part A. New York: Marcel Dekker, 1974, p. 225.

Such classifications are of limited value since a more or less continuous spectrum of types of damage appears to be evident.

The postulated types of host idiosyncrasy that cause liver injury include hypersensitivity or allergic reactions and aberrant metabolism. This type of liver injury is observed only in uniquely susceptible individuals and has been reported with chlorpromazine, sulfonamides, hydrazine derivatives, and other drugs.

18.5. Role of Toxicant Biotransformation in Hepatotoxicity

18.5.1. Metabolism of Toxicants

Most hepatotoxicants are biologically inert per se. They are converted to highly reactive hepatotoxic products primarily by the liver microsomal mixed-function oxidase system. This system consists of the terminal oxidase cytochrome P-450 and a flavoprotein NADPH–cytochrome P-450 reductase, an enzyme required for the transfer of electrons from NADPH to the hemoprotein. Substrate oxidation requires the presence of molecular oxygen and NADPH (see Chapter 4).

The formation of reactive metabolites from the administered toxicant was first suspected from their covalent binding to subcellular components. Further credence was obtained from in vivo studies in which metabolic rates were altered by pretreatment with known inducers or inhibitors of the mixed-function oxidase system. The resulting change in the magnitude of covalent binding correlated with changes in the incidence and severity of liver damage. The fact that newborn animals and adults on hypoproteic diets exhibit tolerance to hepatotoxicants can be correlated with the fact that metabolism of xenobiotics is low or absent because of the depressed levels of mixed-function oxidase activity in these animals. Chickens do not metabolize carbon tetrachloride either in vivo or in vitro and are insensitive to carbon tetrachloride hepatotoxicity. It is now clearly established that biotransformation of the parent compound is the initial biochemical event in the development of hepatotoxicity.

The synthesis of reactive metabolites in biological systems occurs by a variety of mechanisms. The necessary evidence, either direct or indirect, for the production of such reactive species and their implication in triggering mechanisms leading to liver injury has been presented for a number of chemicals. These reactive species include the following: $\cdot CCl_3$ radicals produced by the homolytic cleavage of carbon tetrachloride and bromotrichloromethane; reactive epoxides from the epoxidation of halogenated benzenes; polycyclic hydrocarbons and furan derivatives; N-hydroxyacetoaminophen and/or N-acetylbenzoquinoimine from the oxidation of acetaminophen; chloroethylene oxide or chloroacetaldehyde resulting from oxidation of vinyl chloride; phosgene from chloroform; 2,2,3-trichlorooxirane from trichloroethylene oxidation; acetyl radicals or acetylonium ions generating from N-hydroxy intermediates of hydrazines; quinones from oxidation of α-methyl dopa; pyrrole derivative resulting from dehydrogenation of pyrrolizidine alkaloids; atomic sulfur released during oxidative desulfuration of carbon disulfide, phosphorothionate insecticides, and others. In all of these cases, the microsomal mixed-function oxidase system plays a central role in generating the reactive hepatotoxins. Several other mechanisms have also been shown to be operative in the process of bioactivation. For example, metabolites of various amines are further activated by their conversion to N-O-sulfate or N-O-phosphate esters. Similarly, nitroaryl compounds, including nitroquinoline, nitrofurazone, and nitrofurantoin, may be reduced by several different enzymes to toxic electrophiles.

Several haloalkanes are metabolized by the microsomal mixed-function oxidase system, but at different rates. It is noteworthy that both the rate of metabolism and liver toxicity depend upon the value of the bond dissociation energy. Thus, bromotrichloromethane, which has a bond dissociation energy lower than that of carbon tetrachloride, is cleaved more rapidly and is therefore a more potent hepatotoxicant, where as chloroform, which has a much higher bond dissociation energy, is less easily cleaved and is therefore less toxic.

Pretreatment with Arochlor 1254 (a polychlorinated biphenyl mixture) has recently been shown to cause relatively low doses of halogenated ethylenes to become hepatotoxic. The acute toxicity of unsubstituted ethylene plus Arochlor 1254 and the lack of effect of ethane plus Arochlor 1254 indicates the importance of the double bond in these toxic interactions. The fact that differences in substituents modify potency can be seen in the bromobenzenes. Based on histological examination and serum glutamate–pyruvate transaminase levels 24 hr after administration of the test compound in sesame oil, it was shown that bromobenzenes bearing electron-withdrawing substituents at the ortho position are very potent hepatotoxicants. Those with electron-releasing substituents are less toxic, and substituents with a less pronounced electronic character elicit an intermediate response.

Reactive intermediates are, in general, considered responsible for hepatic injury. However, the widely accepted role of the $\cdot CCl_3$ radical in carbon tetrachloride–induced liver toxicity has recently been challenged. Since highly reactive species usually have extremely short biological half-lives, theoretically they cannot be transported to distant loci to exert their toxic action, and therefore damage arising from such entities could only be localized. Incubation of carbon tetrachloride with NADPH-supplemented microsomes in the presence of EDTA inhibits lipid peroxidation yet permits carbon tetrachloride metabolism. Although production of $\cdot CCl_3$ proceeds, there is no destruction of cytochrome P-450, which occurs extensively in the absence of EDTA. Furthermore, large quantities of some product(s) of lipid peroxidation have been shown to leak out of microsomes into the medium. The hemolytic agent in peroxidized microsomes can survive sedimentation, extraction with organic solvents, and drying and reconstitution procedures, and therefore is unlikely to be a free radical.

18.5.2. Modification of Metabolism

Because hepatic injury results when an accumulation of toxic metabolites overwhelms the capacity of the detoxication pathways, a deliberate alteration in the balance of toxication–detoxication mechanisms induced by chemical pretreatment should yield valuable information. Such techniques have in fact been successful in (a) demonstrating the importance of bioactivation and covalent binding, (b) evaluating the relative importance of various metabolic pathways, and (c) elucidating the underlying biochemical mechanisms in the genesis of hepatotoxicity. These experiments have also provided a sound basis for the design of reliable diagnostic tests as well as the development of appropriate therapeutic procedures.

Over 200 chemicals are known to be inducers of the hepatic microsomal mixed-function oxidase system, but, except for phenobarbital, little is known about the alterations in hepatotoxicity they induce. Phenobarbital treatment causes a large increase in the amount of microsomal cytochrome P-450 and other components of the mixed-function oxidase system. This increase accelerates biotransformation rates and usually reduces the biological half-life of the administered chemical. Thus, it has been claimed that the intensified hepatotoxicity of carbon tetrachloride, bromotrichloromethane, carbon disulfide, bromobenzenes, halogenated ethylenes, halothane, acetaminophen, isoniazid, trielin, and pyrrolizidine alkaloids seen in phenobarbital-pretreated animals is due to the increased production of toxic metabolites and/or increased covalent binding. In addition to phenobarbital, pretreatment of animals with ethanol, isopropanol, DDT, or lindane synergizes liver injury evoked by carbon tetrachloride.

However, observations of apparently anomalous effects have revealed that the enzymatic and pharmacokinetic relationships are not necessarily straightforward. For instance, pretreatment of mice with phenobarbital increases their susceptibility to liver necrosis induced by acetaminophen but has little effect on the metabolic clearance of the drug in vivo. In contrast, phenobarbital pretreatment of hamsters accelerates acetaminophen metabolism in vivo but has little or no effect on its hepatotoxicity.

It has been suggested that epoxidation of the furan ring of the hepatotoxicant furosemide is an activation step. Phenobarbital administration causes a shift in the zone of necrosis produced by furosemide and hydroxymethylfuran from centrilobular–midzonal to entirely midzonal without increasing the size of the necrotic area. A similar effect of phenobarbital administration on hepatic necrosis produced by ngaione, a furanosesquiterpene, has also been reported. In both cases it appears that phenobarbital induced both detoxication and intoxication pathways. This view is further supported by the fact that phenobarbital greatly enhances covalent binding of furosemide to hepatic microsomes in vitro but not in vivo.

Ethylene and its halogenated derivatives, such as vinyl chloride, are hepatotoxic only at very high doses. However, pretreatment of animals with Arochlor 1254 significantly elevates serum alanine-α-ketoglutarate transaminase and produces severe degeneration and necrosis of the liver.

In contrast to phenobarbital-type inducers, pretreatment with polycyclic hydrocarbons induces synthesis of a different species of cytochrome P-450 (cytochrome P-448) without significant alteration in NADPH–cytochrome P-450 reductase activity. Some of the results reported with this class of inducer are not easily explained. For example, 3-methylcholanthrene pretreatment provides protection against the deleterious effects of carbon tetrachloride, whereas administration of 3,4-benzpyrene enhances carbon tetrachloride–induced hepatotoxicity. A shift in the metabolic pattern may also be observed. Pretreatment with 3-methylcholanthrene induces the formation of the relatively nontoxic 2,3-bromobenzene oxide from bromobenzene via an alternative oxidative pathway, while the production of the hepatotoxic metabolite 3,4-bromobenzene oxide is reduced. In addition, the detoxication enzyme epoxide hydrase is also induced. Thus, both of these factors contribute to the protection from bromobenzene toxicity by 3-methylcholanthrene.

Several inhibitors of the microsomal mixed-function oxidase system are known to afford protection against the deleterious effects of hepatotoxicants. This protection is brought about either by depressing the level of hepatic microsomal cytochrome P-450, e.g., with cobaltous chloride, or by rendering the mixed-function oxidase system nonfunctional by forming irreversible complexes with cytochrome P-450, e.g., with piperonyl butoxide or SKF-525A. As a result, lower amounts of injurious metabolites are formed in vivo, reducing both covalent binding and the incidence and severity of poisoning.

In this way cobaltous chloride pretreatment decreases carbon tetrachloride binding to liver proteins and lipids and lowers its toxicity. Similar protection from the hepatotoxicity of acetaminophen and hydrazine derivatives has also been reported. Piperonyl butoxide also reduces the toxicity of acetaminophen and hydrazines. Aminotriazole protects from carbon tetrachloride, acetylhydrazine, and isopropylhydrazine toxicity, probably by inhibiting catalase in peroxisomes. Cycloheximide induces hypothermia, reduces binding, and prevents polysome dispersion in carbon tetrachloride poisoning. SKF-525A protects from the toxicity of orally administered carbon tetrachloride, but not from that administered by inhalation, indicating possible interference in absorption. Similarly, α-naphthyl isothiocyanate prevents covalent binding and liver necrosis by acetaminophen. Protection against hepatotoxicity by small doses of either carbon tetrachloride, ethanol, or phenobarbital administered just prior to carbon tetrachloride treatment has also been reported. In the case of carbon tetrachloride, induction of a cytosolic inhibitor of lipid peroxidation may be an additional protective mechanism. Similarly, prior exposure of animals to vinyl chloride protects against a subsequent toxic dose of vinyl chloride.

Pretreatment with diethyl maleate, a compound that drastically depletes the level of glutathione in the liver, intensifies the toxicity of both acetaminophen and bromobenzene by reducing detoxication based on glutathione S-transferases. According to a recent report this compound also stimulates mixed-function oxidase activity by an unknown mechanism, and therefore its synergistic effect may be due, in part, to increased production of toxic metabolites. Conversely, supplementation of protective mechanisms by glutathione, L-cysteine, methionine, and cystamine lowers hepatotoxicity. Antioxidants such as α-tocopherol, silymarin, catechol, and pyrogallol derivatives all provide protection against hepatotoxicity to a varying degree. Some of these chemicals and diethyldithiocarbamate reduce carbon tetrachloride hepatotoxicity by inhibiting lipid peroxidation in vivo. Both selenium and phenazine methosulfate protect against carbon tetrachloride toxicity. Salicylamide suppresses glucuronidation and sulfation activities, with a resultant increase in the biological half-life of acetaminophen. This increased proportion of dose metabolized by the intoxication pathways results in severe liver necrosis.

18.6. Effects of Hepatotoxicants on Liver Function

In addition to the various biochemical mechanisms of hepatotoxicity previously discussed, several other alterations in the normal metabolic functioning of the liver occur during the course of poisoning by hepatotoxicants.

Relatively few investigations have been carried out on the effects of hepatotoxicants on the microsomal electron transport system. Carbon tetrachloride, the only well-studied chemical in this respect, stimulates lipid peroxidation in hepatic microsomes in vivo as well as in vitro. As a result, cytochrome P-450 and the heme content of microsomes is drastically reduced. However, the level of microsomal cytochrome B_5 and the activities of NADH–ferricyanide dehydrogenase and NAD(P)H–cytochrome C reductase are not affected. Microsomal glucose 6-phosphatase and inorganic pyrophosphatase show a dramatic reduction in their activities. No alteration in epoxide hydrase activity is usually noticed; however, a stimulatory effect on UDP glucuronyltransferase and monoesterase is observed. This effect may be due to partial dissolution of microsomal membranes exposing the active sites of these enzymes. A concurrent rapid decay of drug-metabolizing capacity is reflected in the very low turnover numbers of mixed-function oxidase enzymes in microsomes isolated from the livers of carbon tetrachloride–treated animals. Thus, a significant reduction in the N-demethylation of aminopyrine and ethylmorphine, deethylation of 7-ethoxycoumarin, and hydroxylation of zoxazolamine and aniline is seen.

In phenobarbital-pretreated rats, trichloroethylene causes a significant depression of both cytochrome P-450 and cytochrome b_5. Interestingly, NADH–but not NADPH–cytochrome C reductase activity increases more than threefold, while glucose-6-phosphatase is unaffected. In contrast to vinyl chloride, trichloroethylene administration to phenobarbital-pretreated rats does not cause alterations in the N-demethylation of aminopyrine and ethylmorphine or the hydroxylation of zoxazolamine.

Some hepatotoxicants cause marked swelling as well as eventual rupture of subcellular organelles other than the endoplasmic reticulum, such as mitochondria, lysosomes, and nuclei. These events ultimately lead to either activation, inactivation, or leakage of the enzymes contained within them. Thus, the release of acid phosphatase, β-glucuronidase, and other hydrolases from lysosomes, tricarboxylic acid cycle enzymes from mitochondria, etc., is known to occur in the liver of poisoned animals.

The efflux of enzymes of either subcellular organelle or cytosolic origin from hepatocytes, either by simple diffusion or filtration, is reflected in their sudden increase in the blood. Therefore, the measurement of serum enzyme levels has proven to be a sensitive index of hepatotoxicity. These serological tests not only help to locate an organ lesion but can also help to identify the subcellular site of damage. Such diagnostic tests include the estimation of one or more of the following enzymes in blood serum: alkaline phosphatase, 5-nucleotidase, leucine aminopeptidase, glutamyl transpeptidase, isoenzymes of lactate dehydrogenase (LDH_5), isocitrate dehydrogenase, malate dehydrogenase, sorbitol dehydrogenase, alcohol dehydrogenase, fructose mono- or diphosphate aldolase, arginase, quinine oxidase, β-hydroxybutyrate dehydrogenase, glutamic pyruvic transaminase, and glutamic oxaloacetic transaminase. More then 24 serum enzymes have been studied in relation to carbon tetrachloride–induced hepatotoxicity.

A recent report describes an 11-fold increase in rat serum glutathione S-transferase 24 hr after carbon tetrachloride exposure. There was a simultaneous decrease in the hepatic cytosolic glutathione S-transferase activity, suggesting that most of the serum enzyme activity was due to enzyme leakage from the liver, and that changes in this enzyme could also be included in serological testing.

Other tests of importance in hepatotoxicity include determinations of the serum γ globulin level and/or albumin/globulin ratios, and the hepatic uptake, storage, and excretion of sulfobromophthalein.

It is noteworthy that carbon tetrachloride induces synthesis of a lipid peroxidation inhibitor in liver cytosol. However, the level of induction is the same at low as well as high carbon tetrachloride doses, probably due to inhibition of de novo protein synthesis. No significant change in liver cytosolic DT-diaphorase activity by allyl alcohol, or in glutathione reductase by carbon tetrachloride, has been noted, but a decreased in glutathione peroxidase follows carbon tetrachloride treatment. In contrast to phenobarbital, exposure to carbon disulfide or cobaltous chloride causes an increased utilization of orotic acid for cytidine nucleotide synthesis and a decreased level of microsomal cytochrome P-450. A number of reports have shown that halogenated hydrocarbons produce an increase in "bile duct–pancreatic fluid" flow by an unknown mechanism, although this phenomenon is presumed to be unrelated to the genesis of hepatic necrosis. Hepatotoxicants such as ethionine, carbon disulfide, carbon tetrachloride, and others cause a loss of control of the hepatocyte permeability mechanism, which results in an increase in hepatocyte water content and abnormal flux of Na^+, K^+, and Cu^{3+} ions between blood and liver.

18.7. Protective Mechanisms

Several mechanisms have evolved that appear to have a protective function in hepatotoxicity; as a result, the generation of free radicals does not always lead to hepatotoxicity nor to pathologically disturbed intermediary metabolism, under these circumstances free radical generation is a normal consequence of naturally occurring electron transport. In the body, intoxiciation and detoxication mechanisms appear to be very delicately balanced, and the same metabolic intermediates may be formed after nontoxic, as well as toxic, doses. However, covalent binding and hepatotoxicity result at doses at which this balance is disturbed by the formation of toxic metabolites to an extent that exceeds the capacity of the detoxication system.

The superoxide anion free radical has been implicated by some authors as the active species that causes peroxidative damage to red blood cells as well as lipid peroxidation. It is also believed that superoxide dismutase affords protection by elimination of this radical. Similarly, the autocatalytic progression of lipid peroxidation can be halted or contained by glutathione peroxidase, which catalyzes the rapid conversion of lipid hydroperoxides to their corresponding alcohols. In addition, liver cytosol contains an inhibitor of lipid peroxidation, and this factor is inducible. Several reactive arene oxides are susceptible to detoxication by epoxide hydrase to yield nontoxic metabolites. Glutathione S-transferases, which are very active in the liver and are also present in several other organs, conjugate a wide range of toxic chemicals and remove them from target sites as readily excretable products. Conjugation with sulfates, phosphates, amino acids, glucuronic acid, etc. is yet another mechanism for the elimination of toxic radicals from the body. In addition to these enzymatic controls, the body also contains several antioxidants and trapping agents, such as glutathione, cysteine, ascorbate, α-tocopherol, viatmin K, and serum albumin, which minimize cellular damage and preserve the functional integrity of cells.

18.8 Conclusions

Much is known about the biochemical toxicology of hepatotoxicants, yet much remains to be learned. Hepatotoxicity resulting in either cell necrosis or fatty infiltration is now known to be a vary widespread phenomenon, potentially of great importance to human welfare. It is caused by numerous drugs and environmental agents, and while a few agents—notably carbon tetrachloride, ethanol, acetaminophen, and chloroform—have been studied in some detail, little is known of the mechanisms involved in most cases. In fact, a consistent explanation of the various effects of hepatotoxicants is not yet complete even for the most extensively studied examples.

It is readily apparent why the liver has been selected for separate treatment while other organs, which may show some similar effects, were not. The importance of activation for the production of active metabolites is now well recognized. The high specific activity of the liver for the enzymes involved, principally but not exclusively those of the microsomal mixed-function oxidase system, ensures that such effects are more extensive and more obvious in the liver.

Hopefully, the studies being carried out on the liver will not only lead to an explanation consistent with all of the manifestations of hepatotoxicity, but also provide a model for studies of similar effects in other tissues.

Suggested Reading

Cohen, S. N., Armstrong, M. F. Drug Interactions, A Handbook for Clinical Use. Baltimore: Williams & Wilkins, 1974.

Eliakim, M., Eshchar, J., Zimmerman, H. J. (Eds.). International Symposium on Hepatotoxicity. New York: Academic Press, 1974.

Gillette, J. R. Formation of reactive metabolites of foreign compounds and their covalent binding to cellular constituents. In Lee, D. H. K., Falk, H. L., Murphy, S. D. (Eds.). Handbook of Physiology, Section 9, Reactions to Environmental Agents. Bethesda, Md.: American Physiological Society, 1977.

Raisfeld, I. H. Models of liver injury: The effect of toxins on the liver. Becker, F. F. (Ed.). The Liver: Normal and Abnormal Functions, Part A. New York: Marcel Dekker, 1974, p. 203.

Recknagel, R. O., Glende, E. A. Lipid peroxidation: A specific form of cellular injury. In Lee, D. H. K., Falk, H. L., Murphy, S. D. (Eds.). Handbook of Physiology, Section 9, Reactions to Environmental Agents. Bethesda, Md.: American Physiological Society, 1977, p. 591.

Zimmerman, H. J. Hepatic injury caused by therapeutic agents. In Becker, F. F. (Ed.). The Liver: Normal and Abnormal Functions, Part A. New York: Marcel Dekker, 1974, p. 225.

Frank E. Guthrie

19

Resistance and Tolerance to Toxicants

19.1. Introduction

Adaptation of organisms to the increasing number and quantity of chemicals in the environment is known for nearly all chemical groupings and classes of organisms, both plant and animal. Such adaptation is the measurable ability of an organism to show insensitivity or decreased sensitivity to chemicals that ordinarily cause physiological effects. Such changes may range from essential immunity to the stressor (as is the case of certain bacteria to drugs or houseflies to DDT) to small adjustments from environmental stress (as shown by city dwellers to a multitude of low-level contaminants). Adaptation to drugs is much better known than adaptation to toxicants because the stressor is more directly administered and the effects are more clearly monitored. Accommodation to toxicants is likely to be more subtle but, ultimately, more important in the total environment for man and other organisms are exposed to a large number of chemicals to which they must adapt.

Although both resistance and tolerance are controlled by the genetic constitution of the individual organism, it is convenient to consider these two separate aspects of the broader term, adaptation, in terms of multigeneration and single-generation phenomena, respectively. Resistance is manifested when the genetic makeup of the *population* allows individual organisms to resist the action of a chemical that previously elicited a marked physiological response. In microorganisms resistance is frequently initiated by mutations, that is, the occurrence of an altered gene or mutant. In other instances of resistance (probably the majority), the action is due to selection of genes already present in the population at low frequencies. They become the primary gene component when the normal genes disappear as a result of the stress. If the gene for resistance to the stressor chemical was present in the original population at a low level and the toxicant was required for selection of the adaptive manifestation, such resistance is termed "acquired." If the original population had genes for resistance to the chemical at a high level *before* chemical stress, resistance is termed "natural." In either case, levels of resistance are usually quite high. In acquired resistance they are tens to thousands of times more than the "normal" population, and resistance is evidenced not only throughout the life of a single individual but also in the generations that follow. Thus, in long-lived organisms this adaptation would be manifested in a fashion normally considered evolutionary, and present-day examples would be relatively rare because stress by synthetic chemicals is of recent origin.

In contrast to resistance, tolerance is a term used for the adaptation of the *individual* rather than the population. Although individual organisms may resist chemicals during a single lifetime (resistance not passed to the next generation), the levels of such adaptations are normally low, on the order of tenfold or less. In this instance, the stressor does not usually operate at a physiological concentration great enough to destroy the organism, whereas in the development of acquired resistance a substantial part of the population must be destroyed for selection to occur. Induction of enzymes is a common mechanism for tolerance, in which metabolic alteration may be increased both for the compound in question and for unrelated compounds affected by the induced enzyme system. Vigor and health of the individual are of obvious importance in tolerance to chemicals.

19.1.1. Cross Tolerance Among Toxicants

In many instances prior treatment with one toxicant confers protection from another agent with a similar mode of action or mechanism of adaptation; this phenomena is called cross resistance or cross tolerance. For example, tolerance to ethanol may be attained by administration of barbiturates without previous exposure of the organism to ethanol. Similarly, houseflies that have developed resistance to dieldrin are also resistant to chlordane and heptachlor, even though these flies have not had prior exposure to these compounds. The administration of ozone causes cross tolerance to a number of deep-lung irritants (NO_2, H_2O_2, and CCl_3NO_2), whereas no such cross tolerance is noted for such gaseous irritants as SO_2 and Cl_2, which act at the deeper recesses of the lung alveoli. In some instances, cross tolerance is difficult to envision. For example, the administration of CCl_4 confers resistance to phalloidin, the toxic principle of white mushroom, which is unlike CCl_4 in chemical structure.

19.1.2. Buildup of Adaptive Mechanisms

The buildup of resistance in a population is not well understood. In some cases, insects or microbes may become resistant to the stress of a chemical within a few generations, whereas in other cases this process may require years of selection. In addition to selection of the specific gene(s) for resistance, other genetic changes must be accomplished to cause appropriate adaptive changes in the population. It is obvious that the organism selected by chemical stress was less well adapted to the environment prior to stress, or it would have been the major component of the population. Tolerance to stress may require appreciable periods of time to become evident when complicated mechanisms of adaptation are required, such as increased phagocytosis or morphological changes in the lung. However, tolerance due to increased levels of enzymes or other protein-associated phenomena is often acquired quickly. For example, increased amounts of metallothionein, a protein that binds cadmium and stores it away from the site of action, are evident within a few hours after stress by an appropriate metal.

19.1.3. Reversal of Resistance or Tolerance

When the stressing chemical is removed, populations of organisms that have acquired resistance do not normally revert immediately into a susceptible population. It may take several weeks in the more rapidly reverting organisms or may require months to years in some cases. It seems likely that the return of the gene pool to a biologically fit, susceptible condition involves not only the gene that confers resistance but also associated genes. Nevertheless, tolerance is seldom manifested for more than a few weeks once the stressor is removed, although an occasional tolerance mechanism may be manifested for a longer period.

19.2. Mechanisms of Resistance and Tolerance

There are many reports of cases of adaptation to chemicals, but the exact mechanisms are known for only a few. For example, studies concerned with reported habituation to arsenic by persons ingesting large quantities of this toxicant have failed to provide any scientific explanation for the adaptation. Studies concerning the adaptation to anticholinesterase pesticides by heavily exposed agricultural workers have not provided a specific explanation for the ability of that group to withstand the normally adverse effects of the nerve lesion.

Those cases in which specific mechanisms seem to have an adequate scientific explanation may be conveniently grouped into biochemical, physiological, behavioral, and morphological categories. Examples are of necessity drawn primarily from microorganisms and insects, in which chemical stress, coupled with rapid development, has been more manifest than in other organisms.

19.2.1. Biochemical Mechanisms

This category includes known alterations of the normal biochemistry of an organism, usually altered enzymes or proteins. It often overlaps with physiological mechanisms, but in the latter case the mechanism may lack biochemical clarity.

19.2.1a. Metabolism

Rates of metabolism are of great importance in determining the amount of the toxicant available at the site of action. In general, a change in the metabolism of a xenobiotic is probably the most important factor in alterating the response to chemical stress.

Detoxication. An organism that acquires the ability to detoxify a xenobiotic more rapidly is capable of tolerating concentrations originally adverse to the individual. Resistant insects have utilized a variety of enzymatic detoxications to overcome the effects of insecticides; some classical examples are DDT dehy-drochlorinase activity in DDT-resistant strains, oxidative metabolism of a number of organophosphate and carbamate insecticides, quantitative difference in the esterases of organophosphate-resistant insects, and selection of transferases in insects resistant to organophosphate insecticides. There are also many examples of this mechanisms throughout the plant and animal kingdoms, and some diverse examples will be presented.

Resistance to mercuric chloride by *E. coli* strains has been attributed to the more rapid metabolism of this compound to volatile mercury derivatives, reducing the metal concentration in cells below the toxic level. As shown in Figure 19.1, approximately twice as much mercuric chloride is metabolized by the resistant strain. The form of volatile mercury (elemental or organic) produced has not been determined.

In plants, metabolic tolerance to herbicides is common as an explanation of selectivity between pest and favored species and between resistant strains of the same species. The discovery of cultivars of Hawaiian sugar beets with significantly different responses to the herbicide diuron necessitated appropriate changes in weed control recommendations to spare the more susceptible sugar beet strains. Roots, stems, and leaves of resistant (R) and susceptible (S) cultivars grown in nutrient solutions were subject to ^{14}C-diruon, and the extent of metabolism was determined after 3 weeks (Table 19.1). Metabolism was more extensive (by twofold in leaf cultures) in the resistant strain. Similar results have

Figure 19.1   Time course of uptake of ^{203}HgCl by susceptible and resistant strains of *E. coli*.
SOURCE: *Modified from Komura and Iazki, J. Biochem. 70 (1971), 885.*

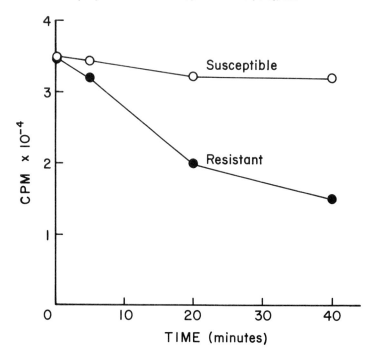

Table 19.1 Metabolism of ^{14}C-Diuron by Roots, Stems, and Leaves of Resistant and Susceptible Cultivars of Sugarcane

| Plant part | Cultivar | Percent of total radioactivity | |
		Parent compound	Metabolites[a]
Roots	R	35	65
	S	50	50
Stems	R	24	76
	S	55	45
Leaves	R	22	78
	S	64	36

Source: Adapted from Osgood et al., Weed Sci. 20 (1972), 537.

[a] Primarily monomethyl and dimethyl diuron.

been shown for the selective action of another herbicide, atrazine, whose main route of detoxication by resistant *Panicum* species is via peptide conjugation.

Tolerance for ethanol can be acquired by induction of ethanol dehydrogenase, which is the rate-limiting step in detoxication. In the example shown in Figure 19.2, human subjects were administered small amounts of alcohol for 4 days, followed by trace amounts of ^{14}C-ethanol. Ethanol blood levels and exhaled CO_2 were determined. The subjects were then given large quantities of ethanol for 7 days and the ^{14}C-ethanol experiment was repeated. The heavy drinkers had a much higher rate of metabolism of alcohol (induction of dehydrogenases), and blood levels declined much faster.

Figure 19.2 Increased metabolism of ethanol by individuals first subjected to low, and then to high, ethanol stress. Traces of ^{14}C-ethanol were provided in each case to monitor CO_2 as a measure of the rate of metabolism.
SOURCE: *Modified from Mendelson et al., Metabolism 14 (1965), 1255. New York: Grune & Stratton, Inc., 1965. Reprinted by permission of Grune & Stratton, Inc.*

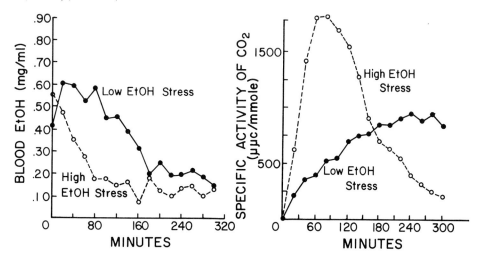

Intoxication. Some compounds require metabolic intoxication before the toxic action can be manifested. In such cases, resistance or tolerance may be noted when the rate of intoxication is depressed, causing less toxicant to be present at the site of action.

An early symptom of injury by CCl_4 is lipid peroxidation, which causes decomposition of the endoplasmic reticulum. The peroxidation reaction is an interaction initiated by free radical formation (intoxication) from metabolism of CCl_4 by oxidative enzymes, a mechanism for which is shown in Chapter 18.

The study shown in Table 19.2 illustrates protection when the intoxication mechanism is reduced. Rats were given 5% of the LD_{50} of CCl_4 for 6 hr. After 24 hr the rats were tolerant to an LD_{95} dose, and the protective effects subsided thereafter. A mechanism of depression of the intoxication reaction involving oxidative enzymes was proposed following examination of two oxidatively metabolized substrates. Whereas both cytochrome P-450–mediated substrate activities were depressed, NADPH–cytochrome c reductase was not implicated in the decrease of intoxicative metabolism. The mechanism is probably due to destruction of cytochrome P-450 in the endoplasmic reticulum. Such a mechanism ultimately causes severe damage to the organism, but in the short term the reduced intoxicative effect is protective.

A second example of reduced intoxication as a mechanism of resistance has been found with 5-fluorouracil, an anticancer agent that mimics thymine and prevents replication of DNA. The agent must first be activated to fluorodeoxyuridylic acid to be incorporated into the genetically important nucleic acids.

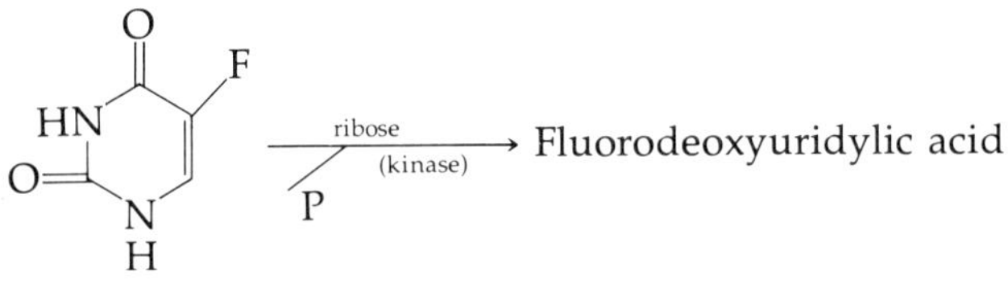

$$\text{(5-fluorouracil)} \xrightarrow[\text{(kinase)}]{\text{ribose}} \text{Fluorodeoxyuridylic acid}$$

In resistant strains of mouse tumor cells, the kinase catalyzing the phosphorylation of fluorouridine to flururidylic acid is markedly decreased in comparison to that in susceptible cells. Therefore, conversion to the active form is inhibited, and little incorporation into the nucleotide is found.

19.2.1b. Alternation of Target Enzyme

When an enzyme whose inhibition is responsible for toxic action is altered, the organism may resist the action of a toxicant. Such changes have been primarily demonstrated by kinetic studies. Specific mechanisms, speculative thus far, might include changes in amino acid sequence, alteration of distances between critical amino acid residues, altered enzyme topography, etc.

Resistance to the action of cholinesterase inhibitors through genetic selection of an altered target enzyme has been shown for both carbamate and organophosphate insecticides in insects, mites, and ticks. Decreased sensitivity of the physiological target has been demonstrated for a number of kinetic parameters of the inhibition scheme. In one report, soluble housefly acetylcholines-

Table 19.2 Decrease in Levels of Oxidative Enzymes Responsible for CCl_4 Intoxication in Rats Pretreated with CCl_4

Time following protective doses	Percent of control		
	Aminopyrine demethylase	Cytochrome P-450 concentration	NADPH–cytochrome c reductase
0 hr	100	100	100
6 hr	65	—	—
12 hr	60	58	—
18 hr	45	38	—
24 hr	38	25	110
4 days	40	30	100
7 days	85	60	80

Source: Calculated from Glende, Biochem. Pharmacol. 21 (1972), 1697.

terases from R and S strains were used in the determination of several kinetic constants in accordance with the following scheme (E represents the enzyme, AX the carbamate or organophosphate, X the leaving group, EAX the reversible complex, and EA the inhibited enzyme:

$$E + AX \overset{K_d}{\rightleftarrows} EAX \overset{k_2}{\to} EA + X$$

where K_d is the dissociation constant of the enzyme–inhibitor complex, and k_2 is the carbamylation or phosphorylation rate constant. These two parameters are related to overall potency by the bimolecular reaction constant $k_i = k_2/K_d$.

In the example shown in Table 19.3, resistant houseflies were stressed during the larval stage with 120 ppm tetrachlorvinphos, while the susceptible strain was not stressed. In this experiment, the phenomenon of cross resistance is demonstrated as flies were resistant to other insecticides although stressed only with tetrachlorvinphos. Ratios between R and S strains for LD_{50} values,

Table 19.3 Dissociation Constants (K_d), Phosphorylation and Carbamylation Constants (K_2), and Bimolecular Rate Constants (k_i) of Housefly Brain Acetylcholinesterase

Compound	Insecticide group	LD_{50} (R/S)	k_i (S/R)	K_d (R/S)	k_2 (R/S)
Tetrachlorvinphos	Organophosphate	>1500	206	573	2.7
Dichlorvos	Organophosphate	17	117	383	3.3
Paraoxon	Organophosphate	16	94	322	3.4
Propoxur	Carbamate	7	62	153	2.5
Dimetilan	Carbamate	6	50	58	1.2

Source: Adapted from Tripathy, Pestic. Biochem. Physiol. 6 (1976), 30.

Note: Numbers shown represent the ratios between susceptible and resistant strains for these parameters.

bimolecular reaction constants (k_i), dissociation constants (K_d), and carbamylation or phosphorylation constants (k_2) are shown.

The potency of the inhibitors (as measured by bimolecular reaction constants k_i) for the enzyme from the R strains was decreased appreciably over the S strain. Higher k_2 values were found in the R strain, the typical increase being about threefold. This small increase in phosphorylation or carbamylation was overwhelmed by tremendous differences in affinity. The K_d values were much greater for the resistant enzymes by factors ranging from 573 to 58. It appears that the reason the R strain enzyme is less sensitive to the inhibitor is probably a change in binding sites (more poorly bound). It has been suggested that a slightly different position of an imidazole residue relative to the serine hydroxyl involved in the inhibition reaction causes the altered activity.

19.2.1c. Alteration of Receptor Protein

Although alterations of the kinetic properties of target enzymes are well known, there are few examples of the alteration of protein receptors (target sites), the kinetic properties of which are less well understood. One recent report involves resistance of certain weeds to the herbicide atrazine.

Both phenylurea herbicides (represented by diuron) and triazine herbicides (represented by atrazine) interfere with the same electron carrier of the photosynthetic electron transport chain in the photosystem II complex. Figure 19.3 shows identical effects of atrazine and diuron on fluorescence transients in susceptible chloroplasts, namely rapid rises in fluorescence, indicating inhibition of electron flow near a photosystem II primary electron acceptor. However, in resistant plants, atrazine had no effect on the fluorescence transient (indicating the loss of an appropriate binding site), whereas diuron induced a rapid fluorescence rise (indicating the presence of an herbicide binding site). It appears that the protein involved in binding has a much lower affinity for atrazine

Figure 19.3 Chlorophyll fluorescence transient changes observed upon illumination of dark-adapted chloroplasts from atrazine-susceptible and -resistant pigweed seedling biotypes. Fo levels of fluorescence determined after 1-msec illumination and F_1 levels after 50-msec illumination. ———control chloroplasts, — — — $+10^{-5}$M atrazine, - - - - - $+10^{-5}$M diuron.
SOURCE: *Modified from Arntzen et al., Proc. Natl. Acad. Sci. 76 (1979), 278.*

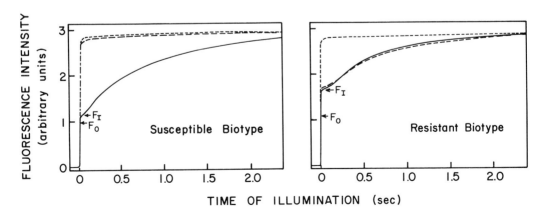

but a near normal affinity for diuron. Furthermore, the ratios of the original fluorescence (F_o), intermediate fluorescence (F_i), and peak fluorescence (F_p), which can be represented as $(F_i-F_o)/(F_p-F_o)$, were always greater in the resistant seedlings. Finally, polypeptide analyses showed that the acceptor proteins of the R and the S strains were slightly different. Only a small change in protein structure would be necessary to affect binding changes of the two classes of herbicides while otherwise permitting normal photosynthetic processes.

19.2.1d. Increased Amount of Target Molecule

Where increased amounts of target molecule can be synthesized to compensate for occupation of the target site, and thus maintain physiological integrity, a lesion may be overcome. Studies on occupationally exposed groups (policemen in heavy traffic and workers in relatively polluted traffic tunnel situations) have shown that an increased amount of hemoglobin provides a partial explanation for tolerance to the adverse effects of CO. Since the affinity of hemoglobin for CO is 250 times greater than for O_2, CO effectively blocks O_2 transport.

When dogs were exposed to 0.08–0.1% CO for 6–8 hr, daily for 36 weeks and compared to controls, a 67% increase in blood hemoglobin was observed (Figure 19.4). This created a greater reserve of the pigment for O_2 transport at a given concentration of hemoglobin–CO. In addition, the number of erythrocytes and the hematocrit also increased over 50%. This mechanism is probably an important factor in tolerance to CO by humans, but there is evidence that additional mechanisms are necessary.

An unusual example of acquired resistance by an increased amount of target enzyme has been shown by *Pseudomonas* for neostigmine. This organism con-

Figure 19.4 Changes in RBC counts during 42 weeks exposure to CO, 0.08–0.10%. SOURCE: *Modified from Wilks et al., J. Appl. Physiol. 14 (1959), 305.*

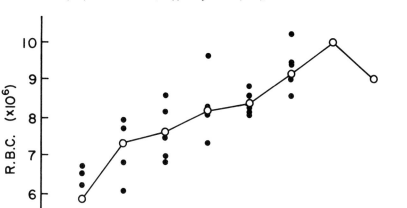

tains a cholinesterase that becomes rate limiting if the organism is furnished acetylcholine, the choline from which serves as the source of carbon and nitrogen. If cholinesterase-inhibiting neostigmine is added, growth is markedly inhibited. Mutant strains have evolved that contain greatly increased levels of cholinesterase that is kinetically identical with the wild-type enzyme. Thus, acquired resistance is attributed to an increased amount of target enzyme.

19.2.1e. Bypass of Receptor

Cases of resistance have been noted in which organisms have evolved mechanisms that bypass the affected site of action. Scale insects in California citrus groves have acquired resistance to hydrogen cyanide (HCN) by utilizing a cytochrome chain sequence that avoids the terminal cytochrome, the site of inhibition by HCN:

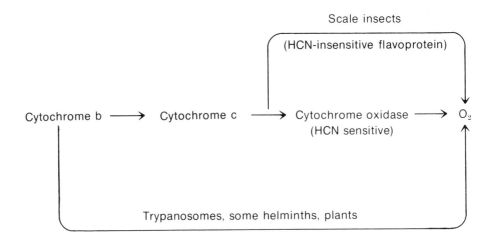

The resistant scales bypass the usual cytochrome oxidase sequence of respiration and utilize an HCN-insensitive flavoprotein. Other naturally resistant organisms have been found (lower part of scheme above) that proceed directly from cytochrome B to molecular oxygen, avoiding both cytochrome c and the HCN-sensitive cytochrome oxidase.

19.2.1f. Repair of Damaged Site of Action

Although repair of genetic material is well known, an appreciable increase in such repair activities has resulted in partial resistance to genetic attack in some cases. The repair of damaged DNA has been established as a mechanism of resistance to bifunctional alkylating agents by *E. coli*. Agents such as mustard gas cross-link at N-7 of guanine to form a diguanine joined by the alkylating moiety

$$-CH_2CH_2\overset{\overset{\displaystyle CH_3}{|}}{N}-CH_2-CH_2-$$

In resistant cells the alkylating agent works similarly, but these strains are capable of repair by excising some of the abnormal diguanyl residues. Normal purines are then permitted to restore functional DNA as shown below and discussed in detail in Chapter 16:

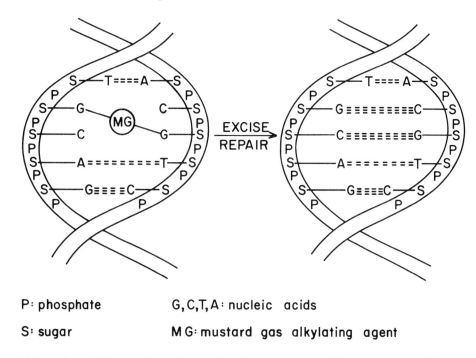

P: phosphate   G, C, T, A: nucleic acids

S: sugar   M G: mustard gas alkylating agent

Although excision and repair mechanisms are normally present in cells, the mutant strains possess much greater repair activity, as shown in Figure 19.5.

19.2.2. Physiological Mechanisms

Although the physiological mechanisms to be illustrated are probably the result of a biochemical change, the mechanism is usually a somewhat diffuse, multicomponent action—hence the term physiological.

19.2.2a. Penetration

Reduced penetration enables adaptation both by decreasing the amounts of toxicant and affording greater opportunity for detoxication during any given period. Reduction in the penetration of arsenic, a dehydrogenase inhibitor, has been show to be an adaptive mechanism in *Pseudomonas*. Cells grown in the presence or absence of arsenite (10^{-2} M) were equilibrated with several concentrations of radioactive arsenite and the uptake of arsenite was determined (Figure 19.6). As shown in the double reciprocal plot, at any given arsenite concentration the uptake by resistant cells was smaller than that by sensitive cells. At very high concentrations, the differences were not apparent as the exclusion mechanism was essentially overwhelmed. Resistance develops in relatively few cell generations and is quickly lost without arsenic stress.

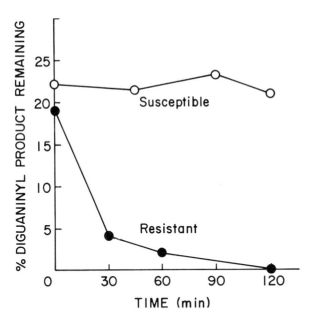

Figure 19.5   Excision of crosslinks in DNA treated with an alkylating agent. Cultures of susceptible and resistant strains of *E. coli* treated with [35] S mustard gas, a bifunctional alkylating agent.
SOURCE: *Modified from Venitt, Biochem. Biophys. Res. Comm.* 31 (1968), 355.

Decreased penetration has been shown as a partial mechanism for resistance in a number of cases in which insects have become resistant to insecticides. In one example (Table 19.4), significantly less insecticide was found to enter the cuticle of the R than the S strain (with exception of DDT in Fc strains). The explanation for this partial adaptation appears to be a function of increased lipids in the R strains rather than a qualitative difference in lipids of R and S strains.

19.2.2b. Storage

Where a toxicant can be essentially immobilized by storage in a reservoir tissue (fat, bone, etc.), physiological levels of exposure can often be offset. Evidence for liver and kidney storage of certain metals (cadmium, mercury, zinc, and copper) combined with a metallothioneinlike protein has been shown in a number of animals, including humans. The protein, not normally present, occurs only when the appropriate metal causes de novo synthesis. Up to 20 μg Cd/g liver may be incorporated into the protein, which may contain 5.9% cadium in extreme cases. Cadmium may be bound for up to 20 months even though there is extensive turnover of protein.

The time course of synthesis of the metallothionein and the content of Cd^{2+} in the liver of rats following administration of Cd^{2+} are shown in Table 19.5. The induction of the metal-binding protein has a short lag period, during which initial binding to a high molecular weight protein is evident. Thereafter, the metal is transferred to the -SH group–rich metallothionein.

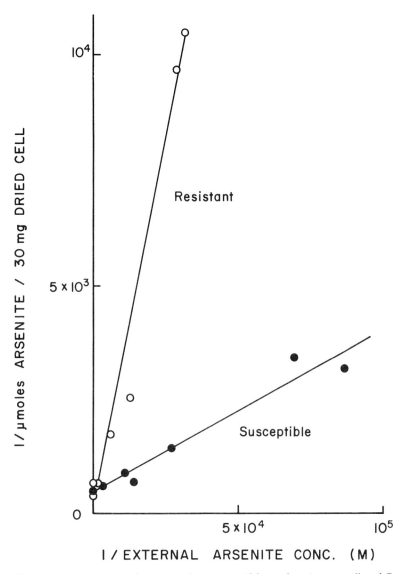

Figure 19.6 Uptake of arsenite by susceptible and resistant cells of *Pseudomonas* as a function of external arsenite.
SOURCE: *Modified from Beppu and Armia, J. Bacteriol 88 (1964), 151.*

Another important example is the storage of lead. Approximately 90% of the total lead in the body of contaminated humans is found in the bone and is not readily accessible to cause damage in the soft tissues, which would be adverse to the individual.

Chlorinated hydrocarbons that are relatively resistant to metabolism (such as highly chlorinated PCB's, DDT, dieldrin, or mirex) tend to be stored in fatty tissues for long periods of time. The half-life of these compounds may be over 100 days and previously exposed animals often retain measurable quantities in

Table 19.4 Reduced Penetration of Several
Insecticides in Susceptible and
Resistant Adult Houseflies

	Percent penetration in 1 hr		
Compound	CSMA(S)	Rutgers(R)	Fc(R)
Dieldrin	42	15	14
Diazinon	48	33	32
Parathion	54	35	47
Carbaryl	80	65	64
DDT	32	18	35

Source: Patil, J. Econ. Entomol., 72 (1979), 416.

fat for several years following removal of the source of contamination. Lactating animals may excrete substantial quantities of these lipid-soluble compounds in milk; this mechanism of resistance (elimination) for the exposed animal could be adverse in the food chain because milk is a substantial component of animal diets.

19.2.2c. Elimination

Rapid elimination of a chemical permits animals to tolerate quantities of toxicant far in excess of the lethal dose. This is the mechanism of adaptation of the tobacco hornworm to the tobacco plant, the leaves of which contain 3–5% nicotine, many times the LD_{50} for susceptible insects. The hornworm survives because the unchanged parent compound is rapidly eliminated (Table 19.6). Although the rapid elimination of the parent toxicant is an important mechanism of adaptation in this instance, an unknown mechanism is also operative which prevents absorbed material from reaching the site of action until elimination occurs.

Table 19.5 Time Course of Synthesis of, and
Content of Cd^{2+} in the Metallothionein
in Liver of Rats Following
Administration of Cd^{2+}

Time after Cd administration (hr)	High MW protein bound to Cd^{2+} ($\mu g/g$ wet liver)	Metallothionein bound to Cd^{2+} ($\mu g/g$ wet liver)
0	0.9	6.9
1	6.7	16.1
3	2.2	21.3
4	1.4	22.0
5	1.4	23.7

Source: Cempel and Webb, Biochem. Pharmacol. 25 (1976), 2067.

Table 19.6 Elimination of Nicotine (μg) by Hornworms Following Ingestion of Treated Tomato Foilage (2500 μg Total Nicotine)

Time after exposure	Blood	Larva	Feces	Not eaten
30 min	70	740	0	1640
2 hr	20	20	1680	700
4 hr	20	60	2400	0

Source: Self et al., J. Insect Physiol. (1964), 907.

Elimination of particles from the upper respiratory tract is also a well-known adaptation. Elimination of SiO_2 was increased by 50% when animals were exposed to trypan blue or TiO_2 1–2 days earlier. Alveolar phagocytosis is the main mechanism preventing penetration of particles into the pulmonary interstitium, and these phagocytes are stimulated by prior exposure. Experiments have shown a greatly increased number of phagocytizing cells to be produced upon appropriate stress. Increased ciliary activity and mucous production in response to low concentrations of irritants in the upper respiratory tract have also been shown. Under stress, there is an increased number of goblet cells which exhibit increased secretion rates. In the pulmonary spaces the mucous response is missing, and increased elimination has been found to be the result of increased production of surfactant along alveolar epithelium.

The alveolar cell turnover rate can be increased by stress particles. When iron oxide was inhaled, increased cellular activity was directed toward the removal of the irritant (Table 19.7).

19.2.3. Behavioral Mechanisms

Although behavioral adaptations to stress caused by toxicants may not properly belong in a consideration of biochemical–physiological resistance mechanisms, brief mention seems warranted. An obvious adaptation to increased pollution has been the movement of a large segment of the human population away from contaminated city air to the suburbs. Acquired resistance attributable to behavior has also been shown by resistant populations of mosquitoes in World Health

Table 19.7 Effect of Particle Inhalation on Alveolar Cell Turnover Rate in the Rat

Group	Iron oxide inhaled (μg)	Cells in metaphase (%)
Control	0	10.2
Dusted	5	14.8
Dusted	10	20.5

Source: Adapted from Casarett and Milley, Health Physics 10 (1964), 1003.

Organization malaria control programs. Normal populations of mosquitoes have the habit of resting on walls of houses between blood meals, and the vector control program is directed to their control by application of insecticides to these surfaces. A strain of mosquitoes developed resistance because the behavior pattern was modified to one of immediately leaving the treated houses following blood meals. Thus, by failure to rest on walls the mosquitoes avoided exposure to the treated surfaces and, in time, became the dominant population even though they had not developed resistance to the insecticide per se.

19.2.4. Morphological Mechanisms

Morphological adaptations to physical stress are obvious. For example, persons indulging in the ancient art of karate experience gradual change of the tissue of the palm until it becomes acclimated (properly calloused) to the stress encountered by severe blows to solid objects.

Although many indications of tissue change as a result of chemical stress have been reported, little evidence has been accumulated. Several types of respiratory particles (asbestos, glass fiber, coal, and quartz) may stimulate the production of fibroblasts and additional production of collagen, as well as stimulate the proliferation of fibroblast stem cells. However, such events tend to have an adverse, antipulmonary action over time, so the result is equivocal as an adaptive mechanism. Morphological adaptations elicited by air-borne toxicants are most often mentioned, but such microscopic changes as thickening of alveolar walls do not appear to be satisfactory explanations for mechanisms of adaptation.

19.3. Biochemical Genetics

The biochemical explanations of events at the gene level have primarily been confined to studies with microorganisms because of the availability of genetic markers and the rapid development of these organisms. Among higher animals, studies have been hampered by the lack of chromosome markers and the long generation time required to manifest genetic change. In recent years, genetic markers have been developed in several insects (especially houseflies). The relatively short life cycle of insects makes genetic studies of resistance mechanisms feasible in these highly evolved animals.

Detoxication, change of target enzyme, bypass of target enzyme, penetration, storage, and elimination have been reported as mechanisms for resistance to a number of insecticides, as discussed above. Genes on chromosomes I, II, III, IV, and V responsible for these mechanisms have been identified in the housefly as follows: oxidative detoxication (I, II, and V); transferases (II); dehydrochlorinases (II); altered target enzyme (II); penetration (III); carboxylesterases (II); and phosphatases (II). Genetic maps for resistance in other species (especially mosquitoes) are also known.

Visible recessive marker genes (homozygous) have been incorporated into a number of housefly strains. In one susceptible strain (designated S or *sbo*), stubbywings (*s* or *stw*) are associated with chromosome II, brown body (*b* or *bwb*) with chromosome III, and ocra eyes (*o* or *ocra*) with chromosome V. The presence of quantitative and qualitative differences in cytochrome P-450 from several housefly strains makes a genetic analysis possible when such strains are crossed with such mutant marker strains as *sbo* to obtain specific combinations of chromosomes. Levels of resistance in the different phenotypes are correlated with enzyme activities and characteristics of cytochrome P-450, such as the type I, II, and III optical difference spectra. In such cases, R strains are normally maintained under stress of an appropriate insecticide at a level that would result in the elimination of the S strain, which is maintained without stress by insecticides.

In two such studies, for example, the susceptible marker strains were bred to a Rutgers diazinon-multiresistant strain. In this case, a series of genetic manipulations resulted in four marker groups. The S strain had all marker chromosomes in the phenotype. A partially resistant strain (R,s^+bo) had all markers in the phenotype, but chromosome II (stubby wing) also had diazinon resistance introduced through crossing-over techniques incorporated with insecticide selection. A third group $(R,+bo)$ had diazinon resistance attributable to chromosome II genes, but other chromosomes were from susceptible parents. The fully resistant strain contained resistance that could be attributed to all three chromosomes.

The data (Table 19.8) showed that diazinon resistance in this strain is controlled by at least three genes since three resistance levels are apparent. The parent resistant strain $(R,+++)$ was most resistant, the strain without contribution of chromosome II $(R,+bo)$ showed partial loss of resistance, and the strain

Table 19.8 Comparison of Substrate and Spectral Reactions for Housefly Strains Derived from Marker (S)[a] and Diazinon-Resistant (R) Houseflies

Parameter	Susceptible S sbo	Partially or fully resistant		
		R s⁺bo	R +bo	R +++
LD$_{50}$ (diazinon, μg/jar)	3.5	40	88	249
Parathion oxidation (pM metabolized/fly)	10	39	72	138
O-Demethylation (p-nitroanisole, nM p-nitrophenol/mg protein)	10	21	30	43
Cytochrome P-450 (OD units/mg protein)	0.015	0.018	0.027	0.044
Type I optical spectrum[b]	Negative	NM[c]	Positive	Positive
Type II optical spectrum[b]	Positive	NM	Positive	Positive
Type III optical spectrum[b]	Positive	NM	Positive	Positive
Transferase activity[d] (nM diazinon metabolized)				
Pyrimidinyl glutathione	0.77	0.53	0.62	0.73
Desethyl	0.22	0.33	1.3	1.7

Source: Adapted from Plapp et al., Pestic. Biochem. Physiol. 6 (1976), 175; and Motoyama and Dauterman, Pestic. Biochem. Physiol. 7 (1977), 443.

[a] Susceptible markers for chromosomes II (*s* or stubby wing), III (*b* or brown body), and V (*o* or ocra eyes).

[b] Optical difference spectra include type I (benzphetamine), type II (pyridine, 4-*n*-octylamine spectra), and type III (ethyl isocyanide). See sources for further details.

[c] NM: not measured.

[d] Glutathione-dependent transferase activity involved dearylation and deethylation of diazinon.

with only a portion of chromosome II, as a result of crossing over, (R,s$^+$bo) showed the least resistance (approximately 10 times that of the S strain). High levels of cytochrome P-450 (apparently controlled by at least two genes, as different levels were found in R,+bo and R,+++ strains) did not appear to be a requirement for expression of either resistance or high oxidase activity. The cytochrome P-450 level of R,s$^+$bo equaled that of S,sbo, even though both resistance and high oxidase activity were present in the former strain. Oxidase activity, as measure by parathion metabolism and O-demethylation of p-nitroanisole, differed in each diazinon-resistant strain and was approximately proportional to total resistance levels. Of the spectral binding differences studied, only type I binding was correlated with resistance; the other spectral differences, although also associated with chromosome II, did not differ in R and S strains.

With respect to transferase activity (data at bottom of table), dearylation (transfer of pyrimidinyl group) reactions did not appear to be involved in the resistance mechanism. Although deethylation (transfer of ethyl group) was a contributing factor to resistance, and is clearly controlled by chromosome II, it appears to be relatively minor when compared to oxidative mechanisms of resistance. In other housefly strains, however, transferases appear to be the major mechanism of resistance.

Based on these findings, expression of oxidative resistance in this diazinon-resistant strain seems to involve more than one gene locus on chromosome II. The most important gene is best measured by O-demethylase, parathion oxidation, and the presence of type I binding. Moreover, total resistance of this strain is controlled by genes not located on chromosome II. Considering the multigenecity of the resistance phenomenon, it is perhaps not surprising to note that other studies have found another diazinon-resistant strain (Fc strain) with genes for resistance and changes in optical spectra on both chromosomes II and V.

Although strains of mammals with acquired tolerance to chemical stress have not been used in biochemical genetic studies, some excellent work has been reported with mice strains that are "responsive" or "nonresponsive" to enzyme induction by certain xenobiotics. In the nonresponsive strains, the toxicity to a number of chemicals (chlorinated hydrocarbons, insecticides, 3-methylcholanthrene, and PCBs among others) is decidedly lower than in the responsive one. Pretreatment with polyaromatic hydrocarbons causes an increase in certain enzymes in the responsive mice which cannot be induced in the nonresponsive strains. Other types of inducers, such as phenobarbital, induce similarly in both groups. The aromatic hydrocarbon induction is inherited as a simple autosomal dominant trait (the Ah locus).

Electrophoretic analysis of liver microsomes of appropriately treated strains has revealed the electrophoretic positions responsible for different types of inductions. Figure 19.7 shows the effects of different inducers on four of the electrophoretic bands in the 49,000–55,000-dalton region. Polycyclic hydrocarbon (PH) induction is associated with band 4 of the responsive, but not the nonresponsive, strain. Inducers of other types of microsomal enzymes such as pregnenolone-16a-carbonitrite (PCN), or phenobarbital (PB) were associated with bands 2 or 3 of both strains. Slight induction of band 4 was also shown by phenobarbitol as well as increased band 1. Administration of 2,3,7,8-

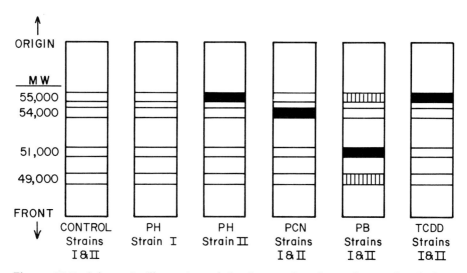

Figure 19.7 Schematic illustration of the four major electrophoretic bands between 49,000–55,000 daltons that change in intensity following treatment of mouse strains with various inducers. PH = polycyclic hydrocarbons; PCN = pregnenolone-16 -carbonitrile; PB = phenobarbital; TCDD = dioxin. Strain I is nonresponsive to polycyclic hydrocarbon induction; strain II is responsive to polycyclic hydrocarbon induction. The solid lined and lightly stippled regions represent decreasing intensities of protein concentration.

SOURCE: *Modified from Haugen et al., J. Biol. Chem. 251 (1976), 1817.*

tetrachlorodibenzo-*p*-dioxin (TCDD) induced band 4 in both responsive and nonresponsive mice. Dioxin is a particularly potent inducer, and it is suggested that the nonresponsive mice fail to recognize less potent inducers (such as 3-methylcholanthrene) but do recognize TCDD. Alternatively, the receptor interactions may be different for these "moderate" and "strong" inducers.

Suggested Reading

DeBruin, A. Biochemical Toxicology of Environmental Agents. Amsterdam: Elsevier, 1976, Chapter 41.

Goldstein, A., Aronow, L., Kalman, S. M. Principles of Drug Action. New York: Wiley, 1977, Chapter 8.

Lee, D. H. K., Falk, H. L. Murphy, S. D. (Eds.). Handbook of Physiology, Section 9, Reactions to Environmental Agents. Baltimore: American Physiological Society 1977.

Oppenoorth, F. J., Welling, W. Biochemistry and physiology of resistance. Wilkinson, C. F. (Ed.). Insecticide Biochemistry and Resistance. New York: Plenum Press, 1977, Chapter 13.

Plapp, F. W. Biochemical genetics and insecticide resistance. Annu. Rev. Entomol. 21 (1976), 179.

William E. Donaldson

20

Natural Toxins

20.1. Introduction

Both the animal and plant kingdoms possess numerous species that produce toxins. In animals these toxins may be classified into two broad categories; (a) those that are actively delivered (venoms), and (b) those that are passively delivered (poisons). Venoms have evolved primarily as a predatory mechanism for obtaining and digesting food, although their value as a protective mechanism cannot be ruled out. However, not all venomous animals are predators, and in some species only one sex possesses venom. Conversely, poisons serve no predatory function since obviously, the eatee cannot become the eater. The protective effect of poisons can be considerable and is exemplified by the bell toad (*Bombina*), which has been raised in the same enclosure with turtles and crocodiles. It has been reported that a voracious turtle will beat a hasty retreat upon touching one of these toads with the tip of its nose.

Plant toxins are widespread, and their biochemistry and modes of action are varied. The purpose of plant toxins is not as clear as that of animal toxins. Protective effects and survival value are obvious possibilities, but in some cases it appears that the toxins exist only as part of the biochemical apparatus for sustaining normal metabolic function.

Microbial toxins, which include mycotoxins such as aflatoxin, are also quite varied in their distribution and effects. However, due to space limitations, microbial toxins will not be discussed here.

20.2. Animal Toxins

Snakes possess the most diverse and the best characterized venoms, and therefore snake venoms will be discussed in more detail than venoms and poisons from other animals. In addition, snake venoms collectively possess most of the toxic principals found in the toxins of other species.

The first clearly recognized toxic components of snake venoms were enzymes, and most research centered upon correlating venom action with enzymatic activity. Recently it has been shown that highly toxic polypeptides are present in the venoms of certain snakes, and this development led some scientists to suggest that polypeptides rather than enzymes are responsible for venom toxicity. The balanced view is that both enzymes and polypeptides have roles in venom toxicity and that these roles assume different importance in various species. It is also becoming apparent that there are synergistic relationships between certain enzymes and polypeptide components of venoms.

20.2.1. Toxic Components and Mechanism of Action of Snake Venoms

20.2.1a. Neurotoxins

Neurotoxins are polypeptides that contain 61–74 amino acid residues. Neurotoxins show no effect on the central nervous system, but rather act as neuromuscular blocking agents by reducing end-plate depolarization by acetylcholine. Neurotoxin effects are additive to curare and are antagonized by anticholinesterase agents. Cobra neurotoxin exhibits no enzyme activity when purified. Conversely, crotoxin, from tropical rattlesnakes, exhibits phospholipase and hyaluronidase activities and inhibits succinate–cytochrome C reductase. Neurotoxins are lethal because they have the ability to cause respiratory failure.

20.2.1b. Cardiotoxins

Cardiotoxins are membrane-active polypeptides. Evidence is mounting that these polypeptides act by causing conformational changes in membranes that expose portions of the membranes to attack by phospholipases. Cardiotoxins act directly on the cardiac muscle and cause lowered blood pressure and permanent systolic contraction. The action of these toxins can be reversed by potassium ions.

20.2.1c. Hemolytic Agents

Hemolytic agents cause the release of hemoglobin from the stroma of erythrocytes by attacking α-lecithin:

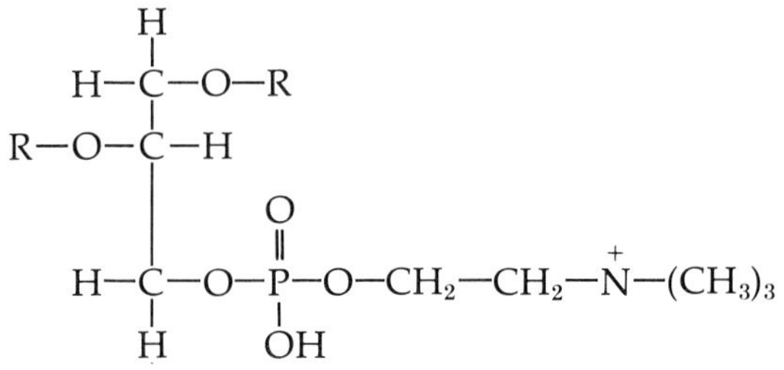

$$
\begin{array}{l}
\quad\quad\ \ \overset{\displaystyle H}{\underset{\displaystyle |}{}} \\
H-\overset{\displaystyle |}{\underset{\displaystyle |}{C}}-O-R \\
R-O-\overset{\displaystyle |}{\underset{\displaystyle |}{C}}-H \\
\quad\quad\ \ \overset{\displaystyle |}{}\quad\quad\quad O \\
\quad\quad\ \ \overset{\displaystyle |}{}\quad\quad\quad \| \\
H-\overset{\displaystyle |}{\underset{\displaystyle H}{C}}-O-\overset{}{\underset{\displaystyle OH}{P}}-O-CH_2-CH_2-\overset{+}{N}-(CH_3)_3
\end{array}
$$

R = fatty acid

α-Lecithin

Lecithinase A is an enzyme (molecular mass approximately 20,000 daltons) that hydrolyzes the fatty acid moiety in the α position to form lysolecithin. The hydrolysis disrupts the conformation of the erythrocyte membrane and results in lysis. Lecithinase B hydrolyzes both fatty acids, and lecithinase C hydrolyzes the choline radical. Lecithinase D is a true phosphatase that hydrolyzes the phosphate ester bond to form a diglyceride. Only A and D are found in venoms, and of these, only A possesses hemolytic activity.

Another hemolytic agent found in venoms is direct hemolytic factor (DLF). This agent is a membrane-active, basic polypeptide with a molecular mass of approximately 2000 daltons. DLF, like the cardiotoxins, is thought to act by inducing a conformational change in erythrocyte membranes that may expose the membranes to attack by phospholipases.

20.2.1d. Blood-Coagulating Agents

Blood-coagulating agents, as the name implies, cause rapid and complete coagulation of the prey's blood in situ. Blood coagulation involves a series of complex biochemical events, however, in the interest of brevity, only a condensed outline of these events will be presented. The blood clotting process begins when factors inside the platelets and in the plasma interact to form an active enzyme called thrombokinase. Thrombokinase and calcium ions catalyze the conversion of prothrombin, a zymogenlike plasma protein, to thrombin, an active enzyme. Thrombin then catalyzes the conversion of fibrinogen, a soluble plasma protein, to fibrin. The strandlike, insoluble fibrin then forms the matrix for the blood clot.

There are two groups of venoms containing coagulating properties. The first stimulates conversion of prothrombin to thrombin, while the second stimulates conversion of fibrinogen to fibrin. The coagulating agents are protein in nature and contain both esterase and protease activities. Their mechanism of action is unknown.

20.2.1e. Crotomine

Crotomine is a proteinlike material found only in the venom of Brazilian rattlesnakes. It is probably a membrane-active polypeptide. It causes paralysis and eventual rigidity of the posterior extremities and respiration difficulties.

20.2.1f. Other Enzymes

Other enzymes are also found in venoms; among these are cholinesterases. Purified acetylcholinesterase from venoms does not show the toxicity of crude venom. This suggests that the neurotoxic effect of venoms are not due to acetylcholinesterase activity alone. However, the cholinesterases, as well as the other enzymes found in venoms that are not toxic per se, may contribute to overall toxicity by interacting with other toxic principles.

Lecithinase D has already been mentioned as an example of a phosphatase found in venoms. In addition, enzymes that catalyze the hydrolysis of phosphoric acid from ATP and NAD are also found in venoms. These phosphatases have not been directly correlated with venom toxicity, however, dilute cobra venom is capable of inhibiting fermentation and glycolysis in yeast cultures. Thus, in more concentrated form, these components of venoms may produce severe localized metabolic distortions in the prey.

Venoms are a variable source of proteolytic enzymes. Viper venoms are a rich source, whereas cobra venoms contain very little proteolytic activity. Proteases contribute to venom toxicity in two ways. First, they destroy tissue integrity, and thus enhance the spread of other toxic principles in the venom. Second, their direct proteolytic action on blood and tissue proteins results in the production of bradykinin, a nonapeptide with the structure Arg-Pro-Pro-Gly-Phe-Ser-Pro-Phe-Arg. This slow-acting peptide produces smooth muscle stimulation, increased capillary permeability with leukocyte migration, pain, vasodilation, and shock.

The action of venom proteases is similar to that of the endopeptidase trypsin. These enzymes hydrolyze the primary structure of proteins on the carbonyl side of lysine and arginine residues. Protein conformation may also be affected by alterations in secondary protein structure. Studies with trypsin inhibitor from soybeans suggest that the active center of venom proteases is identical to the active center of trypsin, however, substrate specificity is different. Venoms do not contain chymotrypsinlike proteases.

Many venoms contain significant quantities of L-amino acid oxidase. Such venoms are distinguished easily by their yellow color, which results from the presence of riboflavin. Venom amino acid oxidase is quite different in its properties from the mammalian enzyme. Snake venom contains FAD, while the flavin component of mammalian enzyme is FMN. Snake venom enzyme attacks only amino acids, whereas mammalian enzyme attacks the α-hydroxy analogs as well. The turnover number of the enzyme is 3100 in venoms versus 6 in mammalian tissue.

The toxicity of venoms does not appear to be related to L-amino acid oxidase content. However, the enzyme may enhance the toxicity of other venom components. The venom oxidase has been reported to activate tissue proteases of the prey, which could enhance the spread of the venom.

Hyaluronidase, or spreading factor, is found in venoms and has the function of rendering the tissue more permeable to large molecules. The substrate is uronic acid–acetylglucosamine (hyaluronic acid), which serves as a viscous, intercellular, cementing substance.

Finally, venoms contain decarboxylating enzymes that produce vasoactive amines, such as histamine, from amino acids. Histamine causes vasodilation, hypotension, and shock.

20.2.1g. Other Venom Constituents

Other venom constituents include large amounts of both organic and inorganic phosphorus, and small amounts of chloride, sodium, potassium, zinc, and ferric ions. Organic constituents include the nucleotides GTP and UTP, the sugars ribose, galactose, mannose, fucose, and glucose, lipids, lipoproteins, peptides, and amino acids. Venoms can also contain low molecular weight compounds with strong pharmacological action such as amines. The primary constituent of venom is protein, which accounts for over 70% of the dry matter.

20.2.2. Animals Possessing Toxins

20.2.2a. Mammals

The male duck-billed platypus can inject a venom by means of spurs located on the hind feet. The venom is protein in nature. It resembles viper venom in that it contains coagulant (thrombin) and hemolytic and cytolytic properties, but no neurotoxic activity. The venom is painful but is not fatal to man.

The anteater and the shrew produce a rapidly acting neurotoxin, which is present in their saliva. The chemical characteristics of the toxin are unknown. Intraperitoneal injections of fresh extract of submaxillary glands from these animals are fatal to mice. The LD_{50} is on the order of 2.9 mg/20 g body weight.

20.2.2b. Reptiles

Snake venoms have been discussed in detail above. Envenomation is by bite from hollow fangs connected to venom sacs.

The Gila monster of the southwestern United States and northern Mexico is the only known poisonous lizard. The author is not aware of any description of the venom in the literature except that it is potent and can be fatal to man.

20.2.2c. Amphibians

Toads, frogs, and salamanders possess potent poisons in the skin and salivary secretions. These are not venoms in that delivery is extremely poor. The poisons are used as a passive, albeit potent, defense mechanism against predators.

Poisonous substances in amphibians include numerous aromatic amines such as the phenylethylamine (catecholamine) and tryptamine (indolethylamine) bases. Included among the former are dopamine, N-methyl dopamine or epinine, noradrenalin or norepinephrine, and adrenalin or epinephrine (N-methyl noradrenalin); the tryptamine bases include 5-hydroxytryptamine or serotonin, N-methyl serotonin, N,N-dimethyl serotonin or bufotenin, and N-methyl-5-methoxytryptamine:

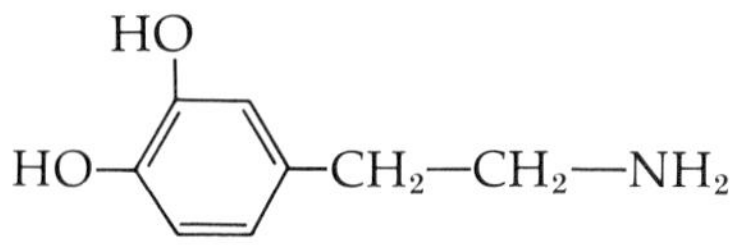

Dopamine

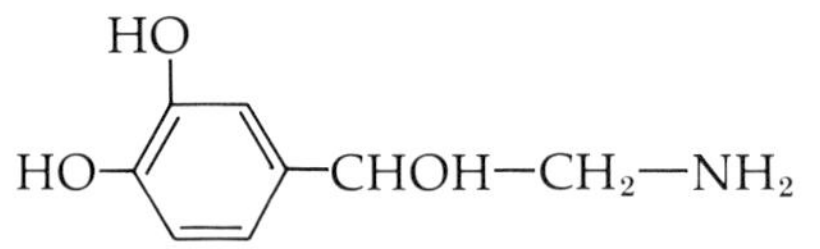

Noradrenalin

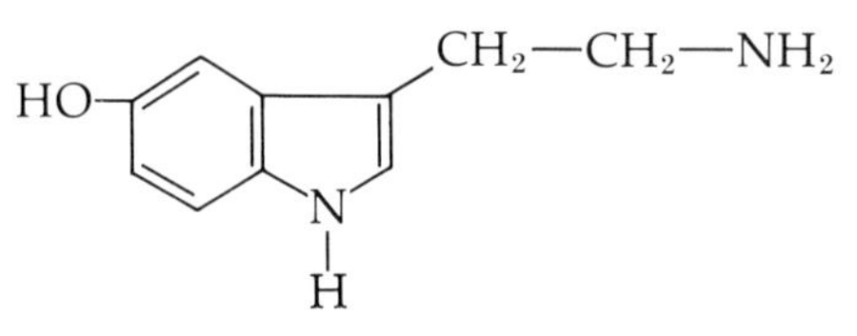

Serotonin

Toad skin can also contain histamine. Whereas histamine is a vasodilator, the aromatic amines act as potent vasoconstrictors and stimulate heart action. As a result, exposure to aromatic amines produces a significant rise in blood pressure.

Amphibians also possess peptides such as bradykinin, the action of which has been described above. Steroidal alkaloids, which cause labored breathing, tachycardia, and hind limb paralysis, are also found in amphibian skin. The European fire salamander possesses a hemolytic protein.

20.2.2d. Fish

Several species of fish are known to possess poisons. The prevalence of these species increases with proximity to the equator. Delivery of the poisons is by fins, spines, or stingers. In many cases, the chemistry of the poisons is very sketchy. Some of the fish used for food by man and animals carry toxicants in parts of their bodies. Some shark livers cannot be eaten safely because of excessive levels of vitamin A, which can be toxic. Toxins occur regularly in the roe, liver, and skin of certain genera of puffer fish. Served regularly in the restaurants of Oriental countries, they call for care in preparation. Errors in cleaning the fish may have fatal consequences to the customers. Clinical signs after ingestion of tetrodotoxin are a tingling sensation in the lips and tongue 10–45 min later. Numbness of the skin and muscle weakness follow. Generalized paralysis, convulsions, and death result in about 60% of the cases. Nontoxic types of fish can become poisonous by taking in "red tide" dinoflagellates containing saxitoxin.

Some shark species can deliver poisons by the dorsal fin, but the pharmacology of the poison is unknown. Sting rays possess a dorsal tail stinger that can deliver a fatal sting to humans. The sting results in intense pain and vasodilation, followed by vasocontriction and ventricular and auricular standstill. Chimaeras deliver a poison by the dorsal fin that causes paralysis of the hind limbs. Catfish deliver a poison by both the dorsal and pectoral fins. The poison causes muscle spasms and respiratory distress and contains a neurotoxin and hemolytic principle.

Weeverfish inhabit beaches in the southeastern United States and are very aggressive. They deliver a poison by dorsal stingers that produces a pain so intense that the victim thrashes about until fainting occurs. The pain cannot be relieved with morphine and is thought to be caused by serotonin. The poison also contains adrenalin, noradrenalin, cholinesterase, and hyaluronidase. In addition to pain, the victim exhibits respiratory paralysis, cardiovascular effects, and hemolysis. The sting can be fatal to humans.

Stargazers deliver poison of unknown pharmacology by means of shoulder spines. Scorpion fish deliver a poison by dorsal, anal, and pelvic stings that causes cardioinhibition, respiratory distress, and hemolysis. Toadfish possess dorsal spines that deliver a poison that causes ascites, paralysis, convulsions, and death in small animals. The poison causes pain but not fatalities in humans. Lamprey eels deliver a strong coagulant by bite. The teeth do not inject venom since the coagulant is secreted by the mucosal cells of the mouth.

20.2.2e. Insects

Insects produce secretions that are toxic to both animals and plants, but only the animal toxins will be considered here. Because relatively minute amounts of venom are communicated, the most serious consequences of insect bites and stings are allergic reactions. The reactions are either immediate (if due to humoral or circulating antibodies) or delayed (if due to cellular antibodies). The antibodies are formed in response to specific protein antigens or haptens (non-protein allergens conjugated to nonantigenic proteins) contained in the insect secretions. Allergic reactions can be quite severe and can be fatal to humans who have developed high antibody titers in response to repeated exposure to the antigens. A single bee sting can result in death in a susceptible individual.

Toxic principles other than antigenic proteins are also found in insect secretions. On a weight basis, these venoms can be as toxic as snake venoms, but because of the amounts involved they usually produce only local irritation in higher animals. The venoms are communicated by urticating (stinging) hairs and spines, by bites, which inject venomous salivary secretions, and by stingers, which envenomate paralyzing venoms.

Urticating hairs and spines are associated with certain types of caterpillars. These hairs and spines produce three types of local reactions. First, a mechanical irritation of the skin is noted that is similar to the irritation produced by the embedding of glass wool fibers. Second, the hairs and spines contain allergens that can precipitate antibody production in the victim. Third, the hairs and spines contain venoms in the true sense and can produce localized lesions and reactions by virtue of their own chemistry.

The reduviid bug is an example of an insect that produces venomous salivary secretions. The secretions are basically digestive in function, although there are toxic elements that can produce local and systemic inactivation in the prey. The saliva is toxic to a wide range of insects and contains at least six proteins. Three of the proteins are trypsinlike proteases. Hyaluronidase is present to supplement the main proteolytic function. The saliva contains weak phospholipase activity but no lipase, esterase, or ATPase activities. Although the saliva can abolish excitability of nerve and muscle tissue, its principal action is to disrupt the cellular matrix and cause a general lysis.

The formicine ant produces formic acid in the saliva. Although this ant is capable of spraying the formic acid solution for distances up to 30 cm, it has no apparatus to deliver the saliva by bite or sting.

Ixodid ticks, fire ants, and army ants produce paralyzing venoms, but unlike those of wasps, bees, and hornets, these venoms are communicated through the saliva rather than by stingers. The ixodid tick injects salivary secretions during feeding that produce an ascending type of flaccid paralysis. The saliva causes neuromuscular block (failure of acetylcholine release), but recovery is rapid if the ticks are removed prior to respiratory paralysis. Fire ants produce a nonprotein, crystalline amine that is strongly hemolytic, and army ants produce a protein toxin that has a histaminelike and cholinergic action.

Parasitic wasp venom contains hyaluronidase, histamine, kinin, and serotonin. Venoms from certain wasps are very specific in terms of the host that they affect, while venoms from other wasps affect various hosts. Wasp venom causes an inactivation of body musculature, probably by means of neuromuscular block. In vertebrates almost all wasp and bee stings, even those of a multiple nature, fall short of gross toxicity and fatal effects. Death in higher animals is commonly the result of hypersensitivity.

Bee venoms contain histidine decarboxylase and histamine per se. Hyaluronidase and lecithinase A are also present. In addition, bee venom contains a protein fraction called melittin, which causes local pain and inflammation, hypotension, and respiratory paralysis. Melittin irreversibly damages the motor end plate, lowers muscle membrane potential by stimulating release of potassium ions, inhibits plasma cholinesterase, and stimulates fibrinogen conversion to fibrin. Sublethal doses in rabbits cause the breakdown of glycogen, which results in hyperglycemia and lowered liver glycogen levels. Whether this is a direct action of melittin or is mediated through epinephrine release from the host adrenal glands is unknown.

It should be noted here that the American honeybee is a rather docile insect and will sting only if directly provoked. In contrast, the African honeybee is more dangerous because it is extremely aggressive and is capable of unprovoked attacks, although its venom is no more potent than that of the American bee. Because of its greater capacity for producing honey, scientists in Brazil used the African bee in breeding experiments with native bees. An African queen bee escaped inadvertently and the African species spread through South and Central America. These bees are migrating slowly northward, and it is predicted that the African bee will reach the United States sometime in the 1980s. The ramifications of this migration on the future of agriculture and the associated toxicological aspects of bee stings in the United States are at best uncertain.

There is a giant bee (*Apis dorsata*) indigenous to India that is capable of inflicting stings fatal to humans. It is even said by Singalese that the giant bee can kill buffalo and elephants and that five stings are the equal of a cobra bite. The components of the venom are unknown.

Finally, hornet venom contains up to 10% acetylcholine. The venom produces intense local pain and inflammation and disrupts nerve function in smaller prey.

20.2.2f. Scorpions

The venom of scorpions contains proteolytic activity and a peptide neurotoxin. Very little serotonin is present, but the venom can contain cateholamines. The venom of some species possesses phosphodiesterase and/or 5-nucleotidase. The venom is delivered by tail stinger. It causes pain, myocarditis, hyperglycemia, and respiratory distress. The cardiac effects resemble an overdose of catecholamines. Scorpion stings can be fatal to humans. Three-fourths of the fatalities from scorpion stings in Mexico occur in children under 4 years of age. The sting of some species can be fatal to children up to 16 years of age or to adults with hypertension.

20.2.2g. Spiders

Several species of spider produce venom that is communicated by biting. As with scorpions, the bite of the spider is more apt to be fatal in young children than in adults. The spider venoms contain neurotoxin, cardiotoxin, and serotonin. Symptoms include a rise in blood pressure followed by shock, tachycardia, cardiac arhythmias, and violent pain as a result of muscle spasms in the lumbar region, thighs, and abdomen.

20.2.2h. Mollusks

Conus geographus and *C. textile* are two species of snail that secrete venoms. These snails possess a sharp appendage, called an operculum, which penetrates the surface of the prey. Toxic secretions enter the host through such openings and can cause intense pain. The pain results from acetylcholine, histamine, kinins, and serotonin. A highly potent protein is present in the secretions that interferes with neuromuscular transmission and results in a flaccid paralysis. The protein effects can be fatal in humans.

The Alaska butterclam contains the most potent nonprotein toxin known. The toxin contains ten carbon atoms and can be chemically degraded to pyrollopyrimidine, which contains eight carbon atoms. It is called saxitoxin and is similar to a material called tarichotoxin, which is found in newts.

The Australian blue octopus possesses a neurotoxin of low molecular weight. The toxin is nonimmunogenic. It results in complete cessation of all muscular activity except cardiac muscle and can cause fatalities in humans.

20.2.2i. Coelenterates

Hydra contain a succinoxidase inhibitor that is protein in nature and a toxic compound, tetramethylammonium, which causes paralysis. Jellyfish possess long tentacles, the cells of which can inject a paralyzing venom. The nature of the toxin is unclear. Encounters with large jellyfish such as the Portuguese man-of-war (*Physalia*) can be fatal to humans.

20.3. Plant Toxins

The medicinal value of plants has been known by mankind for thousands of years. A special branch of the pharmaceutical sciences, pharmacognosy, deals exclusively with the pharmacological effects of plants. Obviously, it is beyond the scope of a single chapter on natural toxins to deal even superficially with so vast an array of pharmacologically active and/or toxic compounds as that found in plants. Therefore, only selected toxins that can find their way into human diets and appear to be normal products of plant metabolism will be discussed. For most of the examples used, an adequate biochemical description of mode of action exists. Mitotic poisons of plant origin are discussed in Chapter 15.

20.3.1. Sulfur Compounds

Members of the cabbage family, such as broccoli, brussel sprouts, cauliflower, and kale, as well as horseradish, mustard seed, and turnips, contain a class of sulfur compounds known as glucosinolates, whose general structure is shown below:

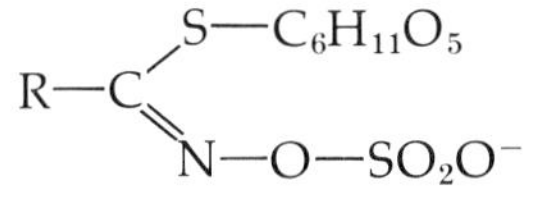

$$R-C\begin{array}{c} \diagup S-C_6H_{11}O_5 \\ \diagdown N-O-SO_2O^- \end{array}$$

R = a variety of alkane and aromatic groupings

The glucosinolates are found in all parts of these plants, but the highest concentration is usually found in the seeds. Glucosinolates can be metabolically converted in animals to thiocyanate and isothiocyanate, which are potent goiterogenic compounds.

Onions, garlic, and chives contain 5-substituted cysteine sulfoxides, which are also goiterogenic. Human consumption of plants containing goiterogenic sulfur compounds poses no threat to human health. However, problems can arise in those areas where iodine intake is low. Iodine deficiency results in hyperactivity of the thyroid gland, with concomitant gland enlargement (goiter). Goiterogenic sulfur compounds can exacerbate the effects of iodine deficiency.

20.3.2. Lipids

Oils of certain plants contain specific fatty acids that interfere with the metabolic processes of the animals that consume them. Rape seed and mustard seed contain a 22-carbon fatty acid with one double bond, *cis*-13 docosenoic or erucic acid, that can cause myocarditis and fatty infiltration of the heart muscle. These oils must comprise approximately 20% of the caloric intake of an animal before problems arise. Rape is grown in large quantities in Canada and is used for animal feeding. The amount of erucic acid in tissues from animals fed rape seed is not great enough to cause problems in humans that consume those tissues.

Oils from plants of the order Malvales contain unsaturated fatty acids called cyclopropenes. The only known exception is cocoa butter. A tropical tree, *Sterculia foetida*, produces a nut whose oil contains up to 50% cyclopropene fatty acids. Cottonseed contains 0.6–1.2% cyclopropenes, and the oil has a correspondingly higher content.

The structure of the most prevalent cyclopropene acid, sterculic acid, is shown below:

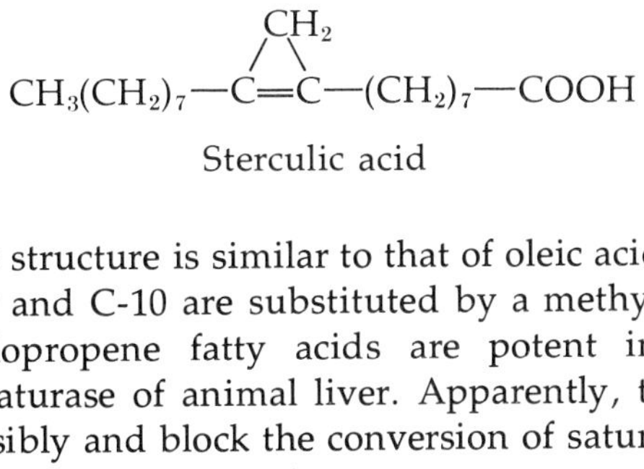

$$CH_3(CH_2)_7 - C = C - (CH_2)_7 - COOH$$

with CH_2 bridging the two central carbons.

Sterculic acid

The structure is similar to that of oleic acid, except that the hydrogen atoms on C-9 and C-10 are substituted by a methylene bridge. Sterculic acid and other cyclopropene fatty acids are potent inhibitors of microsomal fatty acid desaturase of animal liver. Apparently, these acids bind to the enzyme irreversibly and block the conversion of saturated fatty acids to the corresponding monoenoic fatty acids. As a consequence, stearic acid levels increase dramatically while oleic acid levels decline in tissues of animals fed cyclopropenes. The changes in ratio of saturated to unsaturated fatty acids may interfere with membrane function. The effects of cyclopropene ingestion can be fatal depending upon dosage and length of exposure.

The cyclopropene acids in cottonseed oil are removed in the refining process, and therefore these acids pose no human health problem unless raw seeds or unrefined oil is consumed. *Sterculia foetida* nuts have been consumed as famine food in parts of southern Africa and South America. No deaths have been reported as being the direct result of such consumption, however, the effects of cyclopropenes could go unreported because they are obscured by the effects of starvation.

20.3.3. Phenolic Compounds

Several plants contain high levels of phenolic compounds. The structures of these compounds vary widely. Examples of phenolic compounds are dicumarol, rotenone, salicylates, tannic acid, and tetrahydrocannabinol, the active psychogenic agent found in marijuana. Phenols can have high acute toxicity to which carnivores are more susceptible than herbivores. Phenols tend, in general, to uncouple oxidative phosphorylation. Polymerized phenols are more lipid soluble, and their ability to penetrate membranes, and therefore their toxicity, is enhanced by polymerization. Phenols can also act as metal chelates. Phenols are commonly detoxified by methylation. Hence, they prolong the effects of adrenalin by serving as competitive inhibitors of O-methyltransferase. One class of phenols, anthocyanins, are mildly goiterogenic because iodine has a greater affinity for these phenols than for tyrosine, the precursor of thyroxine. Some phenols have an estrogenic effect.

Tannins can cause liver and kidney toxicity in humans. Such toxicity has been observed occasionally in burn patients treated with 3–5% solutions of tannic acid. Repeated subcutaneous doses of tannins are carcinogenic in rats. In humans, increased oral carcinoma is observed in betel nut chewers. The nuts contain up to 26% tannins. An increased incidence of esophageal cancer in South Africa has been correlated with consumption of high-tannin sorghums. There is some evidence that tannins in tea can promote the effects of other carcinogens. Acceptable tannin intake in humans is on the order of 560 mg/day. However, heavy coffee and/or tea drinkers may consume up to 1000 mg/day.

Cottonseed meal is a high-protein material used in animal feeds. Cottonseeds contain a phenol, gossypol, most of which is removed during processing of the seeds. Although it is not usually a problem in human nutrition, gossypol ingestion can cause difficulty in animals fed cottonseed meal. Gossypol toxicity leads to impaired growth, weight loss, and loss of appetite. Among the other symptoms of toxicity are hypoprothrombinemia from inhibition of prothrombin synthesis and anemia from chelation of iron. Gossypol can bind with proteins and render certain amino acids unavailable during the digestive process.

20.3.4. Cyanogenic Compounds

A large variety of plants contain cyanogenic glycosides. Included in this group are lima beans, sorghums, elderberries, cassava, manioc (tapioca), white clover, trefoil, and the seeds of almond, apple, apricot, cherry, peach, pear, plum, and quince. Cyanogenic glycosides yield mono- or disaccharides, aldehydes or ketones, and HCN upon hydrolysis. Cyanide is released by either acid hydrolysis or by appropriate hydrolytic enzymes. The plant glycosides are β linked. Plants possess β-glucosidases, while the digestive enzymes of animals are α-glucosidases. Therefore, cyanide release does not occur as the result of digestive processes. However, the bacteria of the lower digestive tract are able to effect the release of cyanide, as are the plant enzymes in the cyanide-bearing food that is consumed.

Cyanide is a potent inhibitor of cytochrome oxidase, which is the terminal respiratory enzyme in aerobic organisms. Toxicity can range from chronic to acute. The lethal dose in a 70-kg human is in the range of 50–250 mg. Several cases of death in both humans and livestock have been reported as the result of consumption of plant material rich in cyanide-containing compounds.

Parts of the plant that contain cyanogenic glycosides vary, and no generalizations can be made. The sorghum seed contains little cyanogenic compounds, but the young seedling is a rich source. Sorghum plants cannot be fed to cattle without toxicity until the plants are approximately 1 m high.

Cassava is a plant whose starchy root is a food staple in many West African countries. The starch can contain considerable HCN, even after extensive boiling and preparation. Chronic cyanide toxicity is prevalent in West Africa, as is a high incidence of goiter. The goiters result from thiocyanate, which is the product formed from HCN by the body's detoxification mechanisms.

Lima beans can contain high levels of HCN. The white American varieties contain approximately 10 mg/100 g seed. Other varieties can contain up to 300 mg/100 g seed. Cyanide poisoning from lima beans in the United States is not a problem since imports are restricted to varieties yielding less than 20 mg/100 g seed.

Laetrile is a cyanogenic compound, isolated from the seed pits of apricots, which is purported to possess anticancer properties. The potency, in terms of cyanide content, is unregulated in the manufacturing process. As a result, several cases of cyanide poisoning have been reported in humans from laetrile ingestion.

20.3.5. Other Toxic Compounds in Plants

Some plants contain high levels of phytates and oxalates. These materials act as metal chelates, and a high intake can cause trace mineral deficiencies. Most greens are good sources of dietary calcium, except for spinach. The high oxalate content of spinach binds calcium.

Plants can contain high nitrate and nitrite levels as a result of overfertilization. The levels of these materials in plants can be toxic. It should be emphasized that toxic nitrate levels are the result of excessive uptake rather than inherent metabolic patterns. Toxic levels of selenium from soil can accumulate in range plants in several western states in the United States.

Many plants contain vasoactive and psychoactive substances, toxic proteins and peptides, aminonitriles, stimulants, depressants, and hallucinogens. Such plants are not usually eaten for food but can and do serve medicinal functions.

Suggested Reading

Buckerl, W., Buckley, E. E., Deulofeu, V. (Eds.). Venomous Animals and Their Venoms, Vol. 1 Venomous Vertebrates. New York: Academic Press, 1968.

Buckerl, W., Buckley, E. E. (Eds.). Venomous Animals and Their Venom, Vol. 2, Venomous Vertebrates. New York: Academic Press, 1971.

Buckerl, W., Buckley, E. E. (Eds.). Venomous Animals and Their Venom, Vol. 3, Venomous Invertebrates. New York: Academic Press, 1971.

Committee on Food Protection, Food and Nutrition Board, National Research Council. Toxicants

Occurring Naturally in Foods, second edition. Washington, D. C.: National Academy of Sciences, 1973.

Ohsaka, A., Hayashi, K., Sawai, Y. (Eds.). Animal, Plant and Microbial Toxins. Vol. 1 Biochemistry, Vol. 2 Chemistry, Pharmacology and Immunology. New York: Plenum Press, 1976.

Russel, F. E., Saunders, P. R. (Eds.). Animal Toxins. Elmsford, N. Y.: Pergamon Press, 1967.

Toxicon. Oxford: Pergamon. A journal dealing with natural toxins, venoms, and poisons.

Edward J. Gralla

21

Chronic Testing in Animals
In Vivo Techniques

21.1. Introduction

21.1.1. Updating a Term

The term "toxicology" has meant, by tradition, the study of poisons and poisonings following drug overdosing or misapplications of toxic chemicals in humans or animals. Recently, the same term has acquired a broader meaning embodying somewhat different concepts and requiring more atypical approaches. This chapter will focus on these newer aspects of toxicology. First, however, an introductory discussion of the conceptual differences between the newer and older features of this science is in order.

Most important have been changes in the degree of dependence upon analytical information and the difficulties in controlling or preventing exposure to potentially toxic chemicals. Classically, a diagnosis of poisoning was usually confirmed by identifying a toxin in any one of various body fluids or tissues. Follow-up measures included preventing further contact with the offending agent. All this remains unchanged in dealing with typical modern-day poisonings. However, our society faces a different kind of chemical hazard, evolved from a dependency and therefore largely unavoidable. Industrial chemicals have become widely disbursed and serve important needs, hence the twin measures of detection and prevention now have reduced usefulness. For example, an attending physician appreciates that most of his patients consume and excrete foreign chemicals, such as prescription drugs and industrial contaminants, due to current social living conditions and therapeutic practices. The concern of the physician and the experimental toxicologist shifts to the question of detecting toxic exposures by identifying those characteristic biological responses that indicate an excess chemical burden is approaching or has been attained. Questions arise that focus on the organ systems affected and have diagnostic implications, and sometimes the answers are helpful in describing the toxic process.

How such questions are framed and answered is the subject of the remainder of this chapter. Gathering this type of information is usually beyond the design of experiments in humans, and so it falls to the research toxicologist to accumulate sufficient and meaningful answers in animal studies, and from these, to estimate the potential risk that similar effects might occur in humans.

21.1.2. Biological Perspectives

Advancing life emerging from the sea eons ago met two terrestrial forces waiting to cause its extinction. One was a multitude of microorganisms, and the second was a score of natural but toxic chemicals. Biological change and adaptation were essential to survival. Man and his companion species are evidence that complete annihilation was averted by evolution, but the process was not flawless. Most bacteria and chemical agents are harmless and even helpful, but a few can cause serious and sometimes fatal diseases by acting through evolutionary imperfections. Moreover, all organisms, including man, have inherent mechanisms for eliminating or otherwise rendering potentially harmful agents innocuous, but such systems have finite capacities and can be overwhelmed by massive challenges. Moreover, since evolutionary development followed divergent pathways, different species frequently have different susceptibilities to chemical toxicities (and infectious organisms). These premises taken together lead to a fundamental conclusion in toxicology: every chemical can cause a toxic effect in some species at some dose level after some duration of treatment. The primary objective of the branch of toxicology under discussion, commonly called "chemical safety evaluation," is to provide the specific information as to which species, what dose level, what duration of treatment, and what specific damage results, and then face the major responsibility of this science—that of reliably extrapolating these findings across species for application in man.

21.2. Objectives of a Safety Evaluation Study

21.2.1. Toxic Event

The decision to call a chemically induced response a toxicity will reflect the study objectives, as it should. However, the scientific interpretation and application of results are also influential. A chemical that destroys wide areas of liver tissue is easily labeled a hepatotoxin with little disagreement. However, more subtle judgmental problems in classification arise elsewhere. For example, anticancer drugs are specifically designed to attack and destroy those tissues having large populations of rapidly dividing cells. Hopefully, this means tumors (a beneficial effect), but it also includes normal bone marrow and intestine (toxic effects). Clearly, the eventual outcome of the chemically induced response largely determines its classification as toxic or nontoxic. Consider, as another example, chemical depression of reflexes or operant behavior. A small reduction in visual motor coordination is likely to be a minor nuisance to a bedridden patient but a serious problem to someone who must perform intricate movements quickly and flawlessly, as for example, an airline pilot.

21.2.2. Objectives Defined

The problems of semantics and terminology notwithstanding, the primary goals of a safety evaluation study usually include the following:

1. Identify the primary target organ(s).
2. Establish the reversibility of the toxic lesion(s).
3. Determine the most sensitive diagnostic method(s) for detecting the toxicity.
4. Indicate toxic mechanisms, if possible.

21.2.3. Target Organs

Virtually every body organ or tissue is susceptible to some form of recognizable damage (Table 21.1) and has the potential to be a primary target organ. Frequently, the toxic lesion can be further localized to a specific organ structure or biochemical pathway, such as the renal glomeruli or tubules, the hepatic parenchyma or bile ducts, or one of the cell layers comprising the mammalian retina. The detection and identification of toxicity can be accomplished by either mor-

Table 21.1   Adverse Responses to Chemical Ingestion or Exposure

Hepatic	*Ocular*	Ataxia
Direct hepatocellular	Corneal opacities	Ototoxicity
Cholestasis	Cataracts	Emesis
Hypersensitivity	Retinal degeneration	Status spongiosis
Porphyria		
	Cardiovascular	*Musculoskeletal*
Renal	Myocarditis	Paresthesias
Glomerular	Arrhythmias	Gingival hyperplasia
Proximal tubular necrosis	Vasculitis	Osteosis
Distal tubular necrosis	Angina	Osteomalacia
Papillary necrosis	Thrombosis	Tooth and bone discoloration
Diabetes insipidus	Vasospasm	
Urolithiasis		*Pulmonary*
Acute renal shutdown	*Dermal*	Fibrosis
	Phototoxicity	Emphysema
Hematopoietic	Photoallergy	Irritation
Hemolysis	Acne	Edema
Bone marrow suppression	Irritation	Bronchospasms
Methemoglobinemia	Allergy	Pneumoconiosis
Granulocytopenia	Excoriation	
Thrombocytopenia	Alopecia	*Endocrine*
Megaloblastosis	Hirsutism	Diabetes mellitus
Iron deficiency anemia	Stomatitis	Gynecomastia
Hypersplenism	Purpura	Infertility
Splenic atrophy	Puritis	
	Melanosis	*Miscellaneous*
Gastrointestinal	Psoriasis	Hypothermia
Focal ulcers	Nodular sclerosis	Hyperthermia
Mucosal erosions		Immune suppression
Malabsorption	*Neurological*	Carcinogenesis
Colonic ulcers	Peripheral neuritis	Fetal malformations
Pseudomembranous colitis	Parkinsonism	

phological or functional observations or both. Under ideal circumstances, chemical laboratory findings and visible tissue changes, discovered either by gross or microscopic inspection of treated animals, should correlate.

Such animal observations pinpoint the exact site of toxic insult to mammalian tissues. Confirming information may or may not be forthcoming from human exposure. Humans may be insensitive or susceptible to different toxic effects. Moreover, establishing toxicities in humans is difficult since the findings are frequently clouded or distorted by background artifacts such as disease, nutrition, exposure to other chemicals, diverse genetic backgrounds, and a host of other variables. Animal safety evaluation studies are performed under controlled conditions that either limit or prevent the introduction of extraneous factors. Moreover, treated or exposed animals are usually killed and tissue specimens are prepared before agonal or postmortem changes occur. For these reasons, suspected toxic reactions in humans are usually confirmed in animals.

21.2.4. Lesion Reversibility

Once the existence of a toxic lesion has been established, the events following withdrawal of the chemical insult are also investigated. Some of the questions asked are as follows: Will it reverse and disappear and the tissues and organ function recover? Is it permanent and therefore unchanged by discontinuation of the treatment? Will there be continued lesion development, such as occurs in chemically induced cancer? A fourth possibility is latency, whereby toxic lesions develop in animals or patients sometime after chemical administration or exposure is halted. The last possibility is the most worrisome to the practicing toxicologist since there are no reliable techniques for estimating the occurrence of latent periods.

The reversibility of toxicity bears on the final hazard assessment in humans. A higher risk level might be acceptable if a damaged organ (e.g., the liver) regenerates and recovers normal function. On the other hand, the willingness to risk permanent toxic impairment (e.g., cataracts or retinal degeneration) must be counterbalanced with important and unique therapeutic or social benefits.

Functional cell regeneration also depends upon the degree and type of organ insult. Bone marrow and testes are organs containing heterogeneous collections of cells in various stages of maturation with relative sensitivities to cytotoxins. Generally, the more mature cell types, e.g., sperm or circulating blood cells, are resistant to toxic effects. Moreover, the same organs contain progenitor cells— stem cells in bone marrow and spermatogonia in testes—which, if undamaged, can repopulate the organs provided that sufficient numbers survive. In other words, irreversible toxicity implies complete destruction of every primordial cell. Such organs incurring something less than complete cell mortality should recover following treatment.

21.2.5. Selection of the Study Parameters

Animal safety evaluation studies establish the sensitivity of clinical parameters for detecting the onset of impending toxicity in animals—hopefully, at an early stage when the lesion might still be reversible. Such indicators take a variety of forms but as a rule employ noninvasive techniques, involve readily obtainable tissues, such as blood or urine, and require common clinical instruments, such as the electrocardiograph and ophthalmoscope. (At the opposite extreme would be surgical biopsies or exotic instruments, such as radioisotope scanners.) Ease, simplicity, and a lack of trauma are important practical considerations since subsequent follow-up studies in exposed humans would probably employ similar approaches.

21.2.6. Mechanisms

The collection of comprehensive data that might suggest underlying mechanisms of toxicity is another goal of a safety evaluation study. For example, anemias are common toxic phenomena that are induced in a variety of different ways. Erythrocytes can be attacked and destroyed either directly in the circulation or by a chemically stimulated hyperactive spleen. Red cell production in the bone marrow can be suppressed or hemoglobin synthesis may be retarded by either chemically depleting tissue iron or chemically inhibiting absorption of this element from the intestine. Clues to such mechanisms may surface if the study design includes a battery of relevant observations such as bone marrow and spleen histology, serum bilirubin, urine hemoglobin, erythrocyte and reticulocyte counts, and tissue deposition of iron-containing substances. Another previously mentioned example is chemically inhibited cell division. These inhibitors universally attack tissues with populations of rapidly dividing cells, including the bone marrow, intestine, testes, buccal membranes, and skin. Treatment with such chemicals will, as expected, induce an array of clinical problems, including anemia, leukopenia, diarrhea, infertility, stomatitis, and alopecia with underlying cell destruction in the affected organs.

21.3. Study Design

21.3.1. Test Material

The hazards engendered by chemicals that are potentially toxic to humans arise from numerous uses, and the nature of the exposure should be considered and incorporated into the plan of a safety evaluation study. Chemical exposures generally fall into two categories, deliberate and inadvertent. Therapeutic drugs are probably the largest class of chemicals that are willfully taken by humans. They are administered over various periods of time, from single doses to entire lifetimes. (Except for a few exceptions, such as the antibiotics, drugs counteract or suppress disease processes and technically do not "cure." Therefore, many require continuous, sometimes lifetime, administration.) Food additives such as flavor enhancers, preservatives, stabilizers, and sweeteners are also intentionally consumed. On the other hand, environmental pollutants and food animal tissue residues of growth promotants, pesticides, and herbicides fall into the category of chemicals that are inadvertently ingested by humans.

Apart from the intended use, certain other basic information about the physical nature of the substance to be tested should be understood and considered before the treatment of animals begins. Chemical purity must be established. Few chemicals are available in a pure state, especially if newly discovered or synthesized. The type and level of impurities should be defined in the interest of precision and reproducibility. Moreover, if it becomes necessary to work with several different lots of a chemical, then each lot of material should be chemically matched. Stability during storage is also important, since chemicals can deteriorate to by-products that may be more or less toxic. This was demonstrated by the discovery that tetracycline HCl, usually a relatively nontoxic drug, hydrolyzes during prolonged storage into two potent renal toxins. For this reason, light- or heat-sensitive compounds require opaque storage containers or refrigeration.

Certain salt cations, particularly potassium or magnesium, are more toxic forms of their anionic moieties, especially if they are administered parenterally. Conversely, changing the salt form may reduce the toxicity of an orally administered compound if the final product is more poorly absorbed. Lipid solubility affects oral toxicity since the nonpolar, fat-soluble compounds are more easily absorbed from the gut. For the same reason, the pKa of ionizable groups can also influence the rate and amount of gastrointestinal absorption. In most animal species, the intestinal contents become more basic during the descent through the tract.

A chemical's density will affect the experimental design. Low-density microparticles may float freely on air currents, and if the test substance is to be fed as a part of the diet, producing and maintaining a uniform chemical–feed mixture can be difficult. Moreover, cross-contamination between experimental groups of animals can occur and lead to spurious results. Conversely, dense material may settle out of a feed mixture, resulting in nonuniform dosing. Test materials that clump, cake, or consist of grossly heterogenous particles can cause the same mixing problems. Hydroscopic materials must be handled under rigidly controlled conditions of humidity to avoid changes in density during storage and handling.

21.3.2. Species Selection, Number of Animals, and Maintenance

The selection of the species and number of animals for a chemical safety evaluation study involves a combination of logistical and scientific considerations. Animals for these studies must be of small size to allow for long-term housing under laboratory conditions. Smallness also reduces the demand for test substance—no minor consideration when a supply is limited. At the same time, the test species must be large enough to provide uncontaminated body fluids (especially blood constituents) in adequate amounts without endangering the animals' health or physiological status. The test animal must be tractable, healthy, and available in large numbers. While complete genetic uniformity is not always possible, nor desirable, the inclusion of at least one or two species with a documented ancestry can be advantageous.

21.3.2a. Rats

As previously stated, the final number of different species to include in a chemical toxicity study is a somewhat arbitrary decision. Usually a single-species study will employ the outbred albino rat, such as the Sprague Dawley, CD, Fischer, and occasionally Long-Evans or Holtzman strains. The albino rat offers several advantages. The normal life span ranges up to 24 months for most strains, and longer in the Fischer strain. Therefore, a 2-year study starting with

3–6-week-old animals covers a complete life span from early adolescence to old age, when spontaneous diseases are prominent. The rat cannot vomit and so emetic agents can be tested at higher dose levels in this species. The rat breathes only through the nose, and for this reason, vapors and gases and other atmospheric contaminates that damage the mucosal lining of the nares and turbinates are easily detected in inhalation studies using this species. Finally, rats are reliably housed in large numbers, up to ten per group cage under laboratory conditions. This is in contrast to mice, which frequently attack each other (especially previously separated males) and cannibalize members that die.

The rat has several limitations in safety evaluation studies. Foremost is the limited amount of blood that can be taken from a living animal and the difficulty in collecting this fluid. Samples are obtained by cutaneous incision in the tail, amputation of the tip of the tail, or puncture of the suborbital (ocular) venus plexus with a heparinized capillary tube. Less than 0.5 ml can be collected by any of these procedures. Cardiac puncture of the anesthesized animal will yield larger volumes but at an increased risk to the animal. The maximum to be collected without physiologically disturbing the animal is usually considered to be 10% of the total blood volume; since the blood volume equals approximately 50 ml/kg, a 0.3-kg rat has 15.0 ml and collection volumes should not exceed 1.5 ml. A rat to be killed for necropsy can be anesthesized and bled from several internal blood vessels, usually the posterior vena cava or the abdominal aorta. A skilled laboratory worker can obtain 10 ml or more from a rat by this technique.

The production of disease-free rats and other rodents for toxicology studies has reached a high level of scientific sophistication. Breeding animals are obtained by aseptic cesarean delivery from near term pregnant females and the offspring are either hand reared in germ-free containers or foster reared by germ-free mothers. After sexually maturing, they are transferred to production units and maintained under conditions that prevent exposure to specific species pathogens and parasites, hence the term specific pathogen free (SPF). Strict disease-control measures are taken, including the following: sterilizing water, feed, and bedding; daily shower bathing by personnel before entering animal areas; wearing of surgical masks and other sterile garments by attending personnel; and sealing all materials in leak-proof containers before passing them into animal rooms through microbiocidal baths. Control measures are instituted to detect disease organisms that might have broken through the barriers. Procedures used include postmortem examination of representative aged animals for organ lesions; culturing of lungs and intestinal contents for microorganisms such as *Mycoplasma, Pasteurella,* and *Salmonella;* and serological titering of serum for antibodies against the common rat virus diseases.

These measures have reduced or eliminated the most serious epidemics among rats, but a few nuisance diseases remain. Intestinal pinworms are occasionally found, apparently because they are transmitted vertically in utero and horizontally by air. The highly contagious viral disease sialodacryoadenitis is frequently seen, causing reddish ocular and nasal discharges, salivary gland swelling, and decreased food consumption with an attendant reduction in the rate of body weight gain. Fortunately, this is a self-limiting and nonfatal disease, and since it is highly contagious, it usually occurs in young rats before shipment to the toxicology laboratory or while in quarantine.

The rooms holding rats in a toxicology study should be equipped with a controlled lighting system that provides equal amounts of light and darkness each day. Constant lighting causes persistent estrus in females, and such animals are atypical specimens. The cages are usually either woven wire or solid plastic, and should provide at least a minimum amount of floor space for each animal (Table 21.2). Cellulose bedding material such as crushed corn cobs, peanut hulls, or hardwood sawdust should be used with closed caging, although this material can be carried into food receptacles by animals and thus interfere with the accuracy of food consumption determinations. Chemicals from softwood products, such as pine or cedar shavings, can affect animal drug metabolism systems and therefore should be avoided.

Despite a uniform background in heredity and environment, a group of rats within the same age range will probably show some variations, especially in body weight. For this reason, random assignment into experimental groups is necessary. Random number tables are useful for this purpose. Each animal is also individually identified by semipermanent methods. When rats are housed singly, a cage card, color coded to identify chemical and/or dose levels, can be used. Relying exclusively on this approach for extended periods is risky. More reliable methods are ear punching in a distinctive pattern or clamping a metal tag with an embossed number to an ear of each animal. Animal identification must be checked periodically since punched ear holes will be obscured by growing tissue and metal tags will occasionally be lost.

Equal numbers of each sex are usually assigned to each experimental group. The total number will depend upon the purposes and the duration of the pro-

Table 21.2   Space Recommendations for Laboratory Animals in Toxicology (Institute of Laboratory Animal Resources, National Academy of Sciences)

Species	Weight	Type of housing	Floor area/animal	Height
Mouse	<10 g	Cage	39 cm^2 (6 in.^{2})	12.7 cm (5 in.)
	10–15 g	Cage	52 cm^2 (8 in.^{2})	12.7 cm (5 in.)
	16–25 g	Cage	77 cm^2 (12 in.^{2})	12.7 cm (5 in.)
	>25 g	Cage	97 cm^2 (15 in.^{2})	12.7 cm (5 in.)
Rat	<100 g	Cage	110 cm^2 (17 in.^{2})	17.8 cm (7 in.)
	100–200 g	Cage	148 cm^2 (23 in.^{2})	17.8 cm (7 in.)
	201–300 g	Cage	187 cm^2 (29 in.^{2})	17.8 cm (7 in.)
	>300 g	Cage	258 cm^2 (40 in.^{2})	17.8 cm (7 in.)
Dog	<15 kg	Pen or run	0.74 m^2 (8.0 ft^2)	
	15–30 kg	Pen or run	1.12 m^2 (12.0 ft^2)	
	>30 kg	Pen or run	2.23 m^2 (24.0 ft^2)	
	<15 kg	Cage	0.74 m^2 (8.0 ft^2)	81.3 cm (32 in.)
	15–30 kg	Cage	1.12 m^2 (12.0 ft^2)	91.4 cm (36 in.)
Primates		Cage		
Group 1	<1 kg	Cage	0.15 m^2 (1.6 ft^2)	50.8 cm (20 in.)
Group 2	2–3 kg	Cage	0.28 m^2 (3.0 ft^2)	76.2 cm (30 in.)
Group 3	4–15 kg	Cage	0.40 m^2 (4.3 ft^2)	76.2 cm (30 in.)
Group 4	16–25 kg	Cage	0.74 m^2 (8.0 ft^2)	91.4 cm (36 in.)
Group 5	>25 kg	Cage	2.33 m^2 (25.0 ft^2)	213.4 cm (84 in.)

posed study. A short-term, 30- or 90-day study, will involve approximately 10 rats of each sex per group. In an extended study expected to last 1–2 years, several contingencies must be considered that demand additional animals. Natural attrition can reduce the initial colony by 20% over 2 years. Moreover, spontaneous disease processes also generate natural changes that resemble chemically induced lesions. Since problems of this nature require statistical resolution, a sufficient number of animals must remain at risk throughout the study to support any mathematically derived conclusions. Furthermore, a common practice is to remove a sample of animals at periodic intervals for tissue and body fluid evaluation, and this will further reduce the final number of animals. While the final number of animals assigned to a chronic toxicology study is a subjective and somewhat arbitrary decision, a good rule is to aim for a minimum of 50 rats/sex/group at the terminal examination. Another popular guideline is to have the number of control animals equal the size of each treated group times the square root of the number of treated groups; e.g., with 100 rats/group and 4 treatment groups, the control group contain 200 rats, or $100 \times \sqrt{4}$.

21.3.2b. Dogs

The beagle dog is the second most popular research animal in evaluating chemical safety. Registered beagles having a documented ancestry, raised totally in a closed environment, and methodically vaccinated against distemper, canine hepatitis, and leptospirosis are infinitely superior research subjects compared to the nondescript dogs that are usually found at municipal pounds. Moreover, beagles, being medium sized, are conveniently housed and yet provide sufficient blood and other body fluids for laboratory analyses. Blood can be taken from the cephalic, saphenous, or jugular veins without trauma, and arterial blood is available from the femoral artery without requiring surgical intervention. In addition, uncontaminated urine can be collected by nonsurgical cannulation techniques. A moderately slow heart rate allows standard electrocardiography, thus revealing a chemical's potential effect on cardiac conduction. The beagle dog's calm nature makes complete physical examinations, including ocular and neurological, meaningful and useful procedures. Test compounds can be administered in capsules by a single trained animal technician.

The systematic manner in which these animals are produced and raised minimizes disease problems. However, several parasitic problems remain, such as intestinal roundworms and lungworms.

Dogs in toxicology studies are identified by an ear tatoo or neck band, supplemented by a cage card. Housing is in individual cages with water and sometimes food provided ad libitum.

21.3.2c. Primates

Simian species have found favor in toxicology studies, sometimes because of the notion that they somehow are more closely related to man. Regardless of the rationale, primates have proven to be a valuable third species whenever a comprehensive, multispecies toxicological evaluation of a drug or other chemical is needed. A major drawback with these species is low numbers with defined health histories. The most commonly available monkeys are animals trapped in the wild and then conditioned to an acceptable state of health.

They can carry a number of diseases that are transmissible to humans, and therefore require careful handling. One of the most important is pulmonary or intestinal tuberculosis. This disease can be routinely tested for by injecting tuberculin intradermally and then examining the site for the characteristic positive responses each day for a period of up to 72 hr. Radiography is a supplementary diagnostic technique. However, neither method is completely reliable, and so the tuberculin injections are continued quarterly throughout an animal's life span. Shigellosis is another important enteric disease of monkeys that is equally difficult to detect, especially in the clinically normal "carrier" state. Fecal isolations of the infectious agent require exacting techniques since the organism is easily killed by drying conditions. Furthermore, several nonpathogenic bacteria residing in the monkey intestine have characteristics almost identical to those of the *Shigella* species. For this reason, pathogenic *Shigella* and culturally similar, nonpathogenic bacteria are differentiated by serological techniques. Amebiasis is a third natural disease of monkeys transmissible to laboratory workers. Identification of the pathogenic ameba from the more innocuous species found in monkeys requires special staining techniques of prepared specimens and skillful interpretation.

Herpes B virus is a natural herpetic disease of monkeys that carries a risk of causing human encephalitis, especially following bites by infected monkeys. Although the overall incidence of herpes B virus encephalitis in primate research workers is low, the fatality rate in infected people is high. Preventative measures include the use of gloves and gauntlets to avoid bites, surgical masks to avoid inhaling infected particles, and the ultimate measure, selecting and maintaining a closed colony of monkeys free of herpes B virus antibody titers.

Lesions from previous, nonfatal infectious diseases are frequently found in monkeys arriving at the toxicology laboratory. Such lesions can confound the interpretation of results from a safety evaluation study. Intestinal parasitism is widespread. The adult forms can be eliminated by treatment with appropriate drugs, but the larvae survive to continue migrating through distant tissues, thereby creating nondescript inflammatory lesions in organs such as the liver, brain, and kidneys. One unavoidable parasite is the lung mite, *Pneumonysuss simicola*, which invades the bronchi and interstitial lung tissues. This parasite, infecting virtually all Old World monkeys, is an integral artifact in all toxicology studies with this species.

Monkeys are usually housed individually in the laboratory under conditions that are similar to those for dogs. However, since they are semiwild, handling and controlling are more difficult problems. Toxicology studies necessitate that each monkey be restrained for treatment, examination, or bleeding at least once each working day. Moreover, struggling during restraint must be minimized to avoid excitement-induced changes in physiological parameters that are usually followed during a toxicology study (a problem that will be discussed in more detail in Section 21.3.6). Several measures are employed for this purpose. One is the use of "squeeze" cages, i.e., cages with false backs that can be pulled forward against the cage front, thus immobilizing the occupant. A second system is to attach a chain to a collar encircling the monkey's neck and then pass the opposite end to the outside. The animal can then be pulled forward and immobilized against the cage front. This approach carries the attendant risk of injuring the monkey if the chain and collar become twisted or entangled. Identification is by neck banding, skin tatooing, or cage cards in various combinations. Blood samples can be collected from the cephalic, saphenous, or femoral veins or femoral arteries.

21.3.2d. Age of Animals

Animal ages in long-term toxicology studies can influence the information that will be collected. Rats usually enter the study at 3–4 weeks of age, which is soon after weaning. For the next 4–5 months these animals grow rapidly and many organ systems undergo further development. Adolescent and postadolescent rats (sexual maturity usually occurs in this species at approximately 3 months) are sometimes more sensitive to toxins than older, fully grown, but otherwise comparable rats. Rapid development ensures that such animals will reach sufficient size to provide adequate samples of blood and other body fluids for laboratory analyses during the course of long or moderately long-term studies.

Beagle dogs are usually selected for short-term studies lasting 0.5–3 months only if sexually mature. Maturity occurs at 6 months, but this event is variable and unpredictable, so an age range of 8–12 months is a conservative, less risky choice. Using dogs with fully developed sex organs provides for an evaluation of toxic effects to ovaries and testes in a second species (the rat is assumed to be the first). Such an assessment cannot be made in immature animals since chemically inhibited gametogenesis histologically resembles the state of sexual immaturity. Monkeys that are obtained from the wild lack a defined history and so exact ages are unknown. Moreover, fully mature specimens, i.e., females at least 3.5 years of age and males older than 5 years, are rare, expensive, and difficult to handle in the laboratory. Consequently, smaller but immature animals are usually employed in toxicology studies; therefore, an accurate assessment of gonadal toxicity cannot usually be made in this species.

21.3.3. Dose Levels and Ranges

Dose levels for toxicology studies should be projected to produce the following effects: at least one dose level that results in overt toxicity, and possibly death; at least one intermediate dose level that induces toxicity but not death; and at least one dose level that is nontoxic. A companion group of control animals receives the same treatment, excluding the chemical under study, and might receive the solvent, suspending agent, or empty gelatin capsule. Sometimes a separate group of so-called environmental controls is added that are exposed only to nonexperimental variables, such as food, water, handling, and room conditions.

The following important terms and abbreviations are frequently used in designating dose levels:

Lethal dose or concentration 50 (LD_{50}, LC_{50}): The dose or atmospheric concentration that theoretically kills one-half (50%) of the treated or exposed animals within a specified period of time (usually 7–14 days) following a single treatment or exposure.

Lethal dose or concentration (LD, LC): The lowest lethal dose that can be directly or secondarily related to the administration of the test chemical.

Toxic dose or concentration high (TDH, TCH): The highest dose or atmospheric concentration inducing overt toxic signs without causing treatment-related deaths.

Toxic dose or concentration low (TDL, TCL): The lowest dose or exposure that induces measurable toxic effects.

Highest nontoxic dose or concentration (HNTD, HNTC) [*also called maximum tolerated dose (MTD)*]: The highest dose under study that fails to produce clinical signs of toxicity, pathological lesions, or death.

An infrequently used term, supratoxic dose level, should also be mentioned. This designates a special study in which the limiting toxic effect is treated or counteracted in an attempt to produce the widest spectrum of adverse effects. For example, some chemicals destroy by increasing the treated animal's susceptibility to infectious diseases, a fatal response that can obscure direct toxic effects. An antibiotic given in combination with such a test agent might overcome infection and amplify the toxic profile by permitting higher doses to be tolerated.

Despite serious efforts to develop systematic methods for predicting chemical toxicity, dose selection for a safety evaluation study remains a combination of science and intuition. The development of a complete profile of toxicity usually requires progression from short studies with single or multiple doses to long-term studies (2 years or more) with prolonged administration. A valuable tool for discovering the toxic levels of unique compounds is the range-finding method. In rodents, this means broad, logarithmically spaced single doses in small groups of animals. The doses are raised higher in fresh animals until eventually death or a distinct toxicity occurs. In larger (and more expensive) animal species, this can be modified by doubling the daily dose to the same animal until severe toxicity or mortality results.

With the general level of toxicity thus identified, a more definitive acute toxicity study follows with larger groups at several dose levels. The number of animals per group and the intervals between dose levels depend upon the toxic potency of the chemical under study. However, a useful guideline for an acute toxicity study is that the most acceptable final results should cover a minimum of five dose levels, i.e., one each at 0 and 100% mortality and three levels of mortality in between. Following treatment, daily observations usually cover a minimum of 7 days and a maximum of 14 days. Then the final LD_{50} is calculated by standardized mathematical formulas. The clinical responses and time-related mortalities offer clues regarding toxic mechanisms. Convulsions, ataxia, and deaths immediately following treatment can point to possible neurotoxicity. Delayed deaths after a period of inactivity suggest renal or hepatic effects. Diarrhea and/or pilorection indicate possible autonomic stimulation. Gross or histological postmortem inspection of internal organs sometimes yields useful information. However, certain organs such as the liver and gastrointestinal tract will recover from chemically induced damage during a latent period between treatment and death of more than 24 hr.

The information from acute and range-finding studies underlies the design of the prolonged multiple treatment or exposure studies lasting from several days to several months and then to several years. Other decisions regarding the length of treatment or exposure are based the intended use of the toxicology data, and the expected human use of the agent. Drug candidates for short-term therapy, such as a mild analgesics, might require a relatively short period (1–3 months) of continuous study in animals prior to human exposure. Other chemicals are consumed or taken by humans for longer periods of time, sometimes entire lifetimes. Among these are food additives, life-sustaining drugs, and contaminants such as pesticides, herbicides, and industrial pollutants. At least two organs and one serious disease, the eye and heart and cancer, can require prolonged exposure to toxic agents before overt lesions are fully developed.

A careful literature search frequently yields useful information and aids in the selection of dose levels. However, published studies frequently have followed a design different from the one being planned. Compound administration might be one area requiring further extrapolation and interpretation. In many rodent studies, test compounds are administered as a portion of the diet, expressed either as a percent of diet or in parts per million. Such published findings are directly applicable if identical techniques are a part of the planned study. If, however, exposure is to be based on body weight (expressed as mg/kg/day), then the published data generally can be converted into this form by appropriate manipulation (Figure 21.1).

Inhalation toxicology studies require fixed and controlled levels of atmospheric gases, vapors, or particulates, such as aerosols or solid particles. The design must include systems for producing the desired atmospheres and confirming that the prescribed conditions have been met. In the case of particulates, the concentration, size, and distribution of particles or droplets are estimated. Because such exposures are performed in sealed chambers under dynamic conditions, including constantly changing atmospheres, measurement of the exact concentration of test substance is an essential part of the study protocol. With gases and vapors, concentrations are usually reported either in parts per million or milligrams per cubic meter. For the former system of measurement, the concentrations of test material are analyzed directly in air samples collected at regular intervals from inside the exposure chamber. The latter system of measurement may also refer to the estimated concentration of a vapor within the chamber based on the rate and amount of a liquid being volatilized into an air stream passing into the exposure chamber. The latter units can be converted into parts per million by an equation that follows the gas laws and accounts for differences in temperature and pressure.

21.3.4. Administration and Scheduling

A general rule in administering a test chemical is that the animals should receive the substance by the same route as their human counterparts. Food additives, food and water contaminants, and oral drugs are usually given to animals by oral administration. Parenteral drugs are difficult to test in rodents, which have no convenient superficial blood vessels or large muscle masses that withstand repeated injection. For these reasons, parenteral drugs are usually tested for

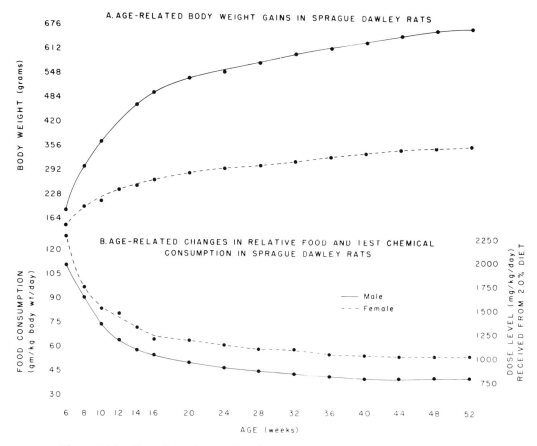

Figure 21.1 The effect of naturally changing growth patterns on relative food intake, and doses received by rats consuming a mixed level of a test chemical. A pair of biphasic curves show that the normal body weight gain of male and female albino rats, during the first year of life, have exponential slopes for the first 14–16 wk, but become nearly horizontal thereafter (**A**). This diminishing rate of growth combined with a relatively stable daily food intake averaging 26.1 g/day for males and 19.1 g/day for females, reduces the relative food intake as a maximum body size is attained (**B**). Therefore a test substance incorporated into the diet at fixed ratios, such as a percent or parts per million, will be consumed at an identically decreasing rate over this portion of the rodents' life span. An example of the outcome of such an experiment is illustrated by the scale on the right. Thus, feeding a diet containing 2% of a test substance will deliver a range of doses with a maximum for males of 2174 mg/kg/day and a minimum of 786 mg/kg/day. The range of doses for females is 2575–1054 mg/kg/day. n = 6500 males; 7800 females.

SOURCE: *Data provided by the Laboratory Animal Data Bank (LABD), Battelle Laboratories, Columbus, Ohio.*

long-term toxic effects in the larger species (dogs and monkeys). Substances that are expected to be inhaled and absorbed by the lungs are appropriately studied by having experimental animals breath air containing fixed concentrations either in chambers or through airtight face masks.

Probably the simplest type of toxicology study design is to offer rodents loose feed or water containing the test material in a fixed concentration, usually as parts per million or a percent of their diet. Large quantities of adulterated diet or drinking water can be prepared and, provided the test material is stable, offered as the animal's food. As demonstrated in Figure 21.1, this technique leads to an uneven level of body exposure in rats, since food consumption relative to body weight will decrease between adolescence and maturity.

A method of uniformly controlling the level of administered compound is to measure the body weight and food consumption of each animal on a fixed schedule, and then compute the amount of test substance required in the diet to cause the animals to consume the desired dose level. The group averages, rather than individual body weight and food consumption, are used for this purpose. More labor is required in this technique since each experimental group will require a weekly diet reformulation by sex, since male and female rats grow and consume feed at different rates. However, additional useful data are collected from such a study in the form of a precise estimate of food consumption. This information will indicate if a depressed rate of body weight gain is related to reduced food consumption. Clearly, a reduction in body weight gain accompanying a lowered food intake is probably caused by unpalatability, and thus is not a true toxic effect.

Surplus feed remaining in the animals' food receptacles from the previous week is discarded and should be destroyed. This wastage must be considered in the initial calculations of the overall amount of test compound required for a study. Diets with either fixed or adjusted concentrations of test materials are usually prepared in mechanical mixers. If the concentration of the test substance is low and the total amount small, then a premix is prepared by mixing equal portions of chemical and feed. This mixture and additional feed are again mixed. This geometric progression is continued until the total amount required is prepared. The actual concentration of a test chemical, uniformity of distribution throughout the feed, and stability in the diet should be verified by appropriate extraction and analytical procedures. This can be time consuming and prohibitively expensive if each individual batch of test diet is examined; random sampling procedures based on quality control theory can be substituted, provided the variance of the concentration is known and is used to determine sampling ratios.

Dietary administration of a chemical to rodents is efficient but loses some precision due to food wastage by the animal and potential loss of volatile chemicals by evaporation. Moreover, the feed dust in an animal room is a source of cross-contamination among experimental groups and could present a hazard to laboratory workers. These problems can be avoided by dissolving or suspending the test chemical in a liquid and administering it by gavage, using either a stomach tube or gavage needle. Each animal then must be handled daily by one or two trained workers. These labor demands increase the cost of this type of research. However, offsetting this disadvantage is a better control and a more precise level of dosing, plus a reduced risk of contaminating workers and other animals.

Dietary administration is not ordinarily practiced when dogs and monkeys are treated for long periods of time because these species waste excessive amounts of food and prefer pelleted feed. Alternative methods are oral dosing by either gelatin capsule or gastric intubation. One daily dose of the test substance is packed into each capsule; usually a 1-week supply is prepared at each filling. The animal's most recent body weight determines the amount of compound to be weighed and placed in each container. Weighing accuracy and filling is improved by diluting the test material with an inert filler, such as lactose. Capsules can be administered to dogs by a single trained individual, who opens the animal's mouth and places the capsule over the arch of the tongue, where it will be swallowed. Capsule administration to monkeys is more complicated and hazardous. In most instances three people are required, i.e., one handler to restrain the animal, another to force the animal's mouth open with a speculum, and a third person to place the capsule in the animal's pharynx with tongs or forceps.

Gastric intubation of dogs and monkeys is both difficult and risky because the tube can be inadvertently misplaced into the trachea and the dose deposited into the lungs—usually a fatal accident. However, it is virtually the only reliable way to deliver large oral doses of a liquid to these species. This procedure also requires two or three highly trained and cautious individuals working together. This technique has been modified successfully in monkey studies by adding sweetening agents to carrier liquids containing the test substances. Monkeys will willingly learn to drink the combination from a syringe.

Chemical solutions given parenterally, e.g., intravenously, intraperitoneally, intramuscularly, or subcutaneously, must be free of bacterial contamination. Heat-stable compounds are sterilized by autoclaving, and heat-labile solutions can be passed through 0.22-μm filters, which will remove most bacteria and fungi. Repeated daily intravenous injections are possible in dogs and monkeys for prolonged periods providing the test material is neither irritating nor toxic to the subcutaneous and intravascular tissues. The latter problem can sometimes be solved by injecting slowly and liberally flushing the injection needles or catheters with a neutral or neutralizing liquid before removing them from the animal's tissues. Dilution is an alternative technique but may produce large volumes; they can be administered by slow infusion but the animal will require prolonged restraint. Continuous daily intraperitoneal injections are an acceptable alternative only as an extreme measure and only with neutral solutions. The chronic intraperitoneal administration of potentially irritating solutions or suspensions carries a high risk of inducing artifactual changes, hence this is a questionable practice.

A chronic dosing schedule is usually determined by the kind of anticipated exposure in humans, sometimes by acute toxic effects, and occasionally by practical necessity. Rodents consuming test diets or adulterated drinking water are theoretically receiving a constant treatment, although in fact these nocturnal animals eat and drink at night. Injections, intubations, or capsules are usually administered once daily, 5 or 7 days/week, unless acute responses, such as emesis, hypotension, respiratory or cardiac depression, anesthesia, etc., necessitate subdividing the total daily dose into smaller fractions administered at equally spaced intervals throughout the day (and night). The duration of inhalation exposure is an individual decision. One widely accepted convention suggests that exposure for 6 hr/day, 5 days/week will simulate conditions in the industrial workplace.

21.3.5. Clinical Observations

With the treatment or exposure planned, the next major consideration becomes the type of data to be collected. Conceptually, laboratory animals might be considered as human surrogates that answer questions centering on the detection of toxic responses at both the clinical and cellular levels. Not surprisingly, the techniques employed in evaluating these animals follow those used in detecting human disease. Physical examinations are performed to search for informative clinical signs and symptoms. Blood samples are collected and analyzed to evaluate internal organ function. Finally, organs are inspected both grossly and microscopically for morphological evidence of damage.

A simple and sometimes meaningful test for toxicity has been briefly discussed, that of measuring body weight gain. Closely associated with this observation is the measurement of food consumption. The relationship between these two parameters, so-called food efficiency, is a mathematical expression of food consumed relative to body weight (or weight gained), or grams of food per kilogram body weight (gained) per day (or week). Such a conversion establishes whether weight losses or inhibited gains are real toxic effects or are due to a distasteful chemical. This technique is easily applied in rodents but is more difficult in dog and monkey studies. The eating habits of the latter species can sometimes signal impending toxicity. Monkeys are usually fed a combination of biscuits and fresh fruit. Frequently, a rejection of the biscuits is the first sign of gastrointestinal distress in this species. A dog with a chemically induced ulcer may appear to be hungry but refuse food past the first mouthful. Presumably, this behavior reflects a painful food-induced gastric acid secretion.

After each treatment in large animals, clinical signs are monitored hourly for the first week and daily thereafter. Rodents being fed or exposed to test substances should be observed at least once each day. Several typical observations are the following: color and consistency of body excretions, color and integrity of skin and mucus membranes, activity patterns, gait, and ocular or nasal discharges. At the same time, an assessment of the nervous system is made. Several general signs such as exophthalmos (bulging eyes) and pilorection (hair standing upright) are detectable without touching the animals. Other types of neurological examinations require handling. Spinal reflexes are evaluated by pinching a toe and assessing the withdrawal reaction. Alternatively, the so-called extensor thrust can be elicited by pressing against the sole of either hind foot. Normally, an animal tested in this manner will push back against the examiner's hand. The strength and degree of pupillary constriction to a strong light shining on the retina yields information on visual acuity. Normally, the iris constricts if the animal is not excessively excited. When the cornea is lightly stimulated with a wisp of cotton or thread, normal blinking follows (the palpebral response), provided eyesight is unimpaired. Spinal and higher center reflexes can be evaluated in various ways. An animal in dorsal recumbency should attempt to roll over into an upright position. If placed on an inclined surface facing downward, it should turn 180° and face upward, the so-called positive geotrophism. Finally, an animal, usually a rodent, can be placed in a narrow corridor that ends in an overhang to evaluate three-dimensional perception. Normally an animal recognizes the dropoff and stops or turns.

Other important clinical observations include an ocular examination of the cornea, iris, vitreous and aqueous humors, and retina with a direct or indirect ophthalmoscope. If a cataractogenic potential exists, then a biomicroscopic examination of the lens with a slit lamp should be made periodically. In dogs and monkeys, the electrocardiograph is an indispensable tool for detecting any adverse effects on cardiac conduction and/or chemically induced electrolyte imbalance. The electrocardiograms should be measured for conduction time intervals, wave amplitudes, and the direction of the mean cardiac vector. The latter is a useful in vivo measure of cardiac dilatation or hypertrophy.

21.3.6. Laboratory Parameters

Blood, urine, and other body fluid analyses are carried out to evaluate organ function and detect chemically induced organ dysfunction. The choice of hematological and biochemical tests should be based on the biological possibilities. Uppermost is a proper evaluation of the function of the liver and kidney, the two major detoxification and excretory organs, which are exposed to foreign substances at high concentrations. The blood elements are another common target organ. Following absorption from the intestine, injection sites, or lungs, chemicals are transported throughout the body in the blood, either bound to plasma proteins or free in plasma, in close contact with the circulating elements. The bone marrow is also sensitive to cytotoxic agents. For these reasons, the various types of blood cells (erythrocytes, leukocytes, and thrombocytes, or platelets) usually found in the vascular system are counted and compared with control animal levels and the normal levels expected to be found in any randomly selected, untreated animal. Different classes of leukocytes are identified by the staining properties of the cytoplasmic granules, if present, and are classified as either neutrophils, eosinophils, or basophils. A second granule-free series includes the lymphocytes and monocytes. The number of circulating cells is determined by counting 100 leukocytes on a stained slide of blood and subclassifying each nucleated cell into one of the above categories. The representative number in each class is thereby calculated as a percentage. Multiplication of the percentages by the total leukocyte count will provide a numerical estimate of the concentration of each type of leukocyte. For example, if the total leukocyte count is 10,000 cells and 50% of these are neutrophils, then the absolute neutrophil count would be 5000/mm^3.

A carefully prepared and stained blood film is essential in order to segregate the leukocytes into separate categories, but the same preparation also contains other useful toxicological information. Variations in the size or shape of the erythrocytes, or the appearance of abnormal structures such as Heinz bodies or Howell-Jolly bodies are significant, especially if accompanying anemia. Similar observations can be made in leukocytes, which might carry "toxic" granules. The separation of neutrophils into stages of maturity is also a standard and helpful practice in differentiating leukopenia resulting from peripheral cell destruction from the same condition following bone marrow suppression. The response to a fall in circulating neutrophils is an increased outpouring from the sites of formation and storage in the bone marrow. Depending upon the severity of demand, the replacement population will include a relative number of immature forms, causing a so-called shift to the left, or leukocytosis of immature forms.

The same type of assessment can be made in the erythrocytes by counting reticulocytes, the immature red cells. These are prematurely released when the demand for replacements is high.

The blood constituents (Table 21.3) selected for analysis provide information on possible alterations in major organ function. Many are circulating by-products of biological reactions that are cleared from the blood by the kidneys (e.g., urea and creatinine) or excreted by the liver (e.g., alkaline phosphatase and bilirubin). Toxic organ dysfunctions, indicated by accumulations in the

Table 21.3 Selected Laboratory Procedures in Chemical Safety Evaluation

Clinical biochemistry	Hematology	Organ tissues for gross and microscopic examination
Albumin	Erythrocyte count	Brain (cerebellum, cerebrum)
Alkaline phosphatase	Leukocyte count with	Spinal cord
Bilirubin (direct and indirect)	differential	Peripheral nerve (sciatic)
Bromosulphalein dye excretion	Hemoglobin	Eyes
Calcium	Hematocrit	Pituitary
Chlorides	Reticulocyte count	Thyroid
Cholesterol	Platelet count	Parathyroid
Creatinine	Nucleated erythrocyte count	Salivary glands (submaxillary)
Glucose	Organs weighed	Heart
Potassium	Adrenals	Lungs
Prothrombin time	Brain	Spleen
Serum glutamic oxaloacetic transaminase	Heart	Liver
Serum glutamic pyruvic transaminase	Kidneys	Pancreas
Sodium	Pituitary	Adrenals
Total protein	Testes	Lymph nodes (mediastinal, cervical
Urea nitrogen	Lungs	laryngeal, bronchial)
		Kidneys
		Bladder
		Prostate
		Testes
		Ovaries
		Uterus
		Tongue
		Esophagus
		Stomach
		Small intestine (three levels)
		Large intestine (three levels)
		Skeletal muscle (thigh)
		Skin (flank)
		Mammary gland
		Gross lesions
		Bone marrow (smear and section)
		Adipose tissue
		Aorta
		Nasal turbinate
		Trachea
		Thymus

blood, are revealed by the analysis of samples collected from treated animals. Another set of parameters that can be measured to detect organ damage are the serum levels of intracellular enzymes that are lost when the cells or cellular membranes are chemically damaged or disrupted. Examples of such enzymes are hepatic transaminases and the heart and skeletal muscle enzyme creatine phosphokinase (CPK). Other common chemical measurements generally reflect the status of the whole body and therefore are less precise. Serum electrolytes, for example, are maintained within a narrow range of levels by complex organ interaction, involving renal function, intestinal absorption, and membrane transport. Glucose levels are controlled by insulin flow, hepatic conversion to other forms, and rate of oxidation.

Organ function can also be evaluated by estimating the rates at which foreign substances are removed from the circulation. The dye bromsulfophthalein (BSP) undergoes hepatic clearance from the blood in direct proportion to liver function. In this test first a baseline blood sample is drawn as a blank. The BSP dye is then injected, and 30 min later the amount of unexcreted dye in a second blood sample is measured. Normal retention is 5% or less at this time. The accuracy of this procedure can be improved by collecting blood samples at other time intervals, for example, 5, 15, and 30 min after injection, and calculating the rate of dye removal. This test is difficult to apply in smaller animals because repetitive bleeding is required.

Another dye, phenolsulfonphthalein (PSP), is employed in a similar manner to judge renal function. This technique requires exact measurements of the clearance rate from the blood and concomitant accumulation in the urine; therefore, the urinary bladder must be catheterized and emptied at the beginning of the test and at timed collection intervals during the procedure. This maneuver can be accomplished with ease only in larger laboratory animals. This restriction, plus the attendant risk of introducing urinary tract infection, has relegated this technique to infrequent use in chemical safety evaluation.

The collection and handling of blood specimens for laboratory analyses deserve serious attention. Erythrocytes are fragile cells and cannot survive trauma or severe osmotic pressure changes. Moreover, since several key elements (e.g., transaminases and potassium) are found at higher levels in erythrocytes than in extracellular fluids, insidious losses can lead to artifactual increases in plasma levels.

The urine can be used to measure renal function and to detect morphological damage. One sensitive indicator of renal function is the concentration of urinary solutes, which are accumulated by water reabsorption from the tubular filtrate. This is estimated by measuring either specific gravity or urine osmolality. This can be made a more exacting test of renal function by including a period of water deprivation. A urine specimen is collected and the specific gravity is measured. Water is withheld for 12–18 hr and then another urine specimen is collected and the specific gravity is measured. Undamaged kidneys should conserve water by reabsorbing it in the tubules, thus inducing a rise in urine specific gravity.

The integrity of the kidney systems can be further evaluated by selective biochemical measurements of urine. For example glucose, albumin, amino acids, and phosphorus are a few substances that are reabsorbed in the proximal tubules, and excesses in the urine will localize the functional lesion to the proximal tubular region. The distal tubules excrete organic acids. The inability of an animal to acidify urine, especially in the presence of an acid load, is a sign of distal tubular dysfunction. Another biochemical test included in the common spectrum of urinalyses is the measurement of urine urobilinogen levels, which can indicate an excessive absorption of bilirubin from the intestine. High ketone levels indicate that high levels of fat are being metabolized, which might occur in starvation or diabetes. Increased urine volume can indicate the presence of a nonspecific polyuria or antidiuretic hormone antagonism.

Little progress has been made in the toxicological application of fecal tests commonly used in human medicine. The potentially most useful test, fecal occult blood, used to evaluate gastrointestinal integrity, is somewhat unreliable because in most animal species there is a high incidence of false positives.

Special attention should be given to the collecting of animal urine because the risk of bacterial contamination is high. At least one bacteria, *Proteus,* is known to produce the enzyme urease, which converts urea to ammonia and leads to an increased urine pH. It is virtually impossible to prevent the introduction of this organism into urine specimens unless collection is by catheterization; therefore, bacteriostatic measures should be a part of collection procedures.

Animal handling can adversely influence the biochemical content of serum samples. Excitation of an animal during catching and bleeding can cause an epinephrine release, leading to hyperglycemia and elevated erythrocytes, the latter from a contracting spleen forcing stored blood cells into the circulation. Skeletal muscles have high concentrations of transaminase enzymes and CPK that are lost during stressful exercise. Therefore, these enzyme levels will rise if an animal such as a monkey is chased before it is caught and bled. The same artifactual changes can occur when an irritating drug or chemical injected intramuscularly causes tissue destruction. The biological activity of a chemical can also influence results. For example, in dogs morphine has been shown to cause a constriction of the sphincter of Oddi, the valve that controls bile outflow from the bile duct into the intestine; this effect mimics biliary obstruction and leads to increases in bilirubin and alkaline phosphatase. Tetracyclines are known to interfere with the later stages of urea formation and thereby cause a prerenal uremia without direct kidney involvement.

21.3.7. Morphology

The last major step in evaluating treated or exposed animals for toxic effects is the visual inspection of all organs and tissues both grossly and microscopically. The most commonly used protocols for investigating chemical effects also include scheduled examinations of small samples of animals periodically, usually at 6- or 12-month intervals, during the study. This approach will determine the status of a study at given points and establish the presence or absence of toxic lesions or the rate at which toxicity is progressing. In addition to these planned events, any animal that is moribund whose survival is doubtful is killed and examined at any time. Such animals are invaluable in pinpointing toxicities, but only if they are purposefully killed and examined, or examined immediately after death. Events that occur during agonal periods, such as a systemic influx of bacteria or bacterial toxins from the gastrointestinal tract, induce lesions that obscure direct chemical effects. Dead animal tissues are self-digested by lysosomal enzymes. This autolysis can erase chemically induced lesions. The

Table 21.4   Special In Vivo Techniques for Studying or Detecting Toxicity

Toxic effect	Procedure
Carcinogenesis	Skin painting; organ implantation
Ototoxicity	Surface preparation of cochlear hair cells
Cataracts	Slit-lamp biomicroscopy
Phototoxicity	Exposure of treated white pigs or nude mice to ultraviolet light
Respiratory irritation	Measurement of respiratory rate and tidal volume; macrophage counts
Porphyria	Examination of fresh hepatic tissues under ultraviolet light
Vasoconstriction	Intraarterial injections
Mutagenesis	Karyotyping of bone marrow cells
Osteoporosis	Skeletal radiography
Teratogenesis	Pregnant animal study
Antifertility	Animal breeding study
Hyperthermia	Rabbit pyrogen test

frequent inspection of severely intoxicated animals plus the efficient, systematic organization of the necropsy laboratory to provide for rapid and comprehensive examination of major organs and rapid excision and fixation of tissue specimens will ensure high-quality tissue slides and more meaningful results.

Organs and tissues are carefully inspected for color, size, shape, and texture in situ. A selected group of major organs are then removed, trimed of accessory tissues such as fat and fascia, blotted dry, and weighed (Table 21.4). These data are usually presented as absolute weight and as related to body and possibly brain weights. The latter can be a useful relationship since the brain weight is usually a stable parameter, unless directly affected by chemical toxicities.

Depending upon the size of the animal, either the organs are excised and immersed in fixing solutions intact, or specimens are selected from representative areas of an organ, excised (always including any grossly visible lesions), and fixed. Some tissues require special attention. Lungs should be inflated and completely distended by intratracheal infusion of fixative. This prevents the alveoli from collapsing and becoming fixed in this position. Skeletal muscles may be fixed in extension by using spreading clamps or by fixing entire muscle groups complete with attached bones. A complete evaluation of bone marrow should include smears, in order to differentiate cell types and determine whether any are selectively affected, and sections, in order to evaluate overall cellularity.

The list of tissues taken and prepared for microscopic examination may reflect individual preferences but should include any organs that are implicated by the toxicological history of the test agent or its congeners. For this reason, it would be difficult to generate a universally appropriate listing. However, the most comprehensive pathological examination in toxicology studies will result in the microscopic examination of 30–40 separate tissues (Table 21.3).

21.4. Concluding Remarks

It should become clear from the preceding discussion that the process of exposing, treating, or otherwise administering a test substance to a large body of animals is only the beginning of an investigation that eventually leads to conclusions regarding hazardous risks in man. Specific toxicities may require special systems and attention (Table 21.4). Moreover, since a host of factors unrelated to treatment are known to influence the outcome of a toxicity study, qualifying questions must be asked about the conduct of the study. These concern disease control, nutrition, husbandry conditions, confirmation of dose levels, detection of human errors, and a paramount and overriding consideration, that of biological similarities and differences between man and the sensitive test species.

Not all the answers to these important questions have been found, but the task of identifying chemical toxicities cannot be postponed. Progress in this field must move on two fronts, the testing of chemicals in animal models, and the development of improvements in the test systems.

Suggested Reading

Ballantyne, B. (Ed.). Current Approaches in Toxicology. Bristol, England: Wright, 1977.

Meyler, L., Peck, H. M. (Eds.). Drug-Induced Diseases. Amsterdam: Excerpta Medica, 1972.

Ministry of Health and Welfare. The Testing of Chemicals for Carcinogenesis, Mutagenesis and Teratogenesis. Ottowa, Canada, 1975.

National Academy of Sciences. Principles for Evaluating Chemicals in the Environment. Washington, D. C., 1975.

Frederick J. de Serres

22

Short-Term Tests
for Mutagenicity in the Toxicological
Evaluation of Chemicals

22.1. Introduction

Exploratory experiments during the past 10 years have shown that there are numerous man-made chemicals in our environment with potent mutagenic activity in experimental organisms. This research has identified an important problem for all of the human population because there is a potential for adverse genetic effects as a result of environmental exposure.

We know that much human disease has a genetic basis and can result from either gene mutations, chromosome rearrangements, or abnormal numbers of chromosomes. There is concern that higher frequencies of genetic disease will result unless exposure to mutagenic environmental chemicals is somehow curtailed. In the Committee 17 Report of the Environmental Mutagen Society on Environmental Mutagenic Hazards, which appeared in the February 14, 1975, issue of *Science,* the hazards to the human population of exposure to such agents were reported, and a strong recommendation was made to initiate screening as rapidly and as extensively as possible.

22.1.1. Correlation Between Mutagenic and Carcinogenic Activity

In the exploratory work mutagenic chemicals have been found in all of the major categories of chemicals in our environment. These include food additives, drugs, pesticides, cosmetics, air and water pollutants, and household and industrial chemicals. Furthermore, research during the past 7 years has shown a high correlation between carcinogenic and mutagenic activity in a wide variety of

Reprinted, with minor editorial changes from: de Serres, F. J., Fouts, J. R., Bend, J. R., Philpot, R. M. (Ed.). New York: Elsevier North Holland, 1977. In Vitro Metabolic Activation in Mutagensis Testing.

assay systems ranging from bacteria, fungi, and insects to mammalian cells in culture [4]. The most extensive study by B. Ames and his colleagues has shown that 90% of chemical carcinogens are also mutagens in *Salmonella* [18]. It is now well established that many carcinogens are mutagens, but we have inadequate data regarding the reverse correlation. The concern is certainly valid, however, that chemicals identified as mutagens in any assay system may not only have potential genetic activity in man but carcinogenic potential as well.

22.1.2. Need for Mass Screening Programs

There is obviously a need to develop a capability to do more than exploratory experiments on environmental chemicals. As a result of these important discoveries there is an urgent need to establish priorities and to start screening on a broader scale. We need not only to be able to test large numbers of untested chemicals—perhaps on the order of tens of thousands— but also their mammaliam metabolites. In many cases, innocuous chemicals are activated by metabolism in the liver or other mammalian organs to form highly toxic derivatives. We also know that metabolic conversion can vary markedly from one animal species to another. In addition, metabolic conversion can also be produced by bacteria in the intestinal flora. In 1975, Plewa and Gentile, at Illinois State University and Yale University, respectively, discovered that the herbicide atrazine can be converted by metabolism in commercially grown corn to a form that is a potent mutagen. The active metabolite in the corn sap is not only mutagenic to yeast and bacteria but also to the corn plant itself [10, 20].

22.2. Types of Assay Systems to Detect Mutagenic Activity

A wide variety of assay systems have been developed to detect mutagenic activity. These include (a) mutation inducation at specific loci, (b) differential inhibition of repair-deficient and wild-type strains of various microbes and (c) unscheduled DNA synthesis in mammalian cells in culture. All of these have potential for use in rapid screening tests because the assays are sensitive and large numbers of compounds can be tested. In addition, many follow-up systems are also available that can better characterize the spectrum of genetic alterations produced. In *Drosophila*, for example, we can obtain information on nondisjunction, chromosome aberration, and recessive lethal mutations occurring in entire X chromosomes [22, 23]. With this approach we can obtain the information that is essential for extrapolation and benefit–risk analysis. Tests for the induction of gene mutations [5] and chromosomal damage in the form of heritable translocations can also be done in mice [9], but the resources required impose serious limitations on their general utility.

Present data suggest that genetic damage can be divided into two main classes: (a) gene mutations and chromosome aberrations, and (b) nondisjunction. Agents that produce the former class do not necessarily produce the latter and vice versa. Furthermore, agents exist that appear to be able to produce gene mutations but not chromosome aberrations, but not vice versa. This suggests that any screen to detect the mutagenicity of environmental chemicals could have assays only for gene mutations and nondisjunction.

22.2.1. Assays for Gene Mutations

In man, gene mutation occurs by point mutation (or alteration of the DNA in a given gene) as well as physical removal of the gene (as well as others in the immediate vicinity) by chromosome deletion.

Most bacterial systems provide assays for point mutation by studying reversion of various auxotrophs to prototrophy. The best known example is the reversion of histidine-requiring mutants of *Salmonella,* which has been used extensively by Ames et al. [2]. Mutants revert either by base-pair substitution or frameshift mutation, and particularly sensitive indicators of this type of damage have been developed by selecting mutants at specific sites within each gene which revert at unusually high frequencies. These are the so-called hot spots, which were first discovered in rII cistron in phage T4 by Benzer [3]. In addition, the sensitivity of the *Salmonella* strains has been enhanced by making them excision-repair deficient and by removing the lipopolysaccharide layer on the cell wall. More recently a resistance transfer factor has also been transferred into the standard tester strains (TA1535 and TA1538) to make even more sensitive derivatives (TA100 and TA98) [2].

Although this approach has provided extremely sensitive indicators of mutagenic activity, there is always the question of significance with regard to the rest of the genome.

Mohn and co-workers [19] have developed a multipurpose strain of *E. coli* K12, in which mutations can be detected simultaneously in several genes by plating the cells on different selective media. The mutation types selected include forward mutation at two loci (5-MTR, gal$^+$) and reverse mutation at two others (nad$^-$, arg$^-$). This assay makes it possible to confirm mutagenic activity at other loci in the same organism as well as to compare reverse-mutation frequencies (based on the analysis of damage at particular sites within the gene) with forward-mutation frequencies (based on the analysis of damage occurring at many sites within the gene).

Since there is no evidence that gene mutations can occur by chromosome deletion and *not* point mutation, it is generally agreed that these simple bacterial systems provide useful assays to detect mutagen activity that will produce gene mutations in man.

22.2.2. Assays for Nondisjunction

At present there are no assays for nondisjunction that are useful for mass screening programs. This is a serious deficiency since nondisjunction is produced by chemicals that interfere with the spindle apparatus, and agents that would produce this type of damage might not necessarily produce gene mutations and chromosome abberrations. A good example of such specificity is that shown by colchicine.

22.2.3. Assays for Differential Inhibition of Repair-Deficient and Wild-Type Strains

Differential inhibition of repair-deficient and wild-type strains of various bacteria has provided a highly sensitive indicator of genetic activity. Among the best known and most widely used are the pol A strains of *E. coli* developed by Slater and co-workers [21] and the rec-assay developed by Kada et al. [11]. Both of these systems have been used to study the mutagenic activity of a wide variety of environmental chemicals. A wide variety of such repair-deficient mutants exist in bacteria, yeast, and fungal strains used as indicator organisms. Much more work should be done to more fully exploit this potential.

22.3. Metabolic Conversion Studies

22.3.1. Need to Consider Metabolic Conversion

The role of metabolic activation, tissue distribution, and metabolic fate and realted problems have become issues of major importance not only in trying to identify mutagenically active environmental chemicals, but also in attempting to make informed benefit–risk analyses. The magnitude of the problems in this area that have been encountered in the past few years has created a need for more extensive communication between toxicologists, pharmacologists, and geneticists.

The geneticists have a new tool to study the mutagenicity of not only the original chemical but also its metabolites in what is referred to in the literature as in vitro metabolic activation.

22.3.2. Techniques for In Vitro Metabolic Activation

By incubating DMN and DEN in a nonenzymatic chemical hydroxylation system, Malling demonstrated the formation of metabolites that were mutagenic in Neurospora [14]. Five years later, Malling used mouse liver homogenates to try to mimic in vitro the type of metabolic conversion that took place in vivo [15]. In the latter paper he showed that nonmutagenic chemical carcinogens could be activated in vitro by mouse liver homogenates to metabolic derivatives that were potent mutagens in *Salmonella*. This technique has been refined by others and widely exploited to try to develop in vitro conditions that would mimic the type of metabolic conversion that occurs in vivo. The advantages of this approach are numerous. It avoids the necessity to use whole animals and the undesirable host reaction against the indicator organism that Malling [16] has found in the host-incubated assay developed by Gabridge and Legator [8]. Furthermore, this approach makes it possible to use organ homogenates derived from man.

Ames et al. first showed that the microsomal fraction derived from rat liver homogenates could be incorporated into a thin layer of agar, along with the bacteria, in their spot test with *Salmonella* on Petri plates [1]. This approach is now used by other investigators with various strains of bacteria and fungi [24] and has made possible the development of rapid, short-term tests for both mutation induction and DNA repair. This has been a remarkable technical achievement because it is possible to test that mutagenic activity of a given chemical, as well as its metabolites, over a wide range of concentrations within a few days. These tests are rapid, sensitive, inexpensive, and entirely suitable for use in screening programs to evaluate the mutagenic activity of large numbers of environmental chemicals.

The primary objective of this approach is to make a meaningful toxicological evaluation on the basis of a simplified test. Although the technique for in vitro metabolic activation is in widespread use, numerous modifications of the procedure proposal by Ames et al. for *Salmonella*, for example, have already arisen, producing confusion in the literature.

The procedure developed by Ames and his colleagues uses rat liver homogenized in 0.15 M KCl which is then centrifuged at 9000 g for 10 min [2]. The supernatant that is decanted and saved is referred to as the S-9 fraction. They have also shown that much higher frequencies of revertants are found with many carcinogens if the rat liver microsomes are derived from rats treated with a polychlorinated biphenyl mixture called Arochlor 1254. In general, these revertant frequencies are higher than with phenobarbital or 3-methylcholanthrene as inducers or with uninduced microsomes. An additional factor for optimum detection of mutagenic activity is the amount of S-9 fraction used. Too much or too little of the S-9 fraction can markedly affect the sensitivity of this assay.

A wide range of factors have been found to affect the sensitivity of the in vitro technique, including purity of the microsomal fraction [13], the organ from which it is derived, sex and species differences [7, 25], and diet [6].

All of these experiments have shown that the utilization of this approach is quite complex; the S-9 microsomal fraction involves a mixture of enzymes that can produce simultaneously both activation and detoxification. The specific activity of any particular enzyme in this preparation can vary markedly.

22.4. Utility of Short-Term Tests for Mutagenicity

Considerable thought has been given to the utilization of this new technology for toxicological evaluation in evaluating the risk of environmental chemicals for man.

A variety of assay systems have been developed in the past few years; many are still in the process of validation. Although many chemicals have been tested, we still do not know what frequency of false negatives and positives will be encountered when we start to screen unknowns. Since various assay systems differ in either the type of genetic damage assayed or the portion of the genome evaluated, it is generally agreed that any prescreen should utilize a battery of tester strains. The advantage of this approach is that evidence for genetic activity can be confirmed readily by means of tests on other organisms.

Since there appears to be a high probability that positive test data will also signal potential carcinogenic activity, this multifaceted approach will provide additional confirmation of activity. It serves no useful purpose to indict falsely any particular chemical or class of chemicals as potential carcinogens. There is no doubt that false indictment would be counter-productive in our attempts to identify and remove harmful chemicals from our environment.

The new technology of short-term tests for mutagenicity has promised a unique opportunity for man to remove disease-causing agents from his environment.

We hope to change the emphasis in treating human health problems from effective treatment to more effective prevention. Prevention can take many forms. Identification of high-risk groups in the human population by epidemiological studies has received widespread publicity in the past few years as a result of the identification of group after group of workers at high risk of cancer [12]. These groups include the following: operating room personnel exposed to anesthetic gases; chemical workers exposed to bischloromethyl ether; rubber workers exposed to benzene, carbon black, and cadmium; metal workers exposed to arsenic, nickel, or chromates; polyvinyl chloride workers exposed to high levels of vinyl chloride; synthetic rubber workers exposed to chloroprene; roofers exposed to benzo(a)pyrene; coke and steel plant workers; and insulation workers exposed to asbestos.

Many of these carcinogenic chemicals have been found to give a positive result in short-term tests for mutagenicity [17, 18]. The widespread use of these tests should certainly provide evidence of potential danger for man where no genetic or carcinogenic risk has as yet been identified.

The problem always has and undoubtedly will be—for a while—one of extrapolation from experimental organisms to man. Unfortunately, this is a new game with rules that have not as yet been correctly deciphered.

22.5. Elimination of Disease-Causing Agents from our Environment

The development of short-term tests has provided man with an unprecedented opportunity to eliminate disease-causing agents from his environment. This approach should not only enable us to reduce genetic disease but also to reduce environmental and industrial carcinogenesis. If there is even the remotest chance of our achieving this goal, research in this area should be given the highest possible priority.

Man's most precious heritage may well be the successful transmission of an unaltered genome from one generation to another. We are now aware of the presence of numerous agents in our environment that have the potential to interfere with this process. As a result of these exploratory studies to evaluate the mutagenicity of chemicals in our environment, we already know that there is extensive human exposure. Many geneticists view this exposure as a serious threat to the future of mankind as we know it.

It will take the combined efforts of all of the disciplines involved in this research to refine this new technology. We must make a concerted effort to determine whether the concern of geneticists is valid by ascertaining as rapidly as possible the extent of the real hazard resulting from exposure of the human population to mutagenic environmental chemicals.

References (*Suggested Reading)

1. Ames, B. N., Durston, W. E., Yamasaki, E., Lee, F. P. Carcinogens are mutagens: Bacterial tester strains as R factor plasmids. Proc. Natl. Acad. Sci. U.S.A. 72 (1973), 979.

*2. Ames, B. M., McCann, J., Yamasaki, E. Methods for detecting carcinogens and mutagens with the Salmonella/mammalian microsome mutagenicity test. Mutat. Res. 31 (1975), 347.

3. Benzer, S. On the topography of the genetic fine structure. Proc. Natl. Acad. Sci. U.S.A. 47 (1961), 403.

*4. Brookes, P., de Serres, F. J. Report of the Workshop on the Mutagenicity of Chemical Carcinogens. Mutat. Res. 38 (1976), 155.

5. Cattanach, B. M. Specific locus mutation in mice. In Hollander, A. (Ed.). Chemical Mutagens, Principles and Methods for Their Detection, Vol. 2. New York: Plenum Press, 1971, pp. 535–539.

6. Cygan, P., Greim, H., Garro, A. J., Hutlerer, F., Schaffner, F., Popper, H., Rosenthal, O., Cooper, D. Y. Microsomal metabolism of dimethylnitrosamine and the cytochrome P-450 dependency of its activation to a mutagen. Cancer Res. 33 (1975), 2983.

7. Felton, J. S., Nebert, D. W. Mutagenesis of certain activated carcinogens in vitro associated with genetically mediated increases in monooxygenase activity and cytochrome P_1-450. J. Biol. Chem. 250 (1975), 6769.

8. Gabridge, M. G., Legator, M. S. A host-mediated assay for the detection of mutagenic compounds. Proc. Soc. Exp. Biol. Med. 130 (1969), 831.

9. Generoso, W. M., Russell, W. L., Huff, S. W., Stout, S. K., Gosslee, D. G. Effects of dose on the induction of dominant lethal mutations and heritable translocations with ethyl methane sulfonate in male mice. Genetics 77 (1974), 741.

10. Gentile, J. M., Plewa, M. J. A bio-assay for screening host-mediated proximal mutagens in agriculture. Mutat. Res. 31 (1975), 317 (abstract).

11. Kada, T., Moriya, M., Shirasu, Y. Screening of pesticides for DNA interactions by "rec-assay" and mutagenesis testing, and frameshift mutagens detected. Mutat. Res. 26 (1974), 243.

12. Lehman, P. Cancer—One in four will get it. Hazard 1 (1976), 4.

*13. Loprieno, N., Barale, R., Baroncelli, S., Bronzetti, G., Cammellini, A., Cinci, A., Corsi, G., Leporini, C., Nieri, R., Nozzolini, M., Serra, C. Microsomal assays in mutagenesis. In Proceedings of the Workshop on Approaches to Assess the Significance of Experimental Chemical Carcinogenesis Data for Man. December 10–12, 1973, Brussels, Belgium. International Agency for Research on Cancer, Scientific Publication 10, 1974, pp. 183–189.

14. Malling, H. V. Mutagenicity of two potent carcinogens, dimethylnitrosamine and diethylnitrosamine, in *Neurospora crassa*. Mutat. Res. 3 (1966), 537.

15. Malling, H. V. Dimethylnitrosamine: Formation of mutagenic compounds by interaction with mouse liver microsomes. Mutat. Res. 13 (1971), 425.

16. Malling, H. V. Mutation induction in *Neurospora crassa* incubated in mice and rats. Mol. Gen. Genet. 116 (1972), 211.

17. McCann, J., Ames, B. N. The detection of mutagenic metabolites of carcinogens in urine using the Salmonella/microsome test. Ann. N.Y. Acad. Sci. 269 (1975), 21.

*18. McCann, J., Choi, E., Yamasaki, E., Ames, B. N. Detection of carcinogens as mutagens in the Salmonella/microsome test: Assay of 3000 chemicals. Proc. Natl. Acad. Sci. U.S.A. 72 (1975), 5135.

19. Mohn, G., Ellenberger, J., McGregor, D. Development of mutagenicity tests using *Escherichia coli* K-12 as indicator organism. Mutat. Res. 25 (1974), 187.

20. Plewa, M. J., Gentile, J. M. Mutagenicity of atrazine. A maize-microbe bioassay. Mutat. Res. 38 (1976), 287.

21. Slater, E. E., Anderson, M. D., Rosenkranz, H. S. Rapid detection of mutagens and carcinogens. Cancer Res. 31 (1971), 970.

*22. Sobels, F. H. The advantages of Drosophila for mutation studies. Mutat. Res. 26 (1974), 277.

23. Sobels, F. H., Vogel E. The capacity of Drosophila for detecting relevant genetic damage. Mutat. Res. 41 (1976), 95.

24. Weekes, V., Williams, J., Butler, P., Roy, G., Brusick, D. Rapid screening techniques for mutagenicity using microbial cells combined with mammalian activation fractions. Mutat. Res. 31 (1975), 310.

25. Weeks, U., Brusick, D. In vitro metabolic activation of chemical mutagens. II. The relationship among mutagen formation, metabolism and carcinogenicity for dimethylnitrosamine and diethylnitrosamine in the livers, kidneys and lungs of BALB/cJ, C57BL/6J and RF/J Mice. Mutat. Res. 31 (1975), 175.

Index